Midnight
in Chattanooga
The game, the team and the dream
behind the rise of JMU football

James Irwin

authorHOUSE®

AuthorHouse™
1663 Liberty Drive
Bloomington, IN 47403
www.authorhouse.com
Phone: 1-800-839-8640

© 2010 James Irwin. All rights reserved.

No part of this book may be reproduced, stored in a retrieval system, or transmitted by any means without the written permission of the author.

First published by AuthorHouse 6/14/2010

ISBN: 978-1-4490-8190-4 (e)
ISBN: 978-1-4490-8189-8 (sc)

Library of Congress Control Number: 2010907803

Printed in the United States of America
Bloomington, Indiana

This book is printed on acid-free paper.

For my mother's father
And my father's father
And for my father

The 2004 James Madison football season

Sept. 4	JMU 62, Lock Haven 7
Sept. 18	JMU 17, Villanova 0
Sept. 25	West Virginia 45, JMU 10
Oct. 2	JMU 31, Hofstra 21
Oct. 9	JMU 28, Massachusetts 7
Oct. 16	JMU 24, Maine 20
Oct. 23	JMU 26, Richmond 20
Oct. 30	JMU 41, VMI 10
Nov. 6	JMU 20, Delaware 13
Nov. 13	William & Mary 27, JMU 24
Nov. 20	JMU 31, Towson 17
Nov. 27	JMU 14, Lehigh 13
Dec. 4	JMU 14, Furman 13
Dec. 10	JMU 48, William & Mary 34
Dec. 17	JMU 31, Montana 21

Foreword

ON A cold winter night in Chattanooga, surrounded by former players, coaches, family and friends, I watched a dream come true. It was a dream that began 32 years earlier on a makeshift football field in Harrisonburg, Va. Fueled by a lifelong passion for football that had been nurtured through my own playing days in high school and college — and an early career in high school coaching — the dream beckoned me forward, and always kept me striving to be the best.

In 1971, I accepted an invitation to come to Madison College — a 3,300-student teacher's school with a 3-to-1 ratio of female to male students. My job was to build the school's track & field and football programs. In July of 1972, the decision was made to field a football team for the upcoming season. The 30 some-odd young men who formed that first Madison College football team were faithful and determined — if not the most skilled players — and the dream was born. From the beginning, our goal was to be the best at whatever level we competed. We knew it would take time, that we were planting trees under which we may never sit.

We competed at the Division III level for most of the decade. Madison began as a JV team but quickly grew into one of the nation's strongest programs. We had a winning record in our first varsity season (1974) and went undefeated in 1975. We began the 1976 season ranked No. 1 in the country and played in the first Division III game televised by a major network. The program continued its success at Division III until we moved to Division I-AA in 1979. Our goals didn't change. We believed JMU football could be one of the country's best programs. By 1982, we were back in the top 10 and on our way to being recognized as one of the nation's strongest teams. My dream was to see a JMU football team win a national championship. It also became a goal of the JMU community.

I left coaching in 1985 and earned my doctorate in sport psychology. I have been fortunate to remain at JMU and I continue to work in areas I find passionate. As an educator, I teach coaching education and sport psychology. As a coach, I have been able to work with many JMU teams and individual athletes in mental training.

During Mickey Matthews' tenure as JMU football coach, he has surrounded himself with good assistants and has proven to be a gifted recruiter. He reached out to me from the very beginning by speaking with me about the history and traditions of the program. Mickey told me he believed JMU football could be one of the nation's top programs and that his goal was to win national championships. Both of those goals became a reality in 2004 when JMU defeated the University of Montana for the I-AA national title. I was fortunate enough to watch and experience this transition. I was present at most of the JMU games during the 2004 season and I was in the stands in Chattanooga the night the Dukes became national champions.

On that star-filled night in December 2004, we — those who had been there in 1972 and the years that followed — knew we had just experienced the rare opportunity to sit in the shade of the tree we planted long ago. Three years after the national championship, I received an e-mail from James Irwin, outlining a project to tell the story of the 2004 Dukes and the rise of the JMU football program. Jimmy is a JMU graduate and a former student of mine, and he has captured the excitement of that season in these pages.

May you, the reader, experience the thrill of *Midnight in Chattanooga*.

— *Challace McMillin, JMU football coach, 1972-1984*

Introduction

TO SOME, this has become a story of overnight success. With no internal precedent, an inconsistent football program broke through a barrier of mediocrity, and a team that showed no signs of greatness became great.

The 2004 James Madison Dukes were not supposed to reach Chattanooga, Tenn. Teams that finish 6-6 one season don't play for national championships a year later. The Dukes weren't even supposed to fare well in their own conference. They didn't earn a single preseason top-25 vote and they barely received any endorsement from their fans when the season began. The idea of a championship was so unbelievable that people who spoke of Madison's playoff potential were mocked by their own friends.

Indeed, what makes this story so remarkable is how it all seemed to unfold at once. How in 13 months, a team that meant so little to so few became a group that meant so much to so many. How a troubled coach could find salvation in fans that once rallied against him. How a team of recent struggle could transform into a group of magic men.

To the casual eye, the 2004 Dukes were an aberration of recent history, a team that suddenly shed the label of underachiever and ushered in the year of purple and gold. To be fair, those with the casual eye are partially correct. Many moving parts came together in 2004 both on and off the field. To call that season an unexpected success might be the understatement of Madison's first century.

Yet an insatiable need for the truth compels this question: How does a team showing no sign of success transform overnight? For that answer, you have to look deeper. And that's where our story begins.

Instantaneous success often is achieved with building blocks that fly under the radar. In reality, JMU's 2004 season wasn't an eleventh-hour occurrence. It was the product of a long process that many people didn't see — a process that began years earlier as the Dukes sputtered through losing seasons and mediocre results. The 2001 JMU football team finished with a record of 2-9. Three years later, more than 30 members of that roster helped spark the program's first run to Chattanooga. Fifteen were starters. They were carriers of the torch, symbols of both the best and worst Madison teams of the past three decades, and the founders of a new era of JMU football that would stretch to the end of the decade. These Dukes were both result and catalyst. They changed the course of the program. While the 2004 season snuck up on us, it certainly did not sneak up on them.

The success of the 2004 Dukes caught everyone off guard except the men who made it happen. Simply put, the majority of us didn't believe what we were seeing until it smacked us in the face on a rain-soaked field in Williamsburg when the Dukes punched their tickets to the national title game. It wasn't random success — even if we thought it was — and while this is a story of a team on the cusp of the unthinkable, it's also the story of a program earning the respect of its inner circle.

This accomplishment will never be diminished because of its historical significance. The Dukes became the first Virginia football team to win a collegiate national championship. They did it without the benefit of a home playoff game — a first in NCAA history. But what's really everlasting is the story of how it happened. This is that story — a truthful and powerful account of a group of men on the doorstep of greatness, the program they changed and the architects of their success.

The story of a team that made believers of us, long after they believed in themselves.

— *James Irwin*

Part I: Chattanooga

Chapter 1

THE GLOWING lights atop Max Finley Stadium were visible from across the Tennessee River as the sun began its descent over Chattanooga. Gusts of sharp wind danced between buildings in the downtown district as another clear December day gave way to a crisp, chilly night in the Scenic City. Evening temperatures were expected to drop as low as 30 degrees, but inside First Tennessee Pavilion the pageantry was reaching a crescendo.

Dr. Linwood Rose strolled across the stadium concourse, leisurely navigating his way through a sea of fans waiting on merchandise and concession lines. First Tennessee Pavilion was the skeleton of an old Ross-Meehan Iron Foundry — an open-air structure characterized by industrial architecture. Exposed beams crisscrossed in the rafters high above the ground and foundation pillars sequentially lined the frame of the pavilion like columns in a parking deck. The building was designed for large crowds, but thanks to vendors, game-day personnel and two university marching bands, it was a noisy cauldron of activity. As Rose continued to weave through the crowd, fans migrated toward the stadium gates. It was championship night in Chattanooga, and the start of the Division I-AA national title game between Montana and James Madison was just over an hour away.

For Rose, the fifth university president in Madison's 96-year history, it was his first national championship game. A month earlier, the 2004 Dukes became only the second JMU team during his eight-year presidency to reach postseason play, and after surviving three road playoff games Madison was playing for its first national title. No team in the history of I-AA football had won a championship without playing at least one postseason game at home, a fitting hurdle for a team whose path through the playoffs had been as unlikely as its success.

Rose was at the helm of a school that had grown from an all-female teacher's college to one of the most recognized masters-level institutions in the South. Mild mannered and impeccably dressed, Rose was every part the academic administrator. His salt-and-pepper hair was neatly combed; his glasses sat balanced on the bridge of his nose; his words spilled forth with the ease of a man who spoke publicly for a living. Except for sporting events, it was hard to remember Rose dressing casually. His attire was politically handsome. Rose almost always wore a dark suit and a light shirt, complete with a tie that was just the right length and a handkerchief in his breast pocket. Tonight, that polished look gave way to informal clothing — black pants, a JMU sweatshirt and a purple Madison cap. Yet Rose still walked with his customary casual importance, a rolling gait that mirrored his character. The 53-year-old president was polite and cordial. He shook hands with a discrete firmness and treated guests with equal respect. It was difficult to look at Rose and not see the administrator. The life, the suit and the walk were part of who he was — assets to the academic persona.

Rose had history at JMU dating to 1975, when he was hired as the assistant director of residence halls at what was then Madison College. For the next 30 years, he would be linked to the university's future. From 1971-1998, under the leadership of Dr. Ronald Carrier, the once-small teacher's college blossomed. And as Rose ascended within the JMU administration, he learned much about the evolution of the Madison identity.

A man with incredible vision, Carrier's tenure as Madison president was marked by tremendous growth. He transformed the institution from a 4,000-student regional college into a 14,000-student university, increasing the size of campus by more than 100 acres and investing more than $200 million in facilities. The only thing bigger than Carrier's foresight was his personality. He was skilled in the art of engaging with people. An eloquent orator, Carrier often outperformed the guest speakers at Madison commencement ceremonies. His delivery was lively and entertaining, completed by a persuasive Southern charm and quick wit. Carrier was a showstopper in front of the crowd. He always knew the best way to reach his audience.

Perhaps Carrier's most important legacy was his ideology. Throughout his tenure, he advanced the idea that the student was Madison's most important figure. This was a focus Rose also embraced. By the mid-90s, many considered Rose to be Carrier's logical successor. Beyond the fiscal and administrative duties he performed, he understood the Madison spirit. And when Rose took over as acting president in 1997, he aimed to build on Carrier's momentum.

One of Rose's first acts was to create a commission to celebrate Madison's 2008 centennial, an executive maneuver that gave rise to a $50 million capital campaign. But most importantly, he pushed the student-centered experience to a new level. With its roots in education and public service, JMU's lineage promoted a hands-on faculty. Madison professors were not as research-oriented as their peers at The University of Virginia or The College of William & Mary. Instead, they understood the university mission to build students at the undergraduate level. History cited James Madison as a champion of knowledge and a man who viewed education as an essential ingredient to democracy. That philosophy fit well with the administration's push to align the university with its namesake. "This is no ordinary organization," Rose said at his inauguration. "It is one filled with hope established from positive momentum. I cannot help but be optimistic about what we can accomplish."

Carrier and Rose's mutual vision spread to JMU's athletics program. Both saw sports as a potential key to the national gateway, specifically football and men's basketball, which by the 1990s had turned into huge vehicles for profitable media exposure. While Carrier helped build the men's basketball program into a mid-major juggernaut by the 1980s, football was his real pet project. Widely heralded as the father of the program, Carrier's quest to bring football to Madison was immediate. Nothing stood in his way when he wanted it badly enough.

From modest beginnings, the program inched forward on the strength of new facilities, Carrier's foresight and coach Challace McMillin's technical prowess. There were hiccups, however. The first Madison College football meeting was held in September of 1972 in a third-floor meeting room in Godwin Hall. Around 60 potential players showed up and listened to McMillin outline the program, the game and the process. McMillin didn't sugarcoat anything. Football, he told them, was a sport with bone-crushing hits; a sport of men, not boys. At the conclusion of the meeting, McMillin instructed his players to go to the ground floor in Godwin and pick up their equipment. "That," JMU centennial director Fred Hilton later wrote, "is when things began to unravel."

When McMillin arrived in the equipment room fewer than 30 players remained. Apparently his pep talk had scared off half the players. "At first I thought they'd gotten lost," he later laughed.

A month after this infamous beginning, the Dukes played their inaugural game on Godwin Field, an adjacent grassy commons that now serves as a prime tailgate location for alumni. McMillin, his coaches and athletics director Dean Ehlers lined the field. Carrier and assorted fans watched the game from folding chairs on the sidelines. The Dukes lost, 6-0.

The team did not stay at Godwin for long. Carrier oversaw the development of a 12,500-seat stadium in 1974. And as investments were made, the program flourished. Madison College did not score a point in its first season, but three years later the Division III Dukes went undefeated, and McMillin was named coach of the year by Kodak and the American Football Coaches Association. In 1980, the Dukes jumped to Division I-AA, and in 1982, JMU earned its first win against a Division I-A opponent, defeating Virginia, 21-17, in Charlottesville. McMillin was the pilot, a smart coach with a focus on positive teaching. Carrier, meanwhile, was the driving force, a relentless visionary with an eye for potential and a magnetic personality. During stadium construction, he encouraged Madison's physical plant supervisor, Lou Frye, to finish the job for the upcoming season. "Rome wasn't built in a day," said Frye, knee deep in wet concrete. Carrier was unfazed. "Lou," he said, "I wasn't in charge."

What Carrier built was a cornerstone for the future. Rose aimed to take that cornerstone and use it as one of several launching pads to take the university to the next level. In eight years he had overseen groundbreaking for a state-of-the-art physics and chemistry research facility, plus the development of a growing health sciences department. Future plans included construction for a performance complex to house one of the largest fine arts programs on the East Coast. And, thanks to several large private donations, groundbreaking on a $10 million student-athlete academic facility began in 2003. With athletics, Rose's philosophy revolved around growth and consistency. "Having consistent winning seasons is our long-term goal," he said. "That's how a program achieves sustained success. New facilities help create an infrastructure to support that."

Yet until the 2004 season, fan support for football remained significantly smaller than its winter counterpart. Throughout the 1980s and into the early 1990s, Madison was a basketball school, characterized by its lively head coach, Lefty Driesell, and its boisterous home fans known throughout the region as "The Electric Zoo." The Dukes reached postseason play nine times between 1981 and 1994, including three consecutive trips to the NCAA Tournament in the early 1980s under coach Lou Campanelli. Even when the football program enjoyed its finest stretch of success — four trips to the NCAA playoffs from 1987 to 1995 — the basketball Dukes still commanded the most attention, as Driesell piloted Madison to five consecutive postseason appearances and a 101-51 record from 1990 to 1994.

The exposure from basketball in the early 1980s benefited both the program and the university, giving Madison its first hint of the national spotlight thanks to televised postseason games. In 1981, '82 and '83, the Campanelli Dukes scored first-round wins in the NCAA Tournament. In the middle year of that stretch, they pushed eventual national champion North Carolina (and confident, skinny shooting guard Michael Jordan) to the brink of elimination before falling to the Tar Heels, 52-50, in the second round. "I think we recognized the potential of a breakthrough [football] season because we had experienced it with basketball in the early 1980s," Rose said. "The media exposure helps bring recognition to the university." Later, with Driesell at the controls, the basketball Dukes had a flamboyant personality, a man who was bigger than the school and buoyed recognition for the university's athletics program into the late 1990s.

By 2003, however, Driesell was long gone and "The Electric Zoo" was in the middle of a prolonged blackout after the Dukes crashed to a 7-21 season. In 10 years since Lefty's final NCAA team, no player in purple and gold had sniffed postseason play. Meanwhile, the Madison football team was in its own drought, reaching the playoffs only one time between 1996 and 2003. JMU's flagship programs were going through a simultaneous identity crisis.

Then came 2004, and the football team's magical run to Chattanooga. As the Dukes began to roll through the season, the response from supporters stretched from current students to prominent local figures. The status of Madison as a basketball school suddenly was up for grabs. "When I learned the team was going to Chattanooga I called [former JMU administrator] Ray Sonner," Carrier told *Montpelier* that spring. "I told him to come with me and lime the field like we had to in the old days." Carrier, of course, was joking, but with basketball on the backburner, the football team certainly had everyone's attention.

In the visiting locker room at Finley Stadium, the men charged with capturing JMU's first football championship waited for their chance to change university history. As fans began pouring through the gates,

Rose dropped down to field level, visiting with the Marching Royal Dukes, fielding a phone call from Virginia governor Mark Warner and finally stopping to wish the team luck before trekking back to his private box atop Finley Stadium. Rose was a case study in contained excitement. His natural saunter and sense of control contrasted the chaotic atmosphere around him. Some joked Rose was the only person at JMU who never seemed rushed. Today was no different. Rose's casual attire may have blended with the fervent JMU fans, but his outward demeanor was calm. Internally, he was counting down to kickoff like everyone else. But at face value, Rose seemed impervious to the game-day buzz.

The Dukes sprinted out of the paddock for warm-ups. Head coach Mickey Matthews, capped in a purple windbreaker and a black JMU football hat, jogged up the sideline and donned a headset for the biggest game of his six-year Madison tenure. Thirteen months earlier, there had been speculation on campus that Matthews might be out of a job after failing to reach the playoffs for four straight years. Even the coach later would admit that while he thought he was safe for 2004, he was one more sub-par season from being fired. Public speculation at the time was cut down the middle, and yet, in the end — after Matthews had been retained — Rose and the administration would say his job had been safe all along, that Madison never had intentions of letting its football coach go. "I was convinced we had hired the right person," Rose declared. "And I can't speak for everyone, but in 2003 I was still convinced we had the right man for the job."

At the time, his conviction was in the minority.

Chapter 2

MICKEY MATTHEWS didn't need anyone to tell him he was on the hot seat in 2004. "I think if we weren't successful, I'd have been fired," he admitted. "I don't think there's any question about that."

Things hadn't always been so tumultuous for Matthews. An Andrews, Texas native, the 45-year-old came to JMU in 1999 and guided the Dukes to a surprising 8-3 record in his first season. With a preference for building with youth and a fiery personality, Matthews vaulted the Dukes to the top of the conference by sparking a fuse under a veteran team that had underachieved the previous two seasons. The result was a conference championship and JMU's first playoff appearance since 1995. Despite using four quarterbacks during an injury-plagued season, Matthews swung a dormant program back into the national spotlight. He was presented with the Eddie Robinson Award as the nation's best I-AA coach. Matthews was a hot commodity, and more importantly, his high-energy approach was a welcome contrast to that of his predecessor.

Linwood Rose hired Matthews in the spring of 1999 to rebuild a program that lacked stability. Alex Wood — the former Madison coach, whose four-year tenure was marked by players and coaches leaving the program — never related well with his athletes, and the team sharply declined during his final seasons. "Alex knew talent," WSVA radio broadcaster and JMU play-by-play man Mike Schikman said. "Players just had difficulty relating to him at times. He thought it was a business deal. The players were labor, and he and his staff were management."

Schikman was one of the few people outside the program who had a solid feel for the locker room temperature. He was heavy-set, in his late 40s, and had Coke bottle-thick glasses and a stubbly gray goatee. A self-described smart-ass Jewish kid from Brooklyn, Schikman was 24 when he arrived in Harrisonburg in the late 1970s. In his early years at WSVA he developed friendships with the athletes and even partied with them on the weekends. As he grew older, Schikman developed into a trusted figure — a pass-down for athletes, grandfathered into the JMU community. Sometimes his inside knowledge gave him access to material that had the potential to hurt a player's reputation. But Schikman never placed his job ahead of his morals. He'd talk to the player about what he knew and might chastise them for the mistake, but he always kept the student's best interest at heart. Eventually, he became a person to go to for advice, both for his honesty and his discretion.

Schikman thought Alex Wood was an intelligent coach. A native of Masillon, Ohio, Wood played for Iowa in the late 1970s before beginning a coaching career that would pass through Kent State, Southern Illinois and Miami. After leaving Madison, he took a job as quarterbacks coach with the Minnesota Vikings. Wood knew football and he knew how to climb the ladder. But, Schikman argued, you couldn't treat 18-to-22-year-old kids like employees. That was Wood's first mistake. External events, like injuries, also fueled Wood's downfall as Madison's head coach.

Perhaps Wood's biggest problem was his desire to go after West Coast recruits. Many of them did not stay at Madison for more than a year. It was a questionable recruiting tactic for a school that drew much of its talent from inside the state. "You have to be making hay at home," JMU sports information director Gary Michael said. "For us to be successful, that's where we have to get kids. And if you look at what happened, we just slipped."

Michael was another man who understood the program. A Madison graduate, he worked at the Harrisonburg *Daily News-Record* in the late 1970s before returning to JMU as an assistant SID. Michael's remarks were backed by underlying currents. During his four-year tenure, Wood employed 11 assistant coaches — including three different defensive coordinators. In total, Madison went through six coaching changes for full-time assistants from 1995 to 1998. The lack of consistency created a gap in Madison's recruiting system. "The further you have to go regionally or nationally, the more difficult it becomes to recruit," said Curt Dudley, director of multimedia communications for JMU Sports. "And why do you have to recruit that way in the first place? Are communications close to home not happening? Are you not able to recruit close to home for some reason? Virginia is a pretty good football state."

Dudley, a Bridgewater College graduate, who lived in nearby Broadway and worked with Schikman in the broadcast booth, believed JMU was plagued by a geographic problem in the late 1990s. The distance between Virginia and California, combined with the coaching flux, kept the program's foundation unstable. Personnel turnover — coupled with Wood's distant relationship with his players — became the primary cause behind JMU's decline in the late 1990s. But to be fair, Michael and Dudley also said Wood's final classes included some of his best recruits, many of whom played an important role in Madison's brief resurrection in 1999. All-America tailback Curtis Keaton and two-time All-Conference safety Ron Atkins committed to JMU during Wood's tenure. Wood also recruited 1999 A-10 defensive player of the year Chris Morant. The problem, Michael noted, was that while Wood was bringing in talent, he wasn't doing it with consistency. And the talent he recruited wasn't enough to mask the glaring holes in the program's long-term plan.

Wood arguably had bigger shoes to fill and bigger expectations than any other JMU coach. His predecessor, Rip Scherer, had guided the Dukes to a 29-19 overall record and two NCAA playoff victories from 1991-1994. In the years since his departure, Scherer's postseason success was credited with exponentially improving the program and building on the growth sustained during the tenures of Joe Purzycki (34-30-2 from 1985-1990) and Challace McMillin (67-56-1 from 1972-1984). Most importantly, Scherer instilled a "team is family" concept that his players embraced — a standard that Alex Wood's business model did not meet. Wood inherited what many believed to be a strong program, and his approach had disastrous consequences. Despite leaving Madison with a winning record — 23-22 over four seasons — popular opinion was that he left the program in disarray. "We inherited a team on the ground floor," Matthews later said, and this for a program that qualified for the postseason three times from 1991-1995. "Alex was one of the most intelligent and well-read coaches I have ever known," Schikman added. "But he came to take over a team with, I believe, a major misconception that plagued him throughout his tenure."

From 1995 to 1998, JMU's offensive production declined, as did the team's victory total — from eight wins to three. As coaches came and went, recruiting connections dried up and JMU's retention of its skilled underclassmen from the West Coast fell sharply in the final two years of Wood's tenure. "Things come in cycles," Michael said. "There were some good players left [in '98 and '99] but [a few years later] we hit a lull because we had almost no seniors. So much of football is a numbers game. You have to get a lot of good players in all your classes."

On March 19, 1999, amidst heightened speculation that he would resign, Wood announced his intention to void the remaining time on his contract and pursue an opening in the NFL. Seven days later, Mickey Matthews was introduced as Madison's fifth head coach. Matthews — a former assistant at Marshall University and the University of Georgia — had been a candidate for the job in 1995, and the JMU coaching search undoubtedly was accelerated by the university's familiarity with its prime candidate.

In the years since his departure, Alex Wood has worked several jobs in the NFL and NCAA, including a brief stint as offensive coordinator of the Arizona Cardinals. Most recently he worked as an assistant coach for the University of Arkansas. Repeated phone calls to Wood's office in

Fayetteville in 2007 were not returned. Still, Mike Schikman believes the former JMU coach understands the dynamic between coaches and players with more clarity. While Wood's methods might have worked better elsewhere, his techniques simply didn't fit JMU during his tenure.

By the time Matthews was brought in, his personality reflected a much-needed changing of the guard. "Alex had burned a lot of bridges," Schikman said. "He didn't realize these are children. He was cold. Mickey came into this terrible situation and brought an air of freshness. He'll yell and scream and cuss at his players but he'll hug them. He treats the kids like his own children."

But while Matthews' energy helped bring JMU's struggling program back to the doorstep of respectability, his fiery temper didn't make him the easiest coach to play for. "When he was younger, his players were scared to death of him," Matthews' son Clayton recalled. "He loves his players more than anything else and he'd do anything for them. But he's not afraid to correct them. He gets to his point quickly."

Clayton Matthews knew this fact better than most. He wasn't just Mickey's son; he was one of his players. And Matthews was just as tough on Clayton as he was on every other athlete. Matthews began assembling a team full of old-fashioned players — hard working kids who valued preparation. He gave them freedom and let them be boys (several players believed Matthews knew he would burn out his kids if he pushed them too hard), but he would not stand for complacency. Laziness was an easy way to earn a ticket out of town. "He was really intense," said Tahir Hinds, who played wide receiver for Matthews from 2001-2005. "If you were soft, you wouldn't make it with coach Matthews. He had to turn the program around. I saw people coming to school, on that beautiful campus, seeing all those ladies and thinking about the parties and I watched Mickey weed out those guys who didn't put football or school first. We knew we had to get better.

"Every day it was get better or get worse."

His ambition and job title made Matthews open to criticism. To some in his first years at Madison, the new coach came off as someone who tried to "big-time" his team, as though his experience at Marshall and Georgia gave him a higher status — and thus elevated his program. But to others, this was an appropriate way for Matthews to boost the mindset of his players. Matthews pushed for an increase in local media exposure and game-day atmosphere. Schikman thought Matthews had a long-term vision for the program. "Mickey has always had this concept of what JMU football could be," Schikman said. "He was far ahead of the curve as to what kind of program they should have and he has built it that way."

However, Matthews managed to rub some people the wrong way, especially those who viewed the program at face value — a I-AA team with fluctuating results. While Matthews had his vision, he often didn't play by the unwritten rules that applied to a premier college football team. Matthews often referred to Madison as "major college football," but his openness often was dictated by the success of his program. "Mickey called it 'major college football,' and that's fine because it creates a mentality," *Daily News-Record* sports editor Chris Simmons said. "But at the same time he did things to counter that."

Simmons referenced JMU's lean years in 2001 and 2002, citing occasions when Matthews would get defensive about why players wouldn't show up for post-game press conferences. "Matthews saw it as protecting his kids," Simmons said. "[But] I think you should be man enough to talk to the media. There's a bit of a dichotomy there as far as how he wants [his players] to think and how he acts."

Simmons believed facing the press was a necessary character-builder for an athlete. He thought Matthews was employing small-time tactics. The players, however, disagreed, especially when it came to young players in overwhelming situations. "Coach Matthews definitely looks out for his players," former free safety Tony LeZotte said. "Reporters want to get their information, but to put a player in a bad situation — like facing the media after making a big mistake to lose a game — it might hurt their career. Some people don't get over that stuff."

LeZotte believed Matthews did not have a blanket philosophy when it came to availability, that it had more to do with the player and the situation. A first-year starter or a freshman with no media experience might need more protection. A senior captain, meanwhile, likely could handle himself.

Matthews was in a precarious situation with the media from the beginning. JMU wasn't big enough for him to shove reporters away without costing his program valuable exposure. And the Dukes weren't small enough to fly completely under the radar. Matthews reluctantly understood the parallel between media exposure and attendance numbers, and unlike his peers at Virginia Tech and Virginia, he gave local reporters almost total access at practice. "The one thing that I have to do at my job that [Virginia Tech coach] Frank Beamer or [Virginia coach] Al Groh don't have to do is sell tickets," Matthews said in 2007. "That means I have to be much more friendly to the media than I'd like to be. I have to keep our team on the front page of the sports section. At JMU we're battling with the Redskins, Virginia and Virginia Tech for the sports pages. I have to be more accommodating as a football coach and it can make my job very difficult."

While this tactic helped keep JMU football on the front page, Matthews knew it opened the door for breaking news he didn't want leaked. "He needs to be in the newspaper every day," *Daily News-Record* assistant sports editor and JMU football reporter Mike Barber said. "Mickey told me, 'If I was at Georgia or Marshall, I wouldn't let you come to practice.' The difference is he needs the coverage. And because I have that access and I give him all this newspaper exposure, I stumble onto some things he doesn't want me to know about. It's the price you pay if you want to have that publicity."

Between Simmons and Barber, the DN-R had a news-breaking sports department. If someone didn't want to talk with them, it peaked their interest. While the two reporters saw investigative journalism as their responsibility, Matthews was tasked with protecting his program and players against negative press. Ninety percent of the time, Matthews said, reporters and coaches get along just fine. The other 10 percent of the time — when suspensions, off-field problems or scandals take place — the two parties butt heads. "We're not paying these kids like they play for the Redskins," Matthews argued. "It's open game on those guys [because] they're like a politician or an entertainer. I get paid a lot of money to coach football and I'm a professional [so] the heat needs to fall on me. I do not agree that when a 19-year-old makes a mistake they should be held to the same public scrutiny as someone who's 25 and making a lot of money."

Like any other coach, if Matthews didn't want the public to know about a problem with his team, he would do everything in his power to keep the word from getting out. This was an impossible goal, and sometimes ended with the story being broken by the papers instead of coming from Matthews — a continual occurrence during his early years at Madison. If a player was involved in an off-field incident, Matthews would deny any allegations unless presented concrete proof by the reporter — partially to avoid leaking information and largely to protect his player. "I do not work for them," he said of the media. And Matthews only would go on the record about the incident when the time was right, if nothing else, to prove that no punishment would be levied based on speculation. Negative press would not dictate what went on in Mickey's shop.

According to Barber, Matthews dramatically improved his ability to handle the media as he grew into the role of head coach — especially once he learned that refusing to comment only peaked a reporter's interest. While Matthews would shield his kids to the best of his capabilities, he also knew that when it was time to talk, nothing good ever came out of "no comment." University personnel saw this as a tactical maneuver by Matthews, who preferred to handle things internally when he could, and would defer the heat away from his players — and onto himself if necessary — to keep his team focused on winning football games. "A good father probably is going to take the heat [off his kids]," Curt Dudley said. "If that's designed intent, you probably have to give Matthews a lot of credit. He may be a sly old Texas fox after all."

It was the Texan in Matthews that made him approachable. He often concluded meetings by outlining the next day's agenda. "This is for mañana," he'd say. "And in Texas, 'mañana' means 'not today.'" Matthews was full-tilt on the sideline but the opposite in his daily activities. He never seemed rushed away from football. Off the field, his rhythmic drawl spilled forth with a relaxing cadence; his athletic stride slowed to a casual shuffle and his mannerisms developed a leisurely quality. Matthews was famous among staff members for sometimes falling asleep during film sessions.

His track record, however, belonged in the fast lane. Before revitalizing the Dukes, Matthews enjoyed consistent success as an assistant coach from 1990 to 1998 at both the Division I-AA and Division I-A levels. From 1990 to 1995, as Marshall University's defensive coordinator, Matthews helped lead the Thundering Herd to four national championship games. When Marshall head coach Jim Donnan was hired at Georgia in 1996, Matthews went with him. The Bulldogs went 24-11 from 1996-1998, and Matthews padded his resume by coaching future NFL star Champ Bailey.

His success and experience (20 years as an assistant coach at the college level) made Matthews an attractive pick when Wood left after the 1998 season. And if nothing else, his fiery and sometimes confrontational approach gave the program a shot of adrenaline. As long as the Dukes won football games, the fans and university officials would tolerate his quirks. His 8-3 debut season ended in the first round of the playoffs, and was followed by his first recruiting class — a group that included quarterback Matt LeZotte, whom Matthews believed would be the cornerstone of a successful program at the turn of the millennium. The 2000 Dukes, a veteran team that outscored its opponents 300-185, missed the playoffs only after losing the final two games of the regular season. "He was winning with a team that no one expected to do much,"

Chris Simmons said. "It was impressive because those kids weren't his. And it gave him huge political capital."

In his first two seasons, Matthews had taken a rock-bottom team to a 14-9 record and an A-10 title. But as he and others expected, the decision to build with young talent — and the fallout from Alex Wood's final years — finally caught up to Madison in 2001. The top-heavy roster from 1999 was bottom-heavy two years later. "I do not blame one person on this Earth except me," Matthews said. "In retrospect I probably should have taken more transfers. College football needs to be played by young men, not old boys."

While Matthews said he inherited the ground floor, it really took him two years to reach its epicenter. In 2001, with a roster comprised of 54 freshman and only 11 seniors, the Dukes plummeted to 2-9, despite LeZotte's emergence as one of the conference's most promising young quarterbacks. They finished 5-7 in 2002, averaging an anemic 16 points per game and tanking in October, losing five straight games in the middle of the season. "You laugh about it now, but when I was a freshman we couldn't run the ball or throw the ball," Clayton Matthews recalled. "Almost every starter we had on offense was either a true freshman or a redshirt freshman. They practically tore my shoulder off at the Maine game [in 2001]. Matt [LeZotte] got hurt four times that year. We couldn't do anything right."

By opening day of 2003, Matthews' political capital was waning. Despite his beliefs that the team was turning into a contender, critics thought the program was mired in quicksand. Matthews had one year remaining on his contract, and already he was running out of excuses. LeZotte, after early promise, had reached a plateau thanks to knee injuries and a patchwork offensive line. After an attendance spike in 1999 and 2000, fan turnout was declining again. And some wondered if Matthews could focus on football, especially after Clayton was badly injured in a horrific car accident just three weeks before the 2003 opener. JMU vice president of administration Charlie King spoke with Matthews that October, and it was clear Matthews was troubled. "Charlie asked me 'Can you do this?' and I told him I could," Matthews recalled. "And I really felt like I could. But the three people I love more than anything else are my two children and my wife, Kay, and they were hurt so badly. I couldn't fix it. It sucks the life out of you."

…

THE PREVIOUS six months had been tumultuous ones for Clayton Matthews. A sure-fire kid, Matthews appeared to have the world at his fingertips when his father took the Madison job. He quarterbacked his high school team to the Georgia state championship in 1999 and had been a versatile player for the Dukes in his first two seasons.

Matthews was Madison's "slash" player. He started four games at quarterback in 2001, throwing for 347 yards, two touchdowns and four picks. In 2002 he pinned teams inside the 20-yard line seven times on 12 punts, kicked two extra points, completed one pass and caught another. Matthews was, by many indications, playing a bit above his talent level. He likely could have been a standout Division II quarterback, but at Madison he was a role player. His talents, however, were useful in a program that was being gutted and rebuilt. Clayton had a coach's brain. He understood the offense and often helped younger teammates better understand schemes.

He and his father were very close. The elder Matthews often called his son "my best friend." They shared a love for football and a passion for golf. They also were similar in their mannerisms, temperament and bravado. Mickey wasn't short on confidence. Neither was his son.

Clayton could be endearing and complimentary one minute, and then flash a mischievous smile the next. He was well known on campus. Clayton had a swagger about him, and there were critics who believed the younger Matthews was full of himself. Much of it, however, could be chalked up to the youthful exuberance of a college kid who saw what he wanted and then went out and got it. Clayton certainly was an alpha personality, but most people thought it was fine. Clayton, they argued, simply enjoyed being Clayton. Mike Schikman remembered sharing an elevator with Clayton and Matt LeZotte during a road trip one season.

The three were heading to the same floor, but the elevator stopped early and two attractive women boarded. "Matt and Clayton grinned at each other," Schikman recalled. The elevator stopped one floor below where the Dukes were staying and the women walked out. LeZotte and the younger Matthews followed, cycling through potential pick-up lines as the doors closed behind them.

On February 2, 2003, Clayton celebrated his 21st birthday with a night on the town. He was arrested for being drunk in public — a foolish but virtually harmless infraction that could have happened to anyone. But Matthews compounded his mistake by assaulting a Rockingham County jailer — a felony offense that later was downgraded to misdemeanor assault and battery charges. He was convicted in May. Mickey Matthews made plans to suspend his son at the beginning of the 2003 season as further punishment, but weeks after the arrest, Clayton injured his back while lifting weights and was forced to shut down his offseason conditioning program. The pain persisted into the summer. "I'd been through injuries my whole life but never anything like that," Clayton recalled. "I couldn't brush my teeth without hurting my back."

Medical evaluations revealed a cracked disc. Doctors told Clayton he could cause permanent injury if he continued playing, and on August 1, Mickey announced that his son's football career was over. "I became aware as a father and a coach in mid-April that he was in intense pain," Matthews told the *Daily News-Record*. "I think he and I both thought it would get better, but it didn't. He didn't take it well at all."

Two days after the announcement, Clayton was driving back to his off-campus apartment when he lost control of his Ford Mustang and plunged down a hill off University Boulevard. The car hit two trees. Matthews was tossed from the driver's seat. A female passenger was in the car with him, and the two lay in the woods for almost an hour before Matthews' former teammate Jerame Southern passed by the accident and heard the girl crying for help.

What happened next has been widely chronicled. When Matthews was taken to Rockingham Memorial Hospital, doctors discovered the extent of his injuries. The former football standout had broken his jaw, his left ankle, his left femur and six ribs. He suffered a puncture in his right lung. His neck was fractured at the T-4 and C-6 vertebrae.

Clayton Matthews was paralyzed. Doctors did not know if he would survive.

It took eight hours of surgery to insert two steel rods and screws into Clayton's broken neck and set the breaks in his leg and jaw. His paralysis was not connected to his initial back injury. For almost three weeks, Clayton was in a drug-induced coma and he spent the majority of the month in intensive care. Only when his conditioned stabilized did he realize he couldn't walk. "I don't remember the wreck at all and I don't remember going to the hospital," Clayton recalled. "You're so drugged it's almost good for you. I had tubes in every hole of my body. It took me two months to get to the rehab center and it wasn't until then that I fully understood the situation.

"You react as expected. You're just waiting to wake up from the nightmare."

Matthews spent several months at the Shepherd Center in Atlanta and began traveling to Mexico for experimental stem cell injections to increase his strength and balance. The physical rehabilitation was bad enough, but the mental rehabilitation was the most demanding. Clayton Matthews was a high school state championship quarterback and a college athlete. His post-graduate plans were rooted in game he loved. Without warning, his future was shattered, and piecing his life back together was a far greater challenge than physical therapy. "I don't think a lot of people went from as high as he was to as low as he was that quickly," Mickey said. "It's just mind-boggling."

Clayton brought his father's observation to a much darker level. "It's almost like alcoholism," he said. "They say recovering alcoholics fight it every day. So when you're in a situation like this you fight it every day. And that's what they talked about, that we all were like recovering alcoholics. I don't have to fight wanting to drink every day. I have to fight thinking that my life is over."

For several months, Clayton alternated his time between Mexico, home and the Virginia Medical Center in Charlottesville. Meanwhile, an outpouring of empathy for his family spread throughout the local community. Clayton's accident had rocked the university at a level that went beyond athletics. In the weeks after the wreck, the family received well wishes and letters of encouragement from throughout the country as members of the Madison community — and friends of the family — rallied to offer support.

As support for Clayton continued to flood the family mailbox, Mickey Matthews prepared for the toughest season of his career. The recovery process wasn't limited to its participant. Mickey's mind was elsewhere. In the weeks following the wreck, his status had shifted. His football program was stuck in neutral and his fan base was turning on him. Yet now, the outpouring of emotion for his family countered his coaching problems, as though the situation caused critics to step back and think of Matthews the father, not Matthews the football coach. "Like most people in the public eye, coach had his fans and detractors," Mike Schikman said. "All fans think losing coaches are being out-coached. Yet everyone tried to be as supportive as possible. It's hard to explain how devastating Clayton's accident was to everyone associated with the Madison family."

As the 2003 season began, it was clear that Matthews was a shell of his former self. His struggling program took a backseat to a much larger problem. Being a father came first. And throughout the season it was the clear the head coach had a lot on his mind that had nothing to do with football. "I was probably more of an adviser [in 2003]," he said. "I probably did less coaching that year than I've ever done.

"I really don't remember that season at all."

...

MICKEY MATTHEWS entered the 2003 season at a professional crossroads. This was year three of the program's rebuilding process, and year three was the year for results. But the snake-bitten Dukes never got on track. JMU opened the 2003 season without All-Conference senior center Leon Steinfeld — who suffered a season-ending knee injury on the first day of contact drills — and split its first six games, alternating impressive and lackluster performances into the middle of the season. Still, the Dukes managed to stay in the playoff hunt until late October, when a seven-point loss to Maine eliminated them from postseason contention.

The final month of the season was fueled by a large segment of fans that wanted Matthews out of Harrisonburg. On the final day of the 2003 season, several JMU seniors walked into Bridgeforth Stadium with shirts reading: "Four years without a playoff game. Hey, Hey Mickey, Goodbye." And with a chance to finish with a winning record for the first time since 2000, the Dukes flopped. LeZotte threw two interceptions and Madison was drubbed by Northeastern, 41-24. "I didn't know they wore them," Matthews said, referring to the shirts. "I don't blame them. I probably would have worn one, too."

As the Dukes finished their 6-6 season, a section of the remaining 2,000 fans broke out in a "Fire Mickey," chant. The critics had cast their vote, and with his contract set to expire in January, Matthews faced the prospect of an uncertain future. As the Madison faithful continued to chant from the Bridgeforth stands and the administration pondered the outlook of the program, Matthews slowly walked off the field. The debate over his tenure was underway.

In previous seasons, the negative rumblings toward Matthews had been relatively minor — largely due to the political capital he built in 1999 and 2000. But now the volume increased. And Madison's performance against Northeastern did nothing to quell those who believed change was necessary. It had been a long season for Matthews, a roller-coaster ride on the field — the Dukes were never more than a game below or above .500 — and a traumatic disaster off it, after Clayton's car accident and subsequent rehabilitation. The last thing Matthews needed was to be in limbo regarding his contract. And for what it was worth, he didn't think he was going anywhere. "I never felt like my job was in jeopardy," Matthews said. "A firing is a lot like a divorce, most of the time when you look back it wasn't a surprise. We just needed to win. And in my discussions with Dr. Rose, Charlie King and Jeff Bourne, that's where we were."

Yet as the 2003 season came to a close, his status was unclear. Regardless of his instincts, his contract had run out. Lots of coaches before him had been fired with better records and more playoff appearances. And for those who supported the program, collective patience was reaching a tipping point. "We had been criticized publicly and privately via a barrage of e-mails to make a change," Madison athletics director Jeff Bourne recalled. "It's tough because you believe in a coach. There comes a time where you make calls that are publicly not popular."

Bourne's instincts were to bring Matthews back. The case for the coach centered on JMU's improvement from 2001 to 2003. Collectively, Bourne and Rose believed Matthews had all the pieces to launch a successful program. The Dukes graduated players, retained assistant coaches and drew average crowds for a I-AA school. And yet the concern was that for all Matthews had done right, he wasn't winning. Each of his predecessors (including the often-criticized Alex Wood) had a winning record through their first four seasons. Matthews was 21-25 after year four. He was 27-31 after year five. For a program that won 55 percent of its games since achieving varsity status, Matthews wasn't measuring up on the score sheet. "I think people who knew Mickey and the program continued to support him," Rose said. "Those on the outside who may have just been attending games were more critical. I don't blame them. We weren't winning."

Publicly, Matthews was on the hot seat. To the decision makers, he probably was safe. Then the Dukes bombed on TV against Northeastern. If ever there was a game that could have provided momentum for next season, this was it. Instead, JMU turned the ball over four times and trailed 38-10 midway through the third quarter. And since the disaster took place on the last day of the season, the bitter taste lingered. Later that offseason, Matthews and one Madison administrator were discussing the outlook of the program. The coach sensed the administrator was frustrated.

"Are you mad about the season or are you mad about the Northeastern game?" Matthews finally asked.

"I'm mad about the Northeastern game," the administrator said.

"Well I'm mad about the Northeastern game, too," Matthews replied. "But are we talking about the future or just one football game?"

Matthews had proven his point, and in the process possibly swung another vote back for Camp Mickey. The personable approach might have helped him more than anything else, because in the end, Bourne, Rose and the administration knew what they were going to get from Matthews — namely, accountability and a clean program. They hoped the results would follow.

Speculation began to break up shortly before the New Year. On Dec. 8, Bourne announced that the university and its beleaguered coach had reached an agreement on a three-year extension at $127,000 per season. For the interim, Matthews was back in purple and gold. But if the new contract gave him more time to build JMU's program, it wasn't an award for a job well done. The contract was merely an extension of his existing deal, with no added benefits thrown in. "We didn't increase the salary for two reasons," Rose said. "When we look at salary increases we look at market value and performance, and I thought it would have been inappropriate to increase compensation without results. The extension was a vote of confidence."

How much confidence is a question that might never be answered. If nothing else, the extension sent a clear message from the administration to its head coach. "I think there was an under-the-table agreement," Mike Schikman said. "If they didn't win, things would have to change."

It might have been a three-year extension, but for Matthews it was a one-year audition. He was walking into the 2004 season with a 27-31 career record and had not taken JMU to the playoffs since his debut season. August training camp was months away and already Madison's head coach was back inside the pressure cooker. Worse yet, after months of physical therapy, Clayton Matthews had suffered a massive setback in his rehabilitation, a turn of events that shook the Matthews family to its core.

…

CLAYTON MATTHEWS grew up with football. And living in a football family, he was accustomed to everything that came with the territory. His voracious interest in the game was an early sign that he would follow his father into coaching. When other kids would go to day care or play with friends after school, Clayton would go to football camp. He began lifting weights as a sixth grader when Mickey was an assistant at Georgia. And Clayton never had a problem finding a place to play. "When you move to a new city and you're the coach's son everyone wants you to play for them," Clayton said. "They don't know anything about you, but the day you arrive in town you've got six messages from local high school coaches. It makes you feel wanted."

It helped that Clayton was good. His football knowledge was incredible. And his intangibles made up for a lack of size. "He studies the game relentlessly," Mickey said of his son.

Clayton was versatile enough to play several different positions. He was tough enough to excel everywhere. Two weeks before his senior year of high school, Clayton ripped ligaments in his right wrist. He played the first few games of the season with a cast on his hand, but the injury prevented him from playing quarterback. So Clayton shifted to wide receiver and led the team in touchdown catches. Moving around, joining new teams and playing different positions were all part of the game to him, and some argued his toughness and work ethic willed him through his first eight months of rehab after the accident. "What happened to him is difficult to emotionally handle as a parent and an adult," Mickey said. "So I think it's almost impossible for a 20-year-old. I think as you go through the realization that you're going to be paralyzed the rest of your life, you come to grips with it."

A few days before JMU's 2004 spring game, Kay Matthews was

driving Clayton home from a doctor's appointment in Charlottesville. It had been raining all day and as Kay piloted her car up Afton Mountain, it hydroplaned and hit a guardrail. The car slid along the rail, then veered and drifted into the median.

Kay shielded her son during the accident, but as the car came to a stop Clayton knew he had broken his neck again. The sudden jolt from the wreck snapped the steel rods in his neck. This time it was a more serious injury. "The biggest difference after my second accident was I was aware of the situation," Clayton recalled. "I remember everything. It was a 'shit, here we go again' thing. And it really did feel like that."

Clayton underwent more surgeries. Doctors replaced the rods in his neck and he was transferred to a rehabilitation hospital in Houston where he began the draining process of starting over. Mickey Matthews faced the media three days later for his spring game press conference. He looked as though he hadn't slept in weeks. The law of averages had played a cruel trick on Matthews, who received the same heart-stopping phone call twice in eight months. He looked mentally and physically shattered. "I thought we had made so much progress after the first accident," he said. "The fact that we were back at square one with more damage just devastated us. You feel so much pressure as a father just to keep everything together."

In the rehab center, there were good days and bad days. The second accident prevented Clayton from using his hands. Mundane tasks like writing and eating became painfully difficult. "They would come in every day and test my grip and I could hardly do anything," Clayton said. "But the weirdest thing was they didn't have to teach me. I had been there before."

His stubbornness was both a catalyst, and at times, a hindrance, especially when Clayton's frustration overtook his desire. The previous fall, it took Matthews three weeks just to learn how to sit upright. And going through the process all over again was difficult. Yet Clayton plowed forward. He built his strength in rehab and eventually improved enough to return home in late June. He also outlined plans to return to campus as both a JMU student and a volunteer coach on his father's staff — opportunities Clayton said helped him take his mind off being depressed. Considering his age and what he went through, Clayton's outlook was remarkably optimistic, a mentality his father attributed to his son's character. In his heart, Mickey believed Clayton's urge to return to football was brought on by his desire to have purpose in his life. Despite his injuries, football remained Clayton's future. In 2004 it also became a life preserver.

...

MUCH LIKE 2003, Mickey Matthews opened the 2004 preseason with a pledge that the program was close to becoming a playoff contender. And while critics dismissed his words, several media members close to the team thought Matthews sounded more confident in his claim, as though the contract extension's implied vote of confidence had given him piece of mind. "It was — as is often the case — the darkest before the dawn," Mike Schikman said. "Dr. Rose and Charlie King had faith in the guy they hired and gave him the opportunity and tools to win. I don't know what would have happened [if they fell apart in '04] but Mickey always told me that if he couldn't win he would leave on his own."

If nothing else, Schikman thought the extension put Matthews firmly in control of his future as JMU's head coach. And it quickly became apparent that Matthews wasn't stretching the truth with his claims. After missing all of 2003, Leon Steinfeld received a medical redshirt from the NCAA and was awarded a final year of eligibility. With a healthy offensive line and a veteran defense that would give up the fewest points in the Atlantic 10, Matthews began to look like the old version of himself.

JMU finished September with a 2-1 record and then reeled off six wins in a row — the program's longest winning streak since 1999. As the season progressed, Madison became known for its run defense and its knack for making big plays in tight games. The Dukes trailed by three late in the fourth quarter of a midseason game at Maine when redshirt sophomore receiver D.D. Boxley made a one-handed catch in the corner of the end zone to give the Dukes a 24-20 win — their first in Orono since 1997. Three weeks later, Cortez Thompson's 87-yard punt return for a touchdown gave the Dukes a 20-13 home win over the defending national champion Delaware Blue Hens. The victory sent the Madison student section storming onto the field in bedlam.

At 8-1 overall, the Dukes rolled into their final regular season home game against 7-2 William & Mary as a playoff-bound football team. With the previous week's win still fresh, the Dukes tied the game with 45 seconds left on another Boxley touchdown catch. Davis Walsh, who worked as a producer for WSVA radio from 2002-04 was sitting in the JMU alumni section and vividly remembered the game's final minutes. The son of a JMU admissions director, Walsh attended Madison as a freshman in 2003 and transferred to W&M before the 2004 academic year. Among his peers, he could measure the pulse of the teams and their fans as well as anyone. And as the stadium rumbled in anticipation of overtime, Walsh — a Madison fan since high school — found himself appraising the reactions of the crowd.

With less than a minute to go in the game, W&M quarterback Lang Campbell quickly drove the Tribe down the field and set up Greg Kuehn for a game-winning 46-yard field goal attempt. In less than 40 seconds the stadium had gone tense. "First, everyone in the stadium thought JMU had done it again," Walsh recalled. "And then W&M picked up some quick yardage but it was still a long field goal attempt."

The snap and spot were good. Kuehn zipped a 46-yard field goal through the uprights and Bridgeforth Stadium went silent. "It was such a long attempt that most of the crowd wasn't worried," Walsh said. "And it wasn't until the kick went through the uprights that it hit everyone. The silence was absolutely brutal."

Kuehn's last-second field goal handed JMU its first loss in two months, and gave W&M the inside track at the A-10's automatic playoff bid. The Tribe secured that trip one week later with a 20-point win over Richmond. As W&M was wrapping up the A-10 title, the Dukes were closing the regular season with a 31-17 win over Towson. Madison would share the A-10 South crown with the Tribe and Delaware, and would earn an at-large bid to the NCAA postseason — but not a home playoff game. Kuehn's field goal had sealed JMU's fate. In order to advance, the Dukes would have to win on the road in the playoffs, something only one Madison team had ever done before.

The Dukes opened the 2004 postseason the Saturday after Thanksgiving with a 14-13 win at Lehigh. It was the program's first road playoff win since 1991 and tied the 1994 team for the most wins (10) in school history. With two weeks remaining in the academic semester, students returned to campus and began preparing for final exams. But they also kept a watchful eye on the NCAA playoff bracket. A win in the second round would put JMU in the national semifinals, and would set up an Atlantic 10 rematch with either Delaware or W&M. If the Dukes could get to the semifinals, a trip to Chattanooga was possible.

On Dec. 4, No. 8 JMU faced No. 2 Furman in the NCAA quarterfinals as a double-digit underdog. Facing a program that had won nearly 80 percent of its home games, the Dukes found themselves down, 13-7, with 5:11 left in the fourth quarter. Madison had the ball at its own 26-yard-line. "The big play was out of the question," JMU offensive coordinator Jeff Durden recalled. "The idea was to move the chains. We weren't ready to go home yet."

Two quick penalties pushed the Dukes back to their 14. Facing second-and-22, Madison embarked on a 12-play drive to save the season, using short passes and timely runs to reach the doorstep of the end zone. On fourth-and-goal from the one, junior tailback Raymond Hines plunged over the line for the game-winning touchdown that made the 2004 Dukes the most successful team in JMU history. "The height of our excitement was after the Furman game because we really didn't know if we could beat them," Clayton Matthews said. "We thought we could play a perfect game and still lose."

The last-minute win against Furman set up an all-Virginia national semifinal. And by the time the Dukes marched into Williamsburg for their highly touted rematch with W&M, even Lang Campbell wasn't enough to stop the Madison machine. By the end of JMU's 48-34 dismantling of the Tribe, chants of "Chattanooga," could be heard from the visiting sections at William & Mary's Zable Stadium. The Dukes were off to the I-AA championship game — a most improbable recovery for Matthews, who had gone from chopping block to coach of the year candidate in a little more than 12 months.

...

LINWOOD ROSE maintains that public opinion regarding Matthews had been split heading into the 2004 season. Regardless, JMU's success achieved a certain amount of validation for the administration's decision to keep its football coach. "It was a vote of confidence in his ability to lead this team," Rose said of the extension. "[After the success of that team] I felt excitement, elation and I guess some validation. Everyone likes to see their decisions play out." In a year where the program was at a crossroads, the controversial decision to retain Matthews made the run to Chattanooga possible.

As Matthews tested his headset, an ESPN camera focused on him pacing the sideline. No team in NCAA history had won three straight road playoff games, and yet the unlikely feat seemed to fit the Dukes. They had overcome the odds all season. Madison was picked to finish fourth in the A-10 South, and was picked to lose both its quarterfinal and semifinal playoff games against Furman and W&M. Yet here were the Dukes — once again double-digit underdogs — 60 minutes away from their first championship. As the pre-game show continued, the Madison faithful showed their appreciation for the coach they booed one year earlier, and the team that few figured would be here when the preseason polls were released in August.

Still, to those who believed in the Dukes all along, the groundwork for this moment could be traced to two things. The first was Matthews' contract extension, which allowed a veteran team to use a familiar system and a coach to work with his own players. The second came in the form of a transfer quarterback from Louisville, who became the face of the program's resurgence.

Chapter 3

NUMBER ELEVEN stretched his right arm, adjusted his helmet and pumped another warm-up throw before the opening coin toss, eye black already smudging from sweat despite temperatures in the low-40s. While the final seconds before kickoff were the most nerve-racking for some, these were Justin Rascati's most relaxing moments. There was no purpose in being uptight before a big game, he thought. If you did the work, you should be able to do the job.

Rascati's unflappable nature was built for pressure. When the meetings were over and the film was put away, his serious demeanor shifted. On game day he was loose, and often goofed around with his teammates in the locker room before kickoff. His production mirrored his composure. In postseason games against Lehigh, Furman and William & Mary, the right-hander completed 74 percent of his passes, threw for three touchdowns and ran for another. In his first season as starting quarterback, he already had a small list of landmark performances. Rascati led JMU to two late-game comeback wins in 2004. And those who witnessed his ability under pressure knew his pedigree. Rascati was a winner. When the Dukes needed him most, he seemed to find a way.

Perhaps Rascati's most important trait was trust. He was a transfer quarterback — a sophomore no less — working in an unfamiliar setting. Yet he demonstrated an uncanny ability to protect the football.

Entering the I-AA title game, JMU had turned the ball over only twice in 202 postseason plays. In 55 pass attempts Rascati had thrown zero interceptions. "Like all the great quarterbacks, Justin had an unbelievable confidence in his ability," Mickey Matthews said. "He didn't turn the ball over. He simply refused to."

At 6-foot-2 and 220 pounds, Rascati's athletic frame was that of a prototype college quarterback. His throwing motion (a rhythmic, over-the-top pump) was remarkably consistent — almost robotic — and yielded high accuracy. His ability to improvise with his legs made him a cross between a pocket passer and a scrambler. His leadership qualities, clean-cut face, polished social skills and laid-back demeanor evoked the franchise poster boy. Rascati had been a JMU student for one semester, and already he was the recognizable face of JMU football, a blend of Joe College and Captain Comeback. "He seemed to have an air of responsibility," Mike Schikman noted. "Justin watched things very seriously. He was a real impressive kid."

Rascati walked with what Schikman called "earnest confidence," just the right mixture for a person in a new environment. He returned phone calls, granted interview requests and treated everyone with respect. More importantly, the Louisville transfer found a way to maintain his competitive swagger without damaging his relationship with teammates. "When you come from a I-A school it's easy to come off as someone who thinks he's better than everyone else," Mike Barber said. "Justin didn't do that. And so when he said things like, 'These are the best receivers I've ever played with, including Louisville,' his teammates took that as a real compliment. I think a lot of guys gained confidence from what he said. In that sense, he used his swagger to elevate them."

At 25, Barber was the senior member of JMU's local media contingent, a group that included Ryan Sonner of *The Northern Virginia Daily*, Joe Downs of WHSV-TV and a revolving door of reporters from JMU's campus paper, *The Breeze*. A Rutgers University alum, Barber covered the Yankees-Mets Subway Series in 2000 for *The Daily Targum*, and worked as an editorial assistant for Major League Baseball before joining the DN-R in 2002. He was a good writer, dogged in his reporting. He had no ties to Harrisonburg or the Dukes and his writing was bluntly factual.

From afar, Barber gave off an air of nonchalance that bugged some in the Madison community. They believed his writing carried a negative slant because he disliked the Dukes. To some ardent JMU fans, Barber wanted to be anywhere but Harrisonburg, and his reporting reflected it. But others pointed out that he inherited the football beat when there wasn't much positive news to write about. They argued that Barber's reporting was centered on an unfortunate reality. "He can come off as a bit aggressive toward JMU," noted former JMU student Brandon Sweeney. "But you have to take the other side because what Barber does is only done by him. He's the reporter for JMU football. He gets it out to the world. It's the hometown team. The hometown writers are not always going to take the side of the team. They will critique. It's their responsibility. Mike's reporting always is based with facts."

Barber and Matthews had an interesting relationship that stemmed from Barber's nearly unlimited access to the football team. By 2004, Barber could do a spot-on impression of Matthews, complete with mannerisms and catch phrases. Likewise, Matthews was never shy about ripping Barber for being a Yankees fan from north New Jersey. Late in the 2004 season, Barber attended night practice in a Yankees windbreaker and began pacing the sideline as the temperature dipped into the high 30s. Matthews ambled over.

"When the hell are you gonna call this practice, Mick?" Barber jawed, only half-kidding.

"Are you cold Mike?" Matthews teased. "I've got a parka in my office [or] maybe you should trade that jacket for a nice Red Sox sweatshirt."

Matthews' open-door policy at practice gave the press plenty of time to talk to players. Early on, Barber noted that Rascati's sensitivity to his teammates was incredible. Above all else, he did not believe his background made him bigger than JMU. He understood he needed to earn the respect he sought. And Rascati gained approval by making plays on the field and acting with class. In a town where JMU football had meant so little for so long, Rascati became the image of the team that made it matter again. "He was the focal point," Barber said. "They had built the program and it was a good 2004 team, but he took it to the next level."

The next level was an atmosphere Rascati was familiar with. As a kid growing up in Gainesville, Fla., his weekends were dominated by football. Friday nights were spent at local high school games, where packed crowds would foreshadow the teenager's future. Saturday was college day, and the Rascati family often would have tickets to the Florida Gators game. Rascati was so excited to watch the Gators he would be nervous the night before the game, as though he was playing instead of watching from the stands.

Rascati considered himself fortunate to grow up in Florida. In the 1990s, with Steve Spurrier at the controls, the Gators were a dominant force, winning five conference championships from 1991-1996. Rascati grew up watching great teams, and those teams often had outstanding leaders. From 1986-2000, five of the nation's 15 Heisman Trophy winners were Sunshine State quarterbacks, including Danny Wuerffel, who led Spurrier's 1996 national championship team at Florida. In a football-crazed state, Wuerffel was a player Rascati looked up to. "You can't describe how big football is in Florida," Rascati recalled. "Everyone plays. Your varsity team has 100 kids on it and people have to share jersey numbers because there aren't enough to go around."

Another role model for Rascati was his uncle, Todd Kirtley, who played quarterback at Virginia from 1978-1981. Ever since Rascati was able to play, he and Kirtley would talk about the quarterback position. Rascati was a quick study. More importantly, he wanted everything that came with being the focal point. In sixth grade, Rascati played fullback and tailback. But by seventh grade he found his home under center.

At Buchholz High School, Rascati lettered in football and basketball. A two-time all-state selection on the gridiron, he threw for 5,033 yards and 45 touchdowns in his career. Those numbers eclipsed the previous school records held by Doug Johnson, who would play for Spurrier at Florida and later spend parts of seven seasons in the NFL. In his senior year, Rascati threw for 2,223 yards and 22 touchdowns, on his way to being named Class 3A-5A player of the year by *The Gainesville Sun*. The performance was enough attract the attention of several coaches from Division I-A programs, including John L. Smith, who was in the midst of developing a national power at the University of Louisville. "I had narrowed my choices to Louisville and N.C. State and I just thought Louisville was the best opportunity for me," Rascati later said. "They had a great quarterback tradition. Coach Smith and his assistants came to my high school games; they sat in my house and explained everything to me. I enjoyed my recruiting visit. I thought it was a perfect fit."

Like most true freshman, Rascati sat out his first season. The Cardinals were 7-5 in 2002 and lost their bowl game to Marshall, 38-15. Smith left Louisville that winter to become the head coach at Michigan State, but the Cardinals remained on the fast track to national prominence. They hired former Jacksonville Jaguars and Auburn University offensive coordinator Bobby Petrino as Smith's replacement, and Petrino shifted the Cardinals into overdrive. By the fall of 2003, Rascati was the heir apparent to one of the nation's most prolific offenses. Louisville averaged 34.6 points per game and finished 9-4 behind the strong play of junior quarterback Stefan LeFors. As the primary backup, Rascati played sparingly. He saw action in five games, threw one touchdown pass and ran for another as he continued to bide his time. With the program about to make a jump to the Big East Conference and Petrino tabbed as one of the nation's most-coveted coaches, Rascati's future was shaping into form.

Then the plan went awry. In the 2003-04 offseason, the Cardinals landed golden quarterback prospect Brian Brohm, the 2003 Gatorade National Player of the Year. In high school, Brohm won three state championships and set a Kentucky high school record for completion percentage. His father and two uncles had played at Louisville, and

Brian's intent to follow their path created an overwhelming response in the commonwealth.

Petrino's popularity as a coach, the program's emergence as a Bowl Championship Series contender and the addition of Brohm were expected to make Louisville a championship threat for years. But the perfect storm for the program also spelled the end of Rascati's days in Kentucky. While he was projected to be a serviceable Division I-A quarterback, Rascati had no chance to beat Brohm. The coveted recruit would be thrown into the quarterback mix as a true freshman. And all signs pointed to Brohm becoming the full-time starter by his sophomore season. "Brian's a great quarterback and LeFors was a great quarterback," Rascati recalled. "I thought I learned a lot under coach Petrino. At the same time, I wanted an opportunity to play."

Faced with what seemed like an unattainable goal, Rascati abandoned any thoughts of starting for the Cardinals and declared his intent to transfer. "I'm not a selfish player," he said. "[But] that was the one time in my career I had to be selfish and put myself before the team."

...

AS RASCATI was looking for a new home, the JMU athletics administration was finalizing a three-year extension for Mickey Matthews. After winning the Atlantic 10 in 1999, Matthews had struggled to rebuild an unstable program. The Dukes were 13-21 from 2000 to 2002. But Madison finished 6-6 in 2003, and those close to the program believed the outlook for 2004 was optimistic. For the first time in four years, the Dukes appeared to be turning the corner. They had depth at every position. The primary exception was quarterback.

In the three seasons since Madison's rebuilding project started, everything on offense began with Matt LeZotte. A 6-foot-1, 210-pound product of Augusta, Ga., LeZotte was the centerpiece of Matthews' first recruiting class, a talented quarterback with a commanding presence. On arrival, he was expected to bring JMU football into a new era of success. He flashed signs of greatness as a redshirt freshman, tossing two touchdowns in his first college game and throwing for 376 yards four weeks later. LeZotte had been a team captain since his sophomore season, but his career had been marked by inconsistency and injuries. The "Diaper Dukes," as they were called, were young and overwhelmed in 2001 and 2002, and LeZotte bore the brunt of the mismatch. "He had taken an inordinate amount of physical punishment," Matthews said. "Sometimes I was astonished at the beating he took."

Still, when he was healthy, LeZotte produced. In 2003 he missed only one game and enjoyed his finest season, throwing for 1,753 yards and 13 touchdowns as the Dukes crawled back to a .500 record. LeZotte was JMU's guy. Yet critics always placed Madison's poor record on the shoulders of its quarterback. LeZotte was the heart of the team both for his leadership and his talent, but fans had learned to be cautious of their optimism. He always seemed to go down with an injury when he was playing his best. And without a suitable backup quarterback, the success of the program hinged on LeZotte's health. "When a team is so dependent on the health of one player it really affects everything," former JMU sports media assistant Jon McNamara said. "Every time Matt dropped back to pass you held your breath a little bit. He had the talent to make great plays, but you also knew he was one big hit from going down with an injury."

Those inside the program believed LeZotte needed to be challenged entering the 2004 season, if nothing else, to improve his production. Matthews had long attempted to find the right person to push his star quarterback. From 2001-2003, JMU's depth chart included a revolving door of backups. Mike Connelly, Jayson Cooke and Clayton Matthews all had played significantly as LeZotte's backups. Dozens of other quarterbacks came to Madison in search of the starting job. But LeZotte was able to swat away all challengers with relative ease. In 2003, former Florida quarterback Pat Dosh expressed his interest in transferring to JMU, a declaration that created buzz among alumni because of his legacy. Dosh's father had been a standout basketball player at Madison under Lou Campinelli and was enshrined in the JMU Athletics Hall of Fame. The addition of Dosh would give the Dukes the player they needed to improve the quarterback position. "JMU Nation was hot over Pat Dosh," Mike Schikman recalled. "And at one spring practice there was Pat and his father. [Dosh] was a big, strong kid and we all thought he wanted to go D I-A, but none of the faithful wanted to hear that because he was a legacy. They wanted Dosh to come to JMU because they thought he belonged here."

Dosh did stay at 1-A, committing to East Carolina. His brief flirt with JMU summed up Madison's quarterback situation. The Dukes wanted security and depth, but they couldn't find the right guy — a testament both to LeZotte's talent and the program's inability to find a suitable backup to push the starter. Jayson Cooke would quit after the 2003 season, and by the spring of 2004 LeZotte was JMU's only experienced quarterback. "Mickey was always talking about how they needed to improve the position," Barber recalled. "I think he wanted to challenge Matt, but I think a big part of it was he did want a better player. Matt was capable, but at the same time Mickey always wanted to get his best 11 on the field."

...

JUSTIN RASCATI was busy that spring. His transfer list included a mix of I-AA and I-A schools — namely Murray State, Tennessee-Chattanooga, Eastern Illinois and Central Florida — and Rascati looked at each program carefully. Of the possible schools, only Central Florida played at the I-A level. If Rascati chose to drop to I-AA he could play immediately, but it would involve smaller crowds and a lower level of football. If he chose Central Florida he would need to sit out the 2004 season as part of the NCAA's transfer eligibility rule — his second season on the bench in three years.

Each university put forth its best sales pitch. Former Eastern Illinois quarterback Tony Romo phoned Rascati and explained the potential success if Rascati committed to the Panthers. Romo was the third-string quarterback for the Dallas Cowboys, and though Rascati was impressed with what Romo had to say, he didn't think the conversation was a big deal. Years later, Romo would become a star in the NFL, and Rascati's girlfriend heard his name in passing. "Wasn't that the guy who called you about transferring to Eastern Illinois?" she wondered. Yes, Rascati replied, it certainly was.

In mid-April, another unfamiliar number appeared on Rascati's cell phone. The caller was Matthews. "To this day I don't know how he got my cell number," Rascati later said. "He introduced himself as coach Matthews from James Madison. The whole time I had no idea where that was. I remember it sounded like he was calling from an emergency room but I didn't want to ask."

Matthews was at the hospital. Days earlier, his son Clayton had been involved in his second car accident. Though Matthews later would explain the situation to Rascati, at the time of the call the quarterback had no idea the coach was at the hospital with his injured son. Matthews and Rascati talked for a few minutes and Matthews invited Rascati to Harrisonburg. When the call ended, Rascati went to his computer to look up information on JMU. Matthews closed his phone and turned to Clayton.

"How'd I do?" Matthews asked his son.

Clayton Matthews had a feeding tube down his throat. Though he could not speak, he was coherent. He looked at his dad and gave him a thumbs up.

Rascati visited JMU that weekend. He had barely researched the university in the three days since his phone conversation with Matthews. The dizzying sequence of events left many questions unanswered. Were the Dukes a competitive team? Would the new facilities Matthews spoke of be operational by the time Rascati graduated? Was Matthews going to give Rascati a chance to play? This was merely a sampling of what the prospective quarterback needed to know. And then there was Matt LeZotte. Unseating the starting quarterback would be a difficult task. "A lot of people thought I was crazy for considering James Madison just because of the quarterback situation," Rascati later said. "Other places I looked at had no one and Matt LeZotte was a three-year starter. He was a great quarterback."

Rascati and his father met Matthews for breakfast that Saturday morning and the three took a walk through campus. Rascati found that the new facilities already were under construction. He learned that Matthews was determined to build a program and that the Dukes played in I-AA's toughest conference. At the spring game that afternoon, Rascati noticed a bumper crop of young talent. He was impressed with the coach's fatherly personality and the university's reputation. Most importantly, Matthews told Rascati he would have a chance to compete for the starting job right away. Rascati — who strongly believed that football was all about competition — was sold. On the plane ride home he told his dad he wanted to transfer to Madison. "As soon as I left the airport at Shenandoah, I knew that I was coming back," he later told Mike Barber.

Rascati's commitment gave the Dukes their quarterback of the future, though for Matthews, the big prize was immediate. There was so much pressure to win in 2004 that Matthews later said he would have taken Rascati even if he only had one year of eligibility remaining. Still, with LeZotte back for his senior season, there was no need to rush Rascati — who missed all of spring practice and had barely played since 2001. Matthews had no preconceived idea about who was going to start in 2004. All that mattered was the Dukes had solidified the quarterback position. "The great thing about it was no matter who started we had a quality backup," Jeff Durden said. "If anything happened we had a guy we weren't afraid to put in the big game."

Durden and Matthews opened the quarterback competition that August. Rascati entered camp with a minor shoulder injury, but his presence did exactly what Matthews expected As the preseason progressed, Rascati and LeZotte pushed each other for the starting job, alternating snaps with the first-team offense into early September. The competition was extremely close. And the ever-cautious Matthews kept it close to the vest, refusing to show his hand until he found what he was looking for. As he put it, the competition would become a controversy only if the team turned it into one, and Matthews held everybody —

even his own players — at arms length until the time was right. "We could see who was getting the majority of the reps and make a judgment for ourselves," Madison receiver Nic Tolley said. "But we were not told who was heading out the competition."

Even LeZotte's brother (freshman free safety Tony LeZotte) was in the dark, leading to the belief that Matthews gave little indication to anyone who his starter would be — including the two men vying for the position. "No one knew what was going on," Tony said. "We were kept on the backburner even heading into the first game. We knew it was a competition and we knew it was close, but that's all we got."

Admittedly, Matthews flipped his opinion dozens of times. The coach could start practice with LeZotte as his starter, only to have Rascati at the top of the list by the end of the day. As camp closed, LeZotte was playing the best football of his life. Meanwhile, Rascati proved he was a cut above former challengers. His athleticism and mobility proved to be the difference. In a move that peaked the interest of many, Matthews gave Rascati the nod on opening night against Lock Haven. And though the two split playing time through the first three weeks, it became clear Rascati would be JMU's quarterback in 2004. As local media swarmed around the early-season story, Matthews deflected much of the attention away from his quarterbacks, choosing to escalate tensions between the coach and the media instead of creating a controversy that could have irreparably damaged the team dynamic.

Matthews made it clear there would be no juicy headlines pitting LeZotte and Rascati against each another. Less than an hour after JMU's 62-7 victory over Lock Haven, *Daily News-Record* sports editor Chris Simmons asked Matthews why he started Rascati over LeZotte, especially when the two quarterbacks were projected to split playing time anyway. Simmons, though usually polite outside of work, was known to be a bulldog when he was digging for information. As the senior member on the sports desk, he fueled the department's inclination to break news. To Simmons, the simple question reflected what many people wanted to know. When Matthews told Simmons it was an arbitrary game-time decision, Simmons pushed harder for a more concrete answer, eventually causing Matthews to snap. "There was no reason," he barked, before telling Simmons to drop the subject. Rascati and LeZotte had just torched Lock Haven for four touchdowns, and yet in the bowels of Bridgeforth Stadium, the coach and the journalist already were trading jabs.

Matthews had long been protective of his players. But this time the logic was clear. LeZotte, despite his experience, easily could have slipped, because this was his team and someone else was at the controls. And Rascati, for all his composure, still was the new kid on the block. "It was one of those cases where both guys kind of said and did the right things from the start," Barber said. "That diffused things. It never became a divisive force in the locker room. And that was good because it could have been a huge, huge problem."

Matthews shouldered the load when it came to the quarterback debate, sparring first with Simmons and then Barber early in the season. He probably didn't need to. LeZotte, who for years had been the unofficial spokesman for JMU football, handled the transition with the professionalism worthy of his captaincy. And if nothing else, Rascati proved he could deal the media as well as his predecessor did.

Rascati was very aware of what to say and how to say it, Barber recalled, and if he had any doubt about the implications of his comments he would revert to a safe statement rather than make a bold declaration. Rascati wasn't candid in his interviews; he was diplomatic. "I always told him he was a great quote when I wasn't quoting him," Barber laughed. "It was always like he was on SportsCenter. He chose his words very carefully, like a politician staying on message. When I flipped off my recorder and we'd walk to the locker room he'd start talking, and some of the stuff he'd say would be great, passionate and interesting. But when the microphones were on, he was very deliberate about what he said."

Though Rascati never flatly rejected a question, his answers were reserved, and at times, very simple. Reporters in New York had long said the same thing about Yankees shortstop Derek Jeter, who would politely answer every question, but would never say anything that made big headlines on the back page. To Barber, Rascati handled himself in the same fashion. He understood his power and made sure he was in complete control of the situation. Accountability became Rascati's trademark. Years later, Simmons wrote that Rascati's character had the potential to help his future as much as his ability. "Leadership, of course, manifests itself in many ways," Simmons wrote. "At Madison, for example, Rascati never failed to meet the press after one of the Dukes' rare losses. And he always did so graciously. People notice leaders, too. A quarterback, after all, is the face of any football team. Keeping him under wraps diminishes him. I'm guessing Rascati won't be diminished."

Rascati's poise was further displayed on the field, specifically in his breakout game. In a 31-21 win against Hofstra in early October, he completed 19 of 22 passes for 188 yards and a touchdown. Perhaps more importantly, fans got their first glimpse of Rascati's ability to create something from nothing. Midway through the second quarter, he turned an eight-yard loss into a seven-yard gain by breaking four tackles in the backfield. When asked about his Houdini escape at the post-game press conference, Rascati shrugged, smiled and deferred the attention to his teammates. To him, enjoying success was as important as being successful. In the huddle, he was serious. In front of the camera, he was tactful. But at heart, Rascati simply was a college kid enjoying his celebrity with casual nonchalance. This opportunity only came along once, and Rascati was set on making it worthwhile. His outlook became the perfect balance for the quarterback of a veteran team that already had its locker room leaders.

Yet while Rascati's stock continued to soar within the conference, he widely was considered nothing more than an efficient game manager outside the Atlantic 10. When it came to the development of his first-year quarterback, Matthews was deliberately conservative. He never asked Rascati to win the game, knowing it would be too much to expect. Instead, he and Durden kept Rascati on tight reins and gave him more rope as he proved himself. Rascati's counterparts in the NCAA semifinals dwarfed him statistically. W&M'S Lang Campbell, Montana's Craig Ochs and Sam Houston State's Dustin Long all threw for more than 30 touchdowns, and each eclipsed 3,000 passing yards in the regular season. Comparably, Rascati tossed 14 touchdowns and didn't reach 2,000 yards passing until midway through the national title game. Part of it was JMU's run-oriented attack, but a big reason was Matthews' refusal to make one player carry JMU's offense.

Much like his team, which would move through the regular season in the shadow of defending national champion Delaware and high octane William & Mary, Rascati coasted under the radar. He seldom attempted more than 25 passes in a game and only once threw for more than 200 yards. With a trio of talented tailbacks behind him and arguably the nation's most physical offensive line guarding his back, Rascati wasn't the marquee player an opponent game planned against. "He wasn't the guy who was going to light you up," Barber said. "You didn't go into the game and think he was going to throw for 350 yards and five touchdowns. But he was the guy who would get seven yards on third-and-six. He was the guy who was going to beat you when the moment came."

To those around the team, the kid from Gainesville was the one player the Dukes couldn't be without. His ability to extend drives set up long runs for Madison tailbacks. His knack for prolonging plays allowed his receivers to get open downfield. He stuck to the game plan, but he also knew how to improvise when necessary.

Rascati was a prime example of a player who was greater than the sum of his parts. He did not have a big arm, but he could make all the required throws. He had a slow release, but rarely threw interceptions. He lacked breakaway speed, but always seemed to elude defenders. Years later, the only criticism Matthews could offer when speaking about his quarterback was that in crucial situations, Rascati never wanted to give the ball to someone else. By the end of his college career, the man who came to JMU to challenge Matt LeZotte would hold a 29-9 record as a starter. His intangibles, people argued, made him indispensable. "Justin was a leader who would guide our team through demonstration," Tolley said, noting Rascati's attention to detail. "His dedication to film and his off-field habits made him irreplaceable. Justin was a winner. [He] would take nothing less than perfection."

In the opening round of the playoffs at Lehigh, Rascati would make a similar jaw-dropping play to the Hofstra scramble, this time changing direction twice in the backfield before knifing into the end zone for a nine-yard touchdown run as the Dukes won their first postseason game since 1994. Through his first 12 games, Rascati accounted for 19 touchdowns and owned a sparkling 10-2 record. But as impressive as those numbers were, JMU's quarterback was about to elevate his game to a near untouchable level. Over the next two playoff games, Rascati would complete 27 of 36 passes for 319 yards and three touchdowns, cementing his legacy as a clutch performer and leading the Dukes to road wins against two of the nation's best teams.

In the NCAA quarterfinals against Furman, with Madison trailing 13-7 and 5:11 left in the game, Rascati brought the Dukes back onto the field, seemingly the season's last line of defense. Seconds earlier, Demetrius Shambley had blocked a Furman field goal attempt, keeping Madison within one score and essentially prolonging the playoff run for one more drive. The Dukes began a slow march for the end zone, and Rascati completed passes to four different receivers, driving JMU to a game-winning touchdown with 28 seconds left in regulation. It was a series that would become a vintage Rascati drive, marked not by 40-yard passes or 20-yard runs, but by simple plays, cold execution and a dash of drama. When Furman quarterback Ingle Martin's final Hail Mary attempt was batted down, the Dukes had their miracle victory. And in the broadcast booth, JMU color commentator Curt Dudley had an ideal view of the drive that marked the arrival of Rascati's national acclaim. "He managed that drive in complete control," Dudley said. "There's anxiety over the situation, but those are drives where someone makes it happen. I think that was a defining game, and a defining series, for him."

One week later against W&M, the Dukes watched a 21-0 second quarter lead evaporate, as Tribe quarterback and Division I-AA player of the year Lang Campbell engineered a 26-point scoring outburst. With momentum swinging against the Dukes, sophomore tailback Maurice Fenner rumbled for 29 yards on first down, and Rascati followed with a 34-yard strike to D.D. Boxley for a touchdown. Just like that, the Dukes were back in front to stay. And if nothing else, Rascati's postseason performance cemented what many close to the team already believed. The Dukes probably were a playoff team from the beginning — their massive offensive line and stingy defense took care of that — but without Rascati, JMU's season likely would have ended somewhere on the road to Chattanooga. When it came to the big game, No. 11 was No. 1, and as long as he was on the field, the Dukes had a chance.

Part II: Same Old Dukes?

Chapter 4

PAUL WANTUCK'S opening kickoff sliced through the cold Tennessee night and bounced three times before Levander Segars fielded the ball and returned it to the Montana 29-yard line. After a week of preparation, the I-AA championship game was underway. The Montana Grizzlies took the field behind senior quarterback Craig Ochs. Of the two offensive leaders, if Justin Rascati was the man with the intangibles, Ochs was the more physically gifted. Montana's catalyst throughout the season, Ochs was a finalist for the Walter Payton Award — given to the nation's best I-AA offensive player — and had piloted the Grizzlies to a 12-2 record in 2004. And of the two programs, if the Dukes were the upstart team striving for respect, Montana was the traditional powerhouse standing in the way.

Since 1995, no team in Division I football had been to as many national championship games as the Montana Grizzlies. With four appearances in nine years and two titles to its credit, Montana was one of the elite programs in I-AA. The Grizzlies had qualified for the playoffs an NCAA-record 12 years in a row and they were making their third trip to Chattanooga since the 2000 season. Montana was the country's most consistent team of the past decade. If the Dukes were to capture their first national championship, they would have to go through I-AA's most prolific program first.

Ochs opened the game's first drive by pitching the ball to Lex

Hilliard. The Montana tailback hit the right side of the line and picked up two yards before being tackled by JMU cornerback Clint Kent. It was a surprising first play for the Grizzlies, who threw the ball almost 50 percent of the time. Still, Montana coach Bobby Hauck said the Grizzlies would keep the Dukes honest. After taking over for starter Justin Green earlier in the season, Hilliard had rushed for 946 yards in 2004. A big game from him would give the Grizzlies the balance they needed to neutralize Madison's strong run defense.

Ochs took the snap on second down and handed the ball to Jefferson Heidelberger. The speedy receiver zipped around the right end, turned the corner near the Montana sideline and picked up a first down before JMU safety Rodney McCarter dragged him to the turf. The Dukes' vaunted rush defense was built on a strong defensive front four, a pair of agile linebackers and a group of hybrid run-stopping defensive backs. By running Heidelberger on the sweep, the Grizzlies aimed to stretch the Madison line horizontally and open the middle for Hilliard. Two plays into the game, the plan appeared to be taking form.

Hilliard picked up five yards on first down from the Montana 39. On second-and-five, Ochs went to the air for the first time, completing a short pass to Segars. A good block from Hillard took JMU free safety Tony LeZotte out of the play and gave the speedy receiver running room down the left sideline. Segars broke cornerback Cortez Thompson's arm tackle before being brought down at the Madison 38. On the JMU sideline, Mickey Matthews barked at the poor tackling. Missed tackles could turn a 10-yard pass into a 30-yard gain, and enough missed tackles against Montana could turn the game into a track meet.

The sloppy defense would continue for JMU, as Ochs connected with Green on the next play for 20 yards and another first down. It was a textbook Montana passing play, as Ochs sent three receivers down the field and stretched the Madison defense, leaving Green room over the middle. The senior tailback broke two tackles before McCarter dragged him out of bounds at the 18. Not two minutes had lapsed in the opening quarter and already the Grizzlies were dictating the tempo of the game.

The Dukes could not afford to get into a shootout with Craig Ochs. And Montana's lightning attack had JMU's proud defense scrambling to keep pace. "I thought we were in for a long night," Tony LeZotte later admitted. "Here we were, we play in one of the toughest conferences in the nation and this team comes out and marches down the field with no problem. No one had done that to us all season."

A one-yard gain for Hilliard, a sack, and a Montana false start brought up third-and-15. For the first time on the opening drive it seemed the Dukes were getting settled. Ochs quickly dismissed that thought, rifling a pass to Tate Hancock for 22 yards and another Montana first down. It was a carbon copy of the Green reception, with Hancock breaking two tackles before McCarter slammed him to the turf at the one-yard line. "Montana looked impressive early," Curt Dudley recalled. "A team with an explosive offense like that has the advantage and what they did certainly wasn't all that unexpected."

The Dukes stuffed Hilliard on first and second down, setting up a third-and-goal attempt from the three. JMU had not allowed a first-quarter touchdown all season, outscoring opponents, 92-3, in the opening period. In September against No. 5 Villanova, the Madison defense gave up a program-low 91 total yards to the Wildcats, pounding Villanova's offense into the ground as the remnants of Hurricane Ivan rolled through Philadelphia. Conversely, the Grizzlies had scored 114 first-quarter points and were 9-0 when striking first.

All week, as predictions for the I-AA title game were made, the one constant opinion was that Montana's offense would be too much for JMU to handle. The Grizzlies would stretch teams to the point of breaking. "When you're around a team you're reluctant to think like that," Mike Barber said. "I went in there thinking JMU could hang with them. And then as I watched that first drive my perspective changed. I started thinking that maybe the experts were right, maybe Montana was too much for this team to handle."

With a chance to cap an impressive opening drive, Bobby Hauck eschewed a third-down run and called for a play-action pass. Ochs faked the handoff and rolled to his right. Heidelberger cut left into the JMU secondary, then broke for the right corner, running along the back of the end zone behind Madison cornerback Clint Kent. As Ochs rolled to the right side of the field, Kent began to drift along the goal line.

In this situation, Kent was responsible for his region of the field — specifically the area Heidelberger was approaching. But with Ochs nearing the line of scrimmage and threatening to run for a touchdown, Kent abandoned his zone and went after the Montana quarterback. True to form, Montana had put Kent in no-man's land. Ochs floated a pass over Kent's head and Heidelberger caught it in stride for a touchdown. Kent flung off his chinstrap and slowly jogged off the field. In less than five minutes, Montana had done what no team could do against JMU all season — find the end zone in the first quarter. Ochs pumped his fists and pointed both index fingers to the sky. The Grizzlies had drawn first blood.

…

DAN CARPENTER'S extra point gave the Grizzlies a 7-0 lead. In the JMU stands, shocked fans stirred with impatience. Montana's electric offense had stretched Madison all over the field, and the Grizzlies had dominated the game's first drive. In the middle of the confused crowd, JMU athletics director Jeff Bourne braced himself against the wind. Tonight, Bourne stood in the elements, not as an administrator of the university, but as a nervous JMU fan. He welcomed the opportunity to sit among the mob. It gave him a chance to experience the moment. And right now the moment was filled with anxiety. "I remember thinking, 'Here we go,'" Bourne said years later. "That opening drive was a sign that this would be a heavyweight fight."

As JMU athletics director since 1999, Bourne had witnessed the best and worst of the Mickey Matthews era first-hand. Yet tonight the Dukes were in uncharted territory. The Grizzlies were frequent guests in Chattanooga. Their dominance and history gave them status in a city 2,000 miles away from home. "I had been in town for two days and had met a lot of people," Bourne recalled. "They all said, 'You're gonna have a tough time with this Montana bunch. They'll beat you by 20 points. It'll be a learning experience.'"

Oddly enough, the Dukes weren't in awe of Montana. Nor did they seem to be overly eager to shock critics by pulling off the upset. Instead, the Madison players carried themselves with quiet confidence. The night before, the two teams were recognized in a pre-game ceremony, and Bourne was pleasantly surprised to see that the Dukes were as large, if not larger, than most of the Grizzlies. He likened it to the movie "Hoosiers," in which the coach of a tiny Indiana high school basketball team quells the intimidation factor at the state title game by measuring the height of the hoop.

At least a few of the Dukes also noticed the symbolism. "It was almost comical when we saw them," defensive end Sid Evans said. "All week people were talking about Montana's high-octane offense. We were expecting this juggernaut. When we saw them in person we realized they were guys just like us."

Now that they had seen their opponent, Bourne believed the Dukes could use their composure to strip away the Montana mystique. "When you looked at our kids the night before you knew someone was going to have to bring their A-game to beat us," he said. Yet true to the collective thoughts in Chattanooga, Montana came out firing and JMU was tight — if not because of who it was playing than certainly because of the stage it was playing on. Madison needed to calm down. To win tonight, the confident Dukes would need to find an extra gear to stop the Montana machine.

...

JEFF BOURNE was hired as JMU athletics director three months after Mickey Matthews was hired as the school's football coach. With 14 years of intercollegiate experience — including three as a senior associate athletics director at Georgia Tech in the late 1990s — Bourne's resume was impressive. And like Matthews, the new AD relished the chance to lead a program after spending years climbing the vocational ladder.

A Salem, Va. native, Bourne received his bachelor's degree in business administration from Bridgewater College. After five years as a public accountant, he took a position as an internal auditor in the athletic business office at Virginia Tech — a move that would jump-start his career in sports administration. Ever patient and deliberate in manner, Bourne served several roles at the university, including a stint as associate athletics director. He completed his master's degree in education and sports management, and by the time Bourne left Blacksburg in 1997, all signs pointed to a future in intercollegiate sports. After three years at Georgia Tech, an opening at JMU allowed the Shenandoah Valley native to inherit a program he could take to the next level. "Here was a place where a lot of changes could be made," Bourne recalled. "[JMU] was like a sleeping giant."

Bourne was a soft-spoken man in his mid-40s and carried a touch of Virginia drawl in his speech. He appeared very meticulous. Every step seemed planned; every answer seemed calculated. Bourne was quite methodical in his public appearances, as though he had rehearsed the event hundreds of times before. His deliberate presence had both positive and negative results. While it gave him a professional public image, it felt very corporate. He looked somewhat staged. Yet when he opened himself to people, Bourne was friendly and passionate. He often stopped at tailgates to grab a beer and chew the fat with alumni, and those informal gatherings were a much better reflection of his true self.

Bourne's arrival at JMU involved an early test of his skills. He acquired a strong but saturated athletics program. As his tenure progressed, he faced the daunting task of providing facilities for these programs with limited funding.

According to Bourne, in the Commonwealth of Virginia, no state-general-fund dollars can be used on upgrades or construction of university athletic facilities. Whereas neighboring states like Maryland allow money from state tourism bureaus to be used for sports, Virginia schools only are allowed to pay these costs through private fund raising or generated dollars in the athletics program.

By the millennium, many of Madison's venues were outdated. Bridgeforth Stadium, Mauck Stadium and Godwin Hall — which combined to house more than 10 programs — all were built in the 1970s. Former athletes recalled Godwin's stifling atmosphere, and Mauck, which hosted a strong baseball program, didn't have lights. Bourne knew that to attract quality athletes, upgrades were necessary. But compared to its peer programs at Virginia and Virginia Tech, JMU's annual donation numbers were small. In the 1980s and 90s, Madison didn't have the infrastructure to support massive fund raising. Since JMU fielded more teams than its neighbors to the south and east, the athletics budget was stretched in more directions. "Funding is a matter of reallocating dollars in the program," Bourne explained. "And for us, we had to make sure we did things deliberately. It's been a sequential process."

Such was the predicament for a young school trying to earn a seat at the adult table. In 2001, five teams shared Bridgeforth Stadium — football, field hockey, women's lacrosse, men's track and women's track. In order to improve the existing facility as a football-only venue, the university first would need to find a new home for its other tenants. As Bourne was arriving at Madison, plans were being designed for a multi-purpose complex across Interstate 81 for the field hockey, lacrosse and track programs. Around the same time, Linwood Rose and the Board of Visitors finalized plans to construct the Robert and Frances Plecker Athletic Performance Center, a $10 million facility anchored to Bridgeforth Stadium's east end zone.

The second move was contingent on the first, as the building's development called for the destruction of the stadium's running track. Yet the Plecker Center did more than transform the functionality of the university's football stadium. It turned JMU into an elite school regarding its athletic-support services. The building included new sports medicine facilities and the McMillin Academic Center (named after

Challace McMillin), available to all JMU student-athletes. "We were in dire need of academic space before the Plecker Center," Bourne recalled. "I can remember going to the offices below mine in Godwin and looking at a little study area with four consoles that was supposed to provide computer support for 600 student-athletes. It was comical but it was also sad and it indicated the level of resources the program needed."

Phase I of construction on the Plecker Center began in the summer of 2003. And while facilities remained an issue as the decade progressed, Bourne approached the problem with the maddening patience of an advanced chemist. Though younger alumni craved construction plans and elaborate announcements, Madison's administration was content to move deliberately — most of the time behind closed doors. As long as they made changes in the correct order, facilities wouldn't be a glaring problem. "I don't deny the fact that we have some weaknesses in our facilities," Bourne said. "I think the day you stop building and enhancing is the day you start falling behind. We're working with that mindset. And that's one of the reasons I came here."

...

FACILITIES DID not keep Jeff Bourne awake at night. That distinction went to a more complicated issue. Like many in his profession, Bourne constantly was challenged to stretch money to fund his program. And early in his tenure, JMU's athletics landscape made that difficult problem an impossible one.

Madison's athletics program brimmed with success in the 1990s. As one of the primary public relations vehicles for the university, JMU sports teams were tremendous recruiting tools. National recognition from Lefty Driesell's men's basketball program increased Madison's visibility. On the soccer field, both teams enjoyed consistent success. Coach Dave Lombardo piloted the women's program to five consecutive NCAA Tournament appearances from 1995-1999. On the men's side, coach Tom Martin's squads won three straight Colonial Athletic Association titles and set a CAA record with a 32-game conference winning streak from 1992-1995. The men's swimming program was a perennial power and won more conference championships than any other university program during the decade. The women's basketball team had a 302-134 record from 1982-1997 under coach Shelia Moorman. The baseball Dukes — which in 1983 became the first Virginia team to reach the College World Series — consistently churned out winning seasons. And in the fall of 1994, the field hockey team captured Madison's first national championship with a double-overtime win over North Carolina.

But by the time Jeff Bourne arrived on campus, JMU's cycle of growth was working against its athletics program. With the addition of softball in 2002, Madison fielded 28 sports — among the highest in the country. It quickly became clear the program's budget could not support its teams equally. In 2001, word quickly spread that JMU was considering cutting several sports to help fix a growing budget and alignment problem. The news galvanized the student body into saving those sports, and in the face of open petitions, the athletics administration proposed an alternative to the cuts, calling for the program to re-allocate existing dollars and establish a tiered system. The new structure would provide funding at different levels, with the top-tier sports receiving maximum funding and the lowest tier receiving almost none.

By nature, the tiered system was flawed. It called for the creation of a double standard in the program. More concretely, it would sink some of JMU's successful programs — notably men's swimming and wrestling — to the bottom of their conferences. Without scholarships, those teams would not be able to perform at the same level. To the athletes, this represented the lesser of two evils. But to the administration, it would dilute the overall program. "You would have this multi-tiered approach and philosophy regarding sports," Bourne explained. "And it obviously wouldn't be the best situation because we would be treating teams differently."

The administration proposed the new plan to the Board of Visitors.

It was hard to believe that the athletics department considered the tiered system a viable option. Colleen Chapman, a member of the Madison track team, had followed the decision carefully. A senior, Colleen had 13 siblings, many of whom also attended JMU. This later included her younger sister Jenn, who followed Colleen onto the track program and would become student-athlete president in 2006. Although she was in high school at the time, Jenn Chapman learned much about the athletics situation from Colleen and Colleen's boyfriend, Eric Post, who later would compete in the Olympic trials. The three often talked about the unfolding dilemma. From conversations with Post, Jenn Chapman learned about the surge of support to save the teams. She also learned about the alternative plan being brought forth by the athletics department.

In later years, Jenn Chapman would decide that the tiered system sounded like a last-ditch effort to put an alternate option on the table. "I think the department came up with that system thinking it would never be accepted," she later said. "Taking money away from programs like that would cause them to fall apart and then why would you even keep those teams around? Anyone would look at that plan and think it was ridiculous. And I think that was the reasoning in the athletics department. They would propose this structure and there was no way the board would accept it. The board would tell them to cut the teams."

But perhaps swayed by the overwhelming student response to the rumored cuts, the BOV voted to implement the tiered system for the 2001-02 academic year. The decision stunned the Madison community, which by now came to recognize the inherent shortcomings of the new plan. It also, Jenn Chapman believed, handcuffed the athletics administration into using a system they knew couldn't last. "Everyone knew the system was flawed," she said. "There's no way a four-tiered system is going to work. A coach for those bottom-tiered sports can't recruit enough talent to compete without money. It's not possible."

The backlash hit the lower tiers hard. For the students on teams that lost funding, the 2000-01 season marked the end of an era. Over the next five years, playing against programs with full scholarships, Madison's lower-tier teams struggled to keep pace. Athletes who arrived before the re-allocation still received scholarships, but their new teammates were mostly walk-ons. The teams weren't even allowed to raise money. "We're not asking for scholarships or financial support," one coach said. "All we're asking is for the ability to use our own money so we can provide a partial scholarship and use the National Letter of Intent."

NCAA regulations, however, prevented this from being an option. And so the tiered system forced JMU to re-examine its teams. Jon McNamara, a JMU student from 2001-05, wrapped himself in the university sports debate by researching documents and talking with coaches impacted by the new structure. As a standout hockey player in high school (McNamara had been invited to try out for the club team at Penn State), he sympathized with the teams impacted by the tiered system and believed that competing without funding was almost worse than not competing at all. McNamara would write a story on the topic for *The Breeze* in the spring of 2004, one of several published over a three-year period by local media. He focused on the re-evaluation of teams in the eyes of the university:

> After an intensive review of the department and the 'goals of intercollegiate athletics' set fourth by the Board of Governors, the University decided that certain programs could, more than others, act as a window to the University at the national and conference level. … The greatest impact the scholarships cuts are having is in limiting the ability of the respective coaches to recruit.

"What I discovered most is coaches constantly were talking about how their once-proud programs were being downgraded to almost club-level status," McNamara said. "That's tough for a coach and players to take, especially when they love the logo on the front of the jersey. It seemed the players cared about the university and the university could not afford to care about them."

Bourne, too, recognized the system's shortcomings, later calling the tiered system "an uncomfortable situation." From 2001-06, the overall success of JMU's program declined. The tiered system may have saved the sports from being cut, but it didn't change the fact that the university was fielding too many teams with too little money. Madison's incredible growth during the Carrier years enabled it to field one of the country's largest athletics programs. But the speed of that growth ensured it could not be sustained. The program had outgrown its fund raising capabilities and the new structure merely prolonged the inevitable. "I remember talking to a lot of coaches," McNamara said with chilling prophecy. "And they were all wondering if this was the day they were going to lose their jobs."

Despite Jeff Bourne's meticulous preparation, he was cornered when it came to the size of his program. Stuck working with a system he knew to be imperfect, Bourne realized any changes would involve significant numbers. According to Bourne, five years after the BOV approved the tiered system, a study of the 337 NCAA-sanctioned universities placed JMU's 28 sports in a tie with the University of North Carolina-Chapel Hill at No. 13 for national program size. And the universities surrounding JMU all had bigger name recognition, larger alumni bases and more money. By late 2006, the administration was preparing to radically change the program's landscape. And the events that would be placed into motion that fall (the cutting of 10 teams, a student-athlete uprising to save the sports, and, later, a lawsuit that would reach the doorstep of the United States Supreme Court) would shake the Madison community to its core.

Yet as Bourne stood among the JMU fans in Chattanooga, the final decisions regarding Madison's athletics infrastructure were still 20 months from being made. In the midst of a crowded landscape, JMU's sleeping football program became the story of 2004. A national championship game featuring JMU had been far-fetched in recent history. Only a year earlier, the Dukes barely drew 7,500 fans for their final home game, and at least a few spent the majority of the day chanting for Mickey Matthews to be fired. The difference between then and now was remarkable and Bourne deserved much of the credit for the turnaround. He stuck with his guy in face of some pretty heavy criticism and it wound up being the best move he could have made.

Bourne easily could have let Matthews walk after the 2003 season; he also could have offered him a one-year contract and forced Matthews to coach for his job. But the collective decision to offer Matthews both time and security (at least immediate security) was a critical move for the 2004 season. It told Matthews that improvement was the desired result. The Dukes likely could have finished 7-4 or 8-3 in 2004 and Matthews would have been retained. And although everyone knew changes would come if the Dukes weren't successful, the collective opinion was the program was on the cusp of something big. "When you have a chance to quell controversy and a lack of confidence in someone you make it," Bourne said. "There's a lot behind a visible sign of support for a coach."

Years later, Bourne pointed to one of his favorite analogies when he spoke of the decision to retain Matthews. In his first three seasons at Duke, basketball coach Mike Krzyzewski was 38-44 and his team was an abysmal 13-29 in conference play. Twenty years later, Krzyzewski became one of just 19 coaches in NCAA Division I history to win 700 games. "After those first few years everyone thought [Krzyzewski] was gone," Bourne said. "And when the administration gave him an extension I'm sure a lot of people thought they were out of their minds. Looking back, I think Duke made a pretty good decision."

Perhaps that type of success wasn't down the road for JMU. But by the end of the regular season the decision to keep Matthews had been validated. As Montana kicker Pete Sloan placed the ball on a tee for the ensuing kickoff, Bourne glanced back at the field. In a year where JMU had done everything right, nothing could put a damper on the program's finest moment. Throughout the offseason, critical e-mails questioned Linwood Rose's intelligence for rehiring Matthews, and the day after the national championship game, Rose and Mike Schikman mused how wrong the critics had been. Though Rose couldn't recall exactly what he said, Schikman remembered with clarity.

"Pretty good hire, huh Lin?" Schikman asked.

"I wish I had kept all those e-mails," Rose is believed to have said. "I would have loved to write back and ask them what they think now."

…

SLOAN'S KICKOFF bounced out of bounds at the JMU 18, drawing a penalty flag, and allowing the Dukes to take over on their own 35-yard line. Justin Rascati led the offense onto the field and set the Dukes in their jumbo package. Maurice Fenner, who would finish the 2004 season with 975 rushing yards, lined up in the backfield. Rascati, with receivers D.D. Boxley and Tahir Hinds split to either sideline, called the cadence, pivoted to his left and extended the ball to Fenner. The sophomore tailback dropped the exchange and fell on the ball at the Madison 34 for a one-yard loss.

After surviving two one-point wins and bulldozing their way through the semifinals, the Dukes suddenly looked awestruck. "Everyone was tight," Jeff Durden said. "We didn't have a great Thursday walkthrough practice and I think everyone was pressing a bit in those opening minutes."

This was neither the time nor the place to freeze under the national spotlight. Madison had to get out of its funk in a hurry. Rascati brought the Dukes to the line on second down, took the snap and fired a pass parallel to the line of scrimmage for Nic Tolley. The junior receiver caught the ball behind the line and immediately was pinned by Montana cornerback Tuff Harris for another loss. The Dukes were in trouble, Tolley thought. They needed to change the way they were approaching Montana. "When we started the game I thought that our locker room presence was a good one and that we were ready to play," he later recalled. "But that did not seem to transfer to the field."

Back-to-back blown plays now left the Dukes 13 yards from the first down marker, exactly where Bobby Hauck and the Grizzlies wanted them. The Madison offensive line outweighed the Montana defensive line by an average of 49 pounds per man. If JMU gained significant yardage on first and second down, it could power the ball all night. In order to slow the Dukes, the Grizzlies would have to keep them in third-and-long situations.

The Montana fans rose to their feet on third-and-13. Rascati lined up in shotgun next to tailback Alvin Banks, deployed four receivers across the line and called for the snap. Immediately he began backpedaling, setting up a screen pass for Banks, who caught the ball at the line of scrimmage and began shifting up the field. Banks danced his way to the 38 before a swarm of Montana defensive backs tackled him seven yards shy of the first down. "That's not a good start for James Madison," ESPN commentator Rod Gilmore noted, as Nick Englehart and the punting unit came onto the field. "They're usually on the board early in the first quarter."

Englehart rocked on the balls of his feet behind the line of scrimmage. Less than eight minutes had lapsed in Chattanooga and the confidant Grizzlies already seemed in firm control of the national title game. Englehart fielded the snap and punted the ball away. The Dukes might have gotten past the Montana mystique, but they still looked overwhelmed on I-AA's largest stage. To beat JMU, Jeff Bourne said, a team would have to come with their A-Game. Now the Dukes would need to find theirs.

Chapter 5

LIKE MANY of his peers in early American politics, James Madison was an activist — a student of both government and change. He promoted religious freedom and civil liberties, both of which became critical to the survival of the United States. Madison believed in an educated citizen. His belief in enlightenment (that knowledge was the path to liberty) became a founding principle of the United States' Constitution. At his core, Madison believed that education, debate and, to an extent, public discourse, was vital for democracy to exist.

Though small and soft-spoken, Madison also was prepared and persistent. The school that bears his name likewise is a prism of opposites. JMU routinely lumps itself into groups with the commonwealth's big boys — Virginia, William & Mary and Virginia Tech — all of which are substantially older and more established. In these conversations, JMU lacks the long-standing ceremonies of its elders. It is the school that named itself after a president who never stepped foot on its campus. William & Mary and Virginia (notably the commonwealth's most illustrious universities) are steeped in traditions and secrets, creating atmospheres of ritual soaked in the lore of Old Virginia. They are institutions created by poets and presidents — environments shaped by classic architecture, secret societies and haunting beauty. Comparatively, Madison lacks the longevity and substance to be as timeless.

At first glance JMU's academic quad mirrors its peers in

Charlottesville and Williamsburg. Lined in columns and bluestone, Madison's quad marks the birth of the university. Yet that form of elegant tradition is merely skin-deep. There are no gravestones or ancient architecture. Parallel to its youth, the rest of campus is rather modern and zoned according to construction dates. It becomes apparent that JMU is radically different from its peer institutions rooted in colonial folklore. Unlike its sister schools, Madison's appearance is neither aristocratic nor traditional.

Yet this tells us very little about JMU's evolution. It is young and aspiring, built on a liberal arts system that is open to both change and growth. Like James Madison (who at 29 was the youngest member of the Continental Congress) the school is built around the concept that public involvement is instrumental to improvement. Ceremony is honored but also created. JMU's "Be The Change" campaign — implemented as part of the university's 2008 centennial celebration — was established to honor the school's first century with profiles of notable graduates and faculty who made a difference in the world. Yet because Madison was relatively young and because some of its notable alumni were continuing their work, "Be The Change" became a celebration of in-progress accomplishment.

That idea was — and continues to be — the beauty of the institution. There is a push to make change and take an active role in society — a vitally important concept of James Madison's vision for the republic. While JMU appears to be a school for the common man, it actually is an institution for the uncommon — a school that places importance on history without living in the past and celebrates tradition by creating it.

In many ways JMU's football program serves as one of several microcosms of the university's history. As it approached its 35th birthday, the program was young, without establishment and appeared to carry few traditions worth mentioning. Yet as the Dukes grew from relative obscurity to a Division III power — and eventually a stable I-AA program — a slow lineage began to form. Most children of first-generation Dukes were still teenagers in the late 1990s, so the program was barely old enough to attract the sons of former Madison players. But JMU wasn't too young to form a pipeline between siblings. In 2001 and 2002, as Mickey Matthews attempted to rebuild the program, the volume of that pipeline increased. It was an advantage Matthews built not by actively recruiting younger brothers, but by treating the older ones well. "We've never lost a brother that we really wanted," Matthews said. "Our players will come by the office and all they want to know is if we think their brothers can play at this level. They will say 'Coach, he's not going anywhere else.' They want their little brothers to come here."

Eventually, the prized second-generation Dukes began to follow their fathers into college football and JMU — like all other programs before it — began battling for legacy recruits. But by then, Matthews had firmly established his own system of family connection. At a school where tradition was honored with the creation of new tradition, Matthews developed a method to gain an edge. Before sons followed their fathers, brothers followed each other.

...

FROM 2000-03, recruiting would bring JMU important pieces to its championship puzzle. Those classes included players like offensive lineman Corey Davis, linebacker Akeem Jordan and cornerback Clint Kent, all of whom helped push the program into the national spotlight. But no player would have the same immediate impact as Tony LeZotte — a scrappy free safety who earned All-America honors as a redshirt freshman. By the middle of the 2004 season, Justin Rascati and LeZotte were the poster boys for the future of JMU football. The understated quarterback made all the right moves with consistency and occasional flair. The freshman defensive back played with reckless energy, doling out punishing hits that hurt him as much as the ball carrier.

Unlike Rascati — who had to search for Madison on Google after his first phone conversation with Matthews — LeZotte's familiarity with JMU was extensive. His older brother, Matt, was a prized Madison recruit when Tony was still in high school, and by his 17th birthday, the younger LeZotte knew campus better than most JMU freshmen. Listed at 6 feet tall and 175 pounds, LeZotte was wiry and tough. He enjoyed a spectacular 2004 season, leading the Atlantic 10 in tackles and earning conference rookie of the year honors, but the punishing nature of his position had taken its toll. LeZotte was bruised and tired as he took the field in Chattanooga, and later admitted he was ready for a couple months of rest after a long first season.

LeZotte came from a busy home in Augusta, Ga., where sports dictated the family calendar and tough love reigned among siblings. The youngest of four, he grew up with competition and spent most of his childhood emulating older brothers Jerry and Matt. For the LeZotte boys, athletic accomplishment hinged on meeting certain standards. As kids, Matt and Tony attended football games at Westside High School, where Jerry played defensive back and older sister Katherine was a cheerleader. By the time he was 10 years old, the youngest LeZotte had an appetite for sports that few could match outside of his own house. The Friday night spotlight cast a powerful spell over the younger brothers and both would follow Jerry on the field at Westside. In the spirit of progress, each LeZotte would be better than his predecessor.

Tony and Matt were closest in age and the brothers enjoyed an active childhood. They played football and church league basketball. They'd hop the fence at a local elementary school and play pick-up baseball games during the summer. Sometimes other neighborhood kids joined, but more times than not those playground contests turned into one-on-one showdowns between the LeZotte boys — games that Matt admitted weren't very fair to Tony. Matt was three years older, possessed a tremendous throwing arm and almost always won the backyard battles. Yet those afternoons and weekends were pivotal to Tony's athletic development, and the future Madison star later would credit some of his success to playing with older kids. "I always wanted to beat my brother," Tony said. "Playing against someone older allowed me to compete against someone with more ability. It taught me a lot about playing to win."

When they were kids, Matt taught Tony how to catch a football by standing 10 feet away and slinging passes until his younger brother started crying. Admittedly, Matt was just looking for another way to pick on his kid brother. Yet events like that also helped shape Tony into the family's most well rounded athlete, so Matt was only partially kidding when he took credit for turning Tony into a standout wide receiver. Under the blazing Augusta sun, Tony LeZotte discovered he could be a football player by shedding tears and catching passes from his rifle-armed older brother. Years later, the siblings laughed at the event. "He was really trying to punish me," Tony recalled. "We fought a lot as kids and there definitely was some tough love between us. But I really just wanted to do whatever he wanted to do."

A bond between brothers is simple. Tony cried when Matt threw too hard, but he also followed Matt everywhere. And while Matt joked that he picked on Tony, he also knew that if his kid brother could handle himself with an older crowd than he'd be ahead of his peers. So Tony trusted Matt — even if it meant getting his ass kicked from time to time. One summer, Matt's high school friend swore he could beat Tony in basketball and Matt — the family trash-talker — decided Tony should come over to settle the argument. Matt knew Tony could hang with anyone. He told his friend that Tony would tear him to pieces, then called his brother and started organizing bets for the game. "Tony is half the size of this guy," Matt recalled laughing. "But we were talking trash about how he could win. I really thought he had a shot."

When 14-year-old Tony stepped on the court, he sacrificed size and years to his opponent, yet he played with such ferocious intensity that he only lost by one basket. "Not the decision I wanted," Tony later recalled. Still the competitive effort was evident. "He's this little fireball," Matt said. "Tony never backed down from a challenge."

…

IN HIGH school, Tony LeZotte made the transition from potential to product, showcasing his talent at both receiver and defensive back as a freshman at Westside. In the third game of the 1999 season, LeZotte — playing free safety and weighing about 125 pounds — planted a punishing hit on a 195-pound tailback that lifted the ball carrier off his feet. The play was the Friday Night Football Hit of the Week, and from that point on, Tony began to move out of his brother's shadow. "Obviously when Tony came here he was Matt's little brother," Westside coach Gerald Barnes said. "He didn't say much. He just went about his business. But he's always been very talented."

Barnes, who took over as Westside head coach in 1997, was one of the few people able to observe the LeZotte brothers through a common, detailed lens. Matt and Tony both played offense and defense in high school, and according to Barnes, they were cut from the same mold. Both were hard working, competitive, athletic kids. Admittedly, Barnes could not say enough good things about the brothers. What he noticed most about Tony was his aggressiveness. And while Matt was the vocal leader, Tony played with quiet determination. "Matt probably talks a bit more than Tony," Barnes later joked. "I guess that's why Tony listens [so well]."

The difference was both inherent and functional. Matt was the senior quarterback who got his picture in the paper and snagged the big headlines. He drew attention because of the position he played. He also was more talkative by nature. Tony enjoyed a certain level of anonymity as a defensive star. He played with reckless disregard for his body, a style that Matt — a tough player in his own right, but also the team's star quarterback — could not afford to play with. They were the same, and yet they were different. In that moment — as Tony was leveling a guy who outweighed him by almost 70 pounds — Matt LeZotte realized his brother had ability unlike his own. "I think that's where it took off for him," Matt said. "To see him run through that guy the way he did — with no physical attributes that should allow him to do that … I was sold on Tony right then and there."

In 2000 — with Matt off at JMU — Tony helped lead Westside

to its first region championship in 15 years. He quickly developed into the area's premier two-way player — one who used his intelligence and competitive drive as much as his talent. His nature pushed him beyond his physical limits. On the gridiron, Tony played with incredible energy, as though he was running on high-octane and everyone else was chugging along on regular unleaded. "He would hit you and sometimes he'd hurt himself," Barnes said.

Autumn became a pattern of certainty. LeZotte totaled more than 100 tackles in each of his four seasons at Westside and finished his high school career with 10 interceptions. He routinely was the team's No. 1 threat at wide receiver and also returned kicks — essentially becoming omnipotent on the football field. He was a star in almost every sport. LeZotte played baseball and batted .400 as a sophomore. He competed in the state swimming meet. He was named Augusta male athlete of the year as a senior. And in 2002, he became the first football player in school history to earn first-team all-state honors from both the *Associated Press* and the *Atlanta Journal-Constitution* in consecutive seasons. "He was heavily recruited by a lot of good college programs for good reason," Mickey Matthews said. "When you watched him play, he was just better than everyone else on the field."

Matthews believed LeZotte was a special player he could build a program around — a hard-working, tough, intelligent kid with talent and confidence. The fact that he was Matt's younger brother only helped because Matt had been a model citizen for the Dukes. In November of 2002, Matthews and his wife, Kay, made the eight-hour drive to Augusta during JMU's bye week to watch Tony play and show him that JMU was interested. Matthews and Barnes discussed Tony's potential as an offensive and defensive player. Both agreed he could be a standout free safety at the college level. By then, Matt LeZotte was entrenched as the Madison starting quarterback and Matthews believed Matt's positive experience, combined with the close bond between the brothers, would steer Tony away from offers at Furman, Wake Forest and Vanderbilt. The only hurdle was Georgia.

…

ATHENS, GEORGIA sits a little more than 100 miles northwest of Augusta, on a path that runs dogleg right along Interstate 20 and Route 22. If you're a football player growing up in the Peach State — raised on the traditions of "Glory, Glory" and the Chapel Bell — then Athens is where you dream of going.

The LeZotte family was familiar with the University of Georgia. Matt LeZotte considered attending UGA as a walk-on player until the Bulldogs signed South Gwinnett High School standout David Greene to a scholarship. Greene became a four-year starter at Georgia and ended his college career with more wins than any quarterback in NCAA Division I-A history. Matt, knowing Greene's pedigree, wisely accepted a scholarship at JMU.

Tony LeZotte's decision appeared to be more difficult than Matt's. Georgia considered the two-time Westside MVP a borderline scholarship player. An offer from Athens likely would negate JMU's aggressive recruiting. Matthews believed Georgia was the only school LeZotte would choose over Madison and thought anything short of a full ride from Athens would put JMU back in the driver's seat. "I thought he and his brother were so close it would make a difference," Matthews said. "If he didn't go [to Georgia] I thought we would get him."

Matthews — who still had many friends and close associates at Georgia — kept a watchful eye on LeZotte's status. In what Matthews called "a heated debate," the Georgia coaching staff voted 5 to 4 not to offer LeZotte a scholarship — a decision that unquestionably changed the future of the Madison football program. Though LeZotte deflected any speculation and though he never questioned his final decision to attend JMU, a scholarship from Georgia likely would have kept him at home. "That probably would have changed things," he later admitted.

His brother was not as diplomatic. "I would have kicked his ass if he chose JMU over Georgia," Matt said laughing. "I would have driven home and signed the letter of intent for him."

But instead, Matt didn't do anything. He let his brother make the decision himself. Matt helped Tony with recruiting questions and gave him guidance when it was asked, but more than anything, he left Tony alone. "It was his decision," Matt said. "I would have loved it if he came here and I would have been supportive if he didn't. I don't think JMU uses older siblings to recruit. I think the experience people have here is the No. 1 recruiting tool. [That's something] the recruit sees himself."

Matt was partially correct. By reducing his direct involvement, he further strengthened Madison's best recruiting tool. Indirectly however, he likely played a large role in his brother's final decision. In high school, Tony would visit Matt a few times every year — hopping in the car after his Friday night game and driving through the night to see his brother play the next afternoon. Tony saw a lot of football. But he also hung out with Matt's friends, walked through campus, was treated well and lived some of the Madison experience before he actually attended the university. By showing Tony what his life was like, Matt unintentionally was selling JMU to his brother.

This was not uncommon among Madison siblings. During his junior season, Rodney McCarter's family visited him when the Dukes faced Virginia Tech and Matthews invited McCarter's younger brother, Rockeed, to watch the game from the JMU sideline. "Instead of sitting way up in the stands with my dad and his girlfriend, coach Matthews let him hang out with the players," Rodney McCarter recalled. "[Rockeed] was in ninth grade, so they didn't know anything about him. They were just being nice. My brother was on the sideline when I came off the field and he had a great time."

In 2006 Rockeed McCarter spurned offers from Syracuse and Cincinnati and accepted a scholarship to come to JMU. His brother had not pushed him on the decision. Instead Rockeed simply went with the place he felt most comfortable. As the Dukes evolved into a formidable program, family ties continued to build. The 2006 recruiting class also included twin brothers Donnell Brown and Ronnell Brown, quarterback Drew Dudzik, fullback Charlie Newman and tight end Jason Dosh. All had family connections to JMU. Matthews later explained that people who enjoy their time at Madison become unofficial recruiters almost by default — a common occurrence at most schools. "When people come here they feel like they've been treated well, that they're important," he said. "It becomes very easy to recommend JMU to your brother, sister, son or daughter. You want your family to experience what you experienced."

Mike Schikman had a more direct take — one that was aimed at the football program. "The fact that we have had so many sets of brothers come play for JMU under Mickey says a lot about him," Schikman said. "Think about it, you may lie to your parents every once in a while; and parents lie to their kids. But brothers don't lie to each other."

LeZotte opened his JMU career in the summer of 2003. He made his presence felt on the field, jumping into the wide receiver rotation by the third preseason practice and impressing Matthews with his athleticism. LeZotte had gained nearly 50 pounds since his freshman year of high school and Matt was shocked at the wiry, muscular body that now complemented his kid brother's scrappy drive. "He was a half second faster and had hands twice as good," Matt recalled. "It amazed me to see the difference."

The 165-pound LeZotte was back in familiar territory that summer — an old boy competing with young men. Still, he was in the receiver mix during training camp and had a legitimate chance to play as a true freshman until he tore his hamstring late in the summer. The Madison coaching staff believed the injury would keep him out for at least half the season. In October, Matthews called LeZotte into his office and suggested a move to free safety. "He told me we really needed help at the safety position," LeZotte said. "He asked me if I was healthy enough to come back [in 2003] if I would consider the switch."

LeZotte agreed. But his hamstring was slow to heal and Matthews ended up sitting him for the entire 2003 season. That winter, LeZotte dedicated himself to building more mass in the weight room. He entered 2004 training camp at a trim 175 pounds and quickly displayed his increased speed and strength. Within a few weeks, Matthews was convinced LeZotte had the tools to be a great defensive back. "Watching him play defense it was obvious his knowledge of the game was so far beyond what a lot of people knew," JMU place kicker David Rabil said. "Mentally he was already there. Physically he just blew up."

Rabil, who roomed with LeZotte for three years, was perhaps his best friend in college. LeZotte, Rabil and sophomore wide receiver Ardon Bransford were almost inseparable. And as LeZotte began to ascend up the JMU depth chart, his two closest friends noticed his potential to do great things on the field. "He had this overall, general desire to win," Rabil said. "That's what he wanted to do every day at practice, in the weight room and in games. You could see it in his eyes every time we played. He was just fired up."

LeZotte won the starting job early in the summer, playing with the tenacious passion that led defensive coordinator George Barlow to call him "a once-in-a-lifetime player." Barlow, an all-league safety at Marshall in the late 1980s, devised a defense aimed at maximizing talent. By the end of preseason practice he noticed that LeZotte's ceiling — his football acumen, physical talent and ability to play through pain — was higher than most. Playing on a defense that would lead the country in sacks and allow just 87 rushing yards per game, LeZotte built immediate recognition, recording 41 tackles, registering a sack and intercepting two passes over a five-game stretch early in the season. His pursuit was relentless, and with linebackers Trey Townsend and Kwynn Walton attacking lead blockers, No. 21 enjoyed free roam to attack the running back from his safety position.

His size betrayed his athleticism. LeZotte still could move throughout campus in relative obscurity, blending in with the rest of the student body at D-Hall thanks to his modest frame. Barlow later joked that a stranger could meet LeZotte on the street and never peg him for an All-American football player. And yet on Saturdays he transformed into the A-10's best rookie defender, the player who always seemed to be around the ball — a heat-seeking missile in cleats.

By the middle of the season the Dukes were a legitimate threat to win the Atlantic 10, and LeZotte was locked in a two-horse race with New Hampshire quarterback Ricky Santos for conference rookie of the year honors. The Dukes took a 4-1 overall record into Maine in mid-October, looking to start 4-0 in conference play for the first time since 1999. Midway through the third quarter, Maine tailback Marcus Williams took a handoff from quarterback Ron Whitcomb and turned up field. The 5-foot-10, 230-pound Williams (who also wore No. 21) was coming off back-to-back 1,000-yard seasons. He was a 2003 Walter Payton award finalist and was three weeks away from becoming the all-time leading rusher in Maine history.

Williams had torched the Dukes the previous year, rushing for 117 yards on 31 carries in Maine's 20-13 win. He was well on his way to another trademark performance when he took Whitcomb's inside handoff and bounced to the outside. As Williams swept toward the JMU sideline, his Madison counterpart closed in for the hit. LeZotte crashed into Williams and the two players went flying out of bounds, landing in a pile near the JMU bench. LeZotte quickly popped up and jogged back toward the field, but as Williams got up, he found himself in hostile territory. The hit super-charged the Dukes, and before Williams could get to his feet, Tony's biggest fan ambled over.

"Yeah baby!" Matt LeZotte yelled. "That's the real No. 21!"

A few series later, an energized Williams took a handoff up the middle and ran over Tony. Matt stood on the sideline for the rest of the game with his arms crossed and his mouth shut. Four years later, the brothers marveled at their own bravado. Williams would finish the game with 166 yards on 29 carries, but LeZotte made nine tackles and intercepted a pass in Madison's 24-20 win, later chalking up the encounter to another butt kicking caused by his big brother's mouth. His hit became another example of the clear message JMU was sending to the rest of the conference: Madison was willing to stand toe-to-toe with anyone. The Dukes were here to stay.

...

AS LEZOTTE'S stock continued to rise, he found a pressing need to crash when he was off the field. Away from the lights he preferred a simple lifestyle. To those who knew him best, LeZotte moved in two gears: warp-speed and slow-mo. He was an entirely different person when he stepped onto the field — a common trait among successful athletes. Yet LeZotte's bi-polar character was almost a necessity. He expelled so much energy in practice and during games that his mind and body needed to slow things to a crawl away from the field so he could recover. "It was real easy to see the difference," Rabil said. "If you hung out with him all the time you saw it easily. It was like Dr. Jekyll and Mr. Hyde."

According to Rabil, laid-back LeZotte was the man behind the facemask. To his closest friends, the standout free safety was a regular college kid who went with the flow. Most conversations were centered on where to eat dinner or what to watch on TV. Having a roommate like Rabil further slowed the tempo. Unlike a lot of kickers, Rabil (Mr. Casual around campus) was a fairly prominent figure in Madison's inner circle. The two became fast friends. LeZotte, who needed to unwind so he could gear himself up for next week's battle, and Rabil, who didn't seem fazed by anything at all, enjoyed kicking back with pizza and a movie as much as they liked to party. LeZotte's star power made him an A-list celebrity. In turn, his friends made sure Mr. A-list had ample servings of humble pie. "He never embraced it to the point where he wasn't humble about it because we didn't let him," Rabil laughed. "We messed with him a lot about the attention he got. I joked with him that they were going to stop the program after he left. So we recognized the celebrity factor, but no one let it get to an extreme."

LeZotte attributed his modest behavior to the company he kept, later saying that competing with teammates and working for a common goal humbles a player. His modesty also could be attributed to his incredible rate of ascent. Despite the hoopla surrounding him, LeZotte usually didn't deviate from his routine. "For a guy who has had that much success, he really hasn't changed," Barlow said. "He's still this humble guy. That's what makes him so affectionate in the eyes of people."

Yet the laid-back, humble boy from Augusta transformed into a wrecking ball on the field, prompting Rabil to call his roommate's behavior, "a complete change in personality." LeZotte was perceptive and vocal on the gridiron, a catalyst for the JMU defense. It was a change that he could summon simply by flicking a switch, and according to Rabil, it was necessary for team success.

In a sport where presence was everything, JMU's freshman free safety was everywhere he was needed. The week after the Maine game, LeZotte made 10 tackles against Richmond — including a touchdown-saving stop of tailback David Freeman with the game still in doubt. He finished the regular season by registering 50 tackles in Madison's final three games. Against Delaware, LeZotte made 19 stops. He also broke up a 40-yard pass by sprinting across the field, launching himself in the air and swatting the ball away as he cart-wheeled over a receiver's shoulder pads. "As the season went on fans began to look at LeZotte as Superman," former JMU sports media assistant Jon McNamara said. "If any play exemplified that concept it was that one. He literally flew."

LeZotte's consistency became more important than his numbers. He was recognized for his big plays but Matthews appreciated him most because he always seemed to be in the right spot, referring to him as "old reliable" later in his career. The moniker likely had a second meaning. Despite a bruising, physical style of play, and despite a host of injuries, LeZotte would start all 50 Madison games in his four-year career — a school record. His media games with Matthews carried enough false drama to start a reality TV series. Matthews, who always seemed to downplay his team and harp on injury problems, often would call LeZotte "questionable" or even "doubtful" in the week leading to a game. When told of his coach's comments, LeZotte shrugged his shoulders, gave a knowing smirk and politely told reporters that nothing was going to keep him from playing.

The whole thing sometimes felt like a choreographed dance. Though

Matthews whole-heartedly believed LeZotte was a game-day decision, he also knew he'd have to barricade his free safety in a storage closet to keep him off the field. In 2006, Mike Barber wrote of LeZotte's perplexing reliability. "What might be most amazing about [LeZotte] is that he's injury prone and durable at the same time. … Admittedly, Matthews worries about injuries to his defensive star. LeZotte plays so physically, and with such wanton disregard for his own health, developing a backup at the position is always on the coach's mind."

The equation with LeZotte was simple: If he could play he would play. And if he played, he played well. LeZotte was a physical marvel because he was so consistent that Matthews always knew what he was getting, later quipping that his free safety never had bad games, just some that were better than others. LeZotte displayed remarkable reliability that the JMU coaching staff came to expect, and at times took for granted. To Barlow, No. 21 played at another level. He routinely referred to his star defensive back as a "special kid," and later spoke of LeZotte in the same breath as Michael Jordan and Tiger Woods. Only after LeZotte graduated could Barlow accurately summarize his free safety's value. "I'll be very shocked if I'm able to coach someone again who is as tough as he was both mentally and physically," Barlow said. "He was the total package."

The high-octane approach helped turn the Madison defense into one of the most physical units in I-AA football. Before the 2004 season, Matthews and Barlow adjusted JMU's 4-3 scheme, changing it to an eight-man front and creating an aggressive unit that could shut down the run. The eight-man front allowed Barlow to disguise his formations and make opposing offenses uncomfortable with the defense they were shown. Safeties Bruce Johnson and Rodney McCarter were used as hybrid players (part cornerback, part safety and part linebacker) giving Barlow the freedom to load-up against the run while still having the athletes available to defend the pass. McCarter and Johnson were critical to this defense (as were cornerbacks Cortez Thompson and Clint Kent) but LeZotte likely was the most important piece of the puzzle. "You need a free safety that can make all the calls and set everything up," Barlow explained. "Tony became the quarterback of our defense. He was like having a coach on the field. His abilities to read keys and tendencies set him apart."

The Madison defense improved as the season progressed. That summer, Barlow went through each projected starter and found that his players were as good — if not better — than the teammates he played with at Marshall. Barlow knew JMU wasn't short on talent. What the Dukes lacked was the swagger of an aggressive, dominating unit. With LeZotte in position as Barlow's new center fielder, the Dukes transformed from a solid group of players into a punishing defense that took away the run and forced teams to become one-dimensional.

Fatigue likely was the only drawback to Barlow's defense. The Dukes played so aggressively and so physically that they often founds themselves as bruised as the ball carrier. This was especially true of LeZotte, who as a freshman was learning how to gut through the long college season. As the Dukes began their playoff surge, he began to buckle. The previous summer, LeZotte sometimes wolfed down five or six meals a day to increase his weight and help absorb hits. Despite this preparation, he was breaking down as he approached the 100-tackle milestone. Nagging injuries slowed his pursuit. By the playoffs, LeZotte — like many of his teammates — was feeling every hit and Matthews began holding him back at practice to save his energy.

LeZotte managed to start each game of Madison's march to Chattanooga but it was obvious the late-season playoff push had left him exhausted. Against Furman, he separated a shoulder while trying to break through a wall of blockers on the game's final kickoff. Matthews limited LeZotte to no-contact drills the next week and LeZotte made seven tackles against William & Mary. But the night before the national title game, he aggravated the same shoulder at practice. There was some doubt whether he would be able to play, and the Madison coaches made tentative plans to go without their star defensive back. LeZotte later called it the only scare he had about not playing a game in his career.

Yet the next day, he found the shoulder was responding. "We played 15 games that championship season and I don't know if I could have done another one," he later admitted. "But when I woke up that morning I knew I was playing."

LeZotte told Matthews he was good to go. Without hesitation, the coach penciled him into the starting lineup. "I don't think I've ever seen him miss a tackle," Justin Rascati later said of LeZotte. "It would take a lot for him to miss a game."

Chapter 6

MONTANA BEGAN its second offensive possession on the nine-yard line (after an illegal block penalty on Nick Englehart's punt). Lex Hilliard tripped on the turf on first down and was stonewalled on second down by the JMU defense. On third-and-11 Craig Ochs went back to work, floating a pass downfield to Jon Talmage for a Montana first down.

Ochs quickly found his rhythm. Back-to-back completions to Talmage and Willie Walden gave the Grizzlies another first down at the 35. Five plays into Montana's second drive and JMU had done nothing to slow the Grizzlies' vaunted passing game. The X-factor was Ochs, who stormed out of the locker room as though prepared to rewrite the record books. As the Grizzlies lined up for their 16th offensive play of the game, Ochs was 7-of-7 for 89 yards and a touchdown.

Montana came to the line with four wide receivers on first down. Ochs surveyed the field from shotgun, fielded the snap and winged a pass over the middle into heavy traffic. Levander Segars, Jefferson Heidelberger, Tony LeZotte and Trey Townsend all were within eight feet of each other and running at full tilt when the ball reached its destination. The play — with Heidelberger and Segars running crossing routes — had all the makings of a giant train wreck.

Heidelberger caught the ball with Townsend on his heels and Segars right in front of him, then instinctively turned his body in self-defense. The two Montana receivers brushed past each other. Somehow Heidelberger avoided contact with Segars, danced to the left and sprinted toward the far sideline. Behind him, LeZotte — who had been covering Segars — ran into Townsend, springing Heidelberger free into the secondary before Cortez Thompson ran him out of bounds at the JMU 34. Even when he threw a poor pass into a crowd, Ochs could do no wrong.

Sitting in the JMU radio booth, Curt Dudley began to wonder if the Dukes could hang with the Grizzlies. "The pressure started to build there during Montana's second drive," he recalled. "That first quarter was all Grizzlies. Maybe because the Dukes played those close games at Lehigh and Furman they weren't worried. But at that point my concern was that we'd flop on the big stage."

Dudley's observation was warranted. Ochs already had completed passes to six different receivers and Montana's elaborate routes had the JMU defense scrambling to keep pace. Yet despite giving up 128 yards to the Grizzlies in the first nine minutes, the Dukes seemed composed. "Our mindset was to be persistent," Townsend said. "A great quarterback will be able to move the ball against a good defense. We knew if we stayed persistent we could stop them in the red zone. We didn't become frustrated."

Inside JMU territory for the second time in as many drives, Montana went back to the ground. Hilliard picked up four yards on first down to the JMU 30. On second-and-six, Ochs threw behind Talmage, his first incompletion of the game. A third-down draw to Hilliard went for one yard and brought up fourth-and-five from the JMU 29-yard-line. The Grizzlies were in no man's land and ESPN analyst Rod Gilmore wondered aloud if Montana would kick the field goal or go for the first down. Bobby Hauck answered by sending his kicking unit onto the field.

Though the evening forecast was for clear skies, the field conditions were about to become one of the night's big talking points. A month earlier, the turf at Max Finley Stadium had been replaced with new sod for the national title game. It was a common step taken by host venues for many championship events. For years, title-game participants practiced at off-site facilities to ensure pristine field conditions on game day. As a community facility, Finley Stadium played host to band competitions, high school football and the University of Tennessee-Chattanooga during the fall. By the end of the 2004 regular season Davenport Field needed a facelift. "Like a lot of Super Bowl venues it was decided to lay down new turf at the end of the regular season," Greater Chattanooga Sports & Events Committee vice president Scott Smith said. "Normally everything is fine. We had turf growing all year and we placed new sod down between the hashmarks. It looked beautiful."

That beauty, Smith later admitted, was superficial. Heavy rain in late November and early December slowed the final step of the installation process. "We had everything down in time," Smith said. "But it rained to much that the turf didn't take root because it wasn't searching for water. Once people got on it and started cutting the turf just came up."

Hours before kickoff, as players and members of the media buzzed around the stadium, Mike Schikman examined the field. From the pressbox, it looked green and immaculate. But on ground level, Schikman thought the turf looked like a wire fence with a carpet over it. He walked to the end zone and lifted the end of the sod. "It looked like you could wave it all the way down the field like a plastic runner," he later said. Schikman turned to Madison center Leon Steinfeld and asked for an observation. "This is gonna be nasty," Steinfeld replied.

By the time Dan Carpenter lined up for his 46-yard field goal attempt, large divots of sod littered the playing field. Montana placeholder Tyson Johnson called for the snap, caught the ball and flipped it through his legs to a running Carpenter. The Grizzlies were going for the first down. Madison was quick to recover however, and even though Carpenter had blockers to his right, Townsend had cut off his path to the corner. Carpenter shifted to his left inside a wall of blockers and turned up the field. Townsend slammed on the breaks and dove to his right as Carpenter scooted by him. "We were all caught off guard," Townsend recalled. "I just wanted to get over there and make him cut back into our defense."

While Madison was not prepared for the fake, Tony LeZotte later admitted that the poor field conditions made it difficult to assume the Grizzlies would kick the field goal. As Carpenter slipped past Townsend and crossed the line of scrimmage, LeZotte swooped in from the left and wrapped his arms around the Montana kicker. Kwynn Walton then grabbed Carpenter at the waist and Carpenter fell forward to the 26. The Grizzlies were short, thanks in large part to the execution of Madison's three best defensive players. Walton, Townsend and LeZotte had accounted for more than 300 tackles during the season. Now they had put the first dent in Montana's armor.

Though Matthews later downplayed the stop as a turning point in the game, his players thought otherwise. The Dukes were fired up as they came off the field, as though the defensive stand had shattered Montana's invincibility. The Grizzlies were dangerous but they were not perfect. "I think it was big," LeZotte later said. "I don't see how it couldn't be. They had just driven down the field like it was nothing the series before, and then they have a great opportunity to go up 14 or 10 early. For them not to get that first down, for us to stop them, I don't know if it was a single turning point, but it was close to it."

...

BOBBY HAUCK tore off his headset and pursed his lips in frustration. The Grizzlies had dominated the first 12 minutes of the game and yet Montana was up only 7-0. Carpenter had made 18 of 27 field goals during the season and his season-long was 49 yards. On a raw, windless night in Chattanooga there was no doubt he had enough leg to make that kick. Hauck called for the fake based on his observations of the field. As early as the pre-game walkthrough, players from both teams were griping about poor footing. Less than five minutes into the telecast, ESPN sideline reporter Rob Stone gave an update on the horrid conditions. Divots were everywhere by the end of the opening quarter and plastic netting — placed under the sod to help it take root — had been torn and brought to the surface. Several players later called it the worst field they ever played on. And as the game progressed, the field continued to wreck havoc. "We faked the field goal because we didn't think our kicker could plant and kick it," Hauck said at halftime. "It's well within his range but he wasn't comfortable kicking the field goal from that distance."

With 32 luxury skyboxes, press facilities for 60 media members and seats for 20,000 fans, Max Finley Stadium's amenities made it an attractive choice for I-AA's biggest game. The venue, constructed in 1997, had hosted the national title game since its inaugural season. The Greater Chattanooga Sports and Events Committee were the caretakers and Scott Smith's crew ran championship week dinners, trips, photo sessions and, as Smith said, game day logistics "all the way down to the towels in the locker room." Combined with First Tennessee Pavilion — which provided a large, functional space to host game-day activities and tailgates — Finley Stadium was the class of its football subdivision. Chattanooga was geographically central to the majority of I-AA programs and the event pumped an estimated $2.5 million into the local economy each year.

For nearly a decade the game had been synonymous with its host city. Yet in the weeks following the 2004 title game, the word used to describe the field was "embarrassing." In front of a national TV audience, the tattered turf had turned Chattanooga's proud facilities into a punch line. "Obviously [the NCAA] was unhappy and said we couldn't field a championship event under those conditions," Smith said. "It was a disaster [and] the negative exposure finally brought it to the attention of the community."

According to Smith, the Greater Chattanooga Sports and Events Committee had been discussing a switch from natural grass to an artificial playing surface for some time. A major producer of synthetic athletic fields — TenCate Grass North America — had a facility located less than 30 minutes from downtown Chattanooga. "The company was looking for a showplace close to their plant," Smith said. "Talks had been going on for some time about Finley Stadium being that showplace. [The 2004 title game] sped up the process."

TenCate donated the grass in conjunction with a synthetic turf resources company in Dalton, Ga. Installation costs were covered by a group headed by Gordon Davenport Jr., a well-known Chattanooga businessman, who sought to eliminate any chance of future embarrassment brought to the field named after his father, the late Gordon Lee Davenport — chairman of the campaign team that developed the plans for Finley Stadium. "It ended up working out in our favor a bit because it was an embarrassing situation for the people in the city and the university," UTC sports information director Jeff Romero said. "It didn't take more than a couple of weeks for a group to get together and find some private donors to get the funding for a new field. The donations were raised rather quickly."

Davenport's group raised more than $260,000 to cover the installation costs. Six months later the new field was installed and in December of 2005 — one year after the Dukes and Grizzlies stumbled on the unstable turf — Appalachian State and Northern Iowa played on a state-of-the-art synthetic surface.

But that game was still a year away. As JMU took over on its own 26-yard-line there was nothing that could be done to fix the turf problem. "You'd move and a sheet of turf would move with you," Madison defensive tackle Brandon Beach recalled. After the game, Matthews would deliver the strongest analogy of all. "It was like playing basketball in socks," he said.

Rascati brought the Dukes back onto the field for their second offensive possession. He took the snap, faked a handoff to Alvin Banks and dropped back to pass. To his left, Montana all-conference defensive end Mike Murphy cut inside JMU tackle Corey Davis and rushed Rascati, who tucked the ball and spun away from the initial hit. His pocket breaking down, Rascati tried to run up the field but Murphy —

who led the Grizzlies with 11 sacks — was quick to recover and dragged the JMU quarterback down at the 21 for a five-yard-loss. Almost 13 minutes of game time had lapsed and the Dukes had minus-2 yards of total offense to show for it.

Rascati's second-down throw sailed over the head of Nic Tolley. On third-and-15 Rascati again dropped back to pass, this time rolling to his right and firing the ball downfield for D.D. Boxley. An undersized but speedy wideout, Boxley was Rascati's most dependable downfield target and led the Dukes in almost every receiving category. As Boxley approached the far sideline, he felt a push on his back. He shuffled his feet to stay in bounds, but dropped the ball as he stumbled across the sideline. Boxley walked up the field motioning for a pass interference call. It never came, and it was another three-and-out for JMU. Boxley, visibly frustrated, took off his helmet and walked toward the bench.

After scoring three touchdowns in the first quarter the previous week against William & Mary, the Dukes looked sluggish and timid. On the Madison sideline, junior tailback Raymond Hines clutched the neckline of his jersey with both hands. Hines had been JMU's most productive tailback in 2004 but he injured his ribs in Williamsburg and could do nothing to help jump-start Madison's struggling offense. It was an unfamiliar setting for Hines, who had never been in a situation where he was needed but could not deliver. Yet as Englehart booted the ball back into Montana territory, Hines — the 1,000-yard runner who carried the Dukes to Chattanooga — could only stand and watch.

Chapter 7

RAYMOND HINES did not command attention. Unlike other star players, his name did not generate tremendous fanfare or acclaim. He led all JMU backs in touchdowns, yards and carries in 2004, yet he was relatively anonymous — a foil to Justin Rascati and Tony LeZotte, both of whom became overnight celebrities during the 2004 season. Instead Hines had a small, intimate following. Fans were not in awe of his talent; they merely appreciated his effort. By the end of the season, however, it would be widely recognized that Hines was the player most responsible for the Dukes' run to Chattanooga.

A 5-foot-9-inch, 175-pound junior, Hines toiled in relative obscurity his first two seasons at Madison. He rushed for 461 total yards as a freshman and sophomore, spending most of his first two years fighting for playing time. In 2002 Hines was the third option behind Rondell Bradley and Brandon Goins. In '03 he was buried on the depth chart behind freshmen Alvin Banks and Maurice Fenner. Opportunity was readily available but it came with harsh reality. "He was always the third best athlete at the position," Mickey Matthews said. "We would look at Alvin, Maurice and Raymond every August and it was the same story. He was a very good back — it wasn't like he was a bad football player — but he was just the third best out of the three."

Hines was quiet. When he did talk, it was with a gentle, mild-mannered and thoughtful tone. Running backs coach Ulrick Edmonds called Hines "a down to earth, calm guy." Hines was friendly in a reserved, almost withdrawn way, and his megawatt smile came with the frequency and impact of a solar eclipse. His demeanor deterred some people, but he was approachable, and his quiet nature was somewhat amusing. "Raymond was something else," said Clayton Matthews, who lived in the same residence hall as Hines when the two were teammates in 2002. "He could take a question that required an explanation and find a way to give you a one-word answer."

The youngest son of Alva and Willie Hines, Raymond grew up in a modest and clean home in Hyattsville, Md. Willie worked for the Washington D.C. Metro Area Transit Authority (WMATA). Alva was an administrative assistant. Neither had the chance to attend college. The Hines family was the product of two driven, intelligent people. Alva and Willie raised their five children on a set of simple principles, the most important of which was to value hard work. "My parents gave me a reason to think that anything was possible," Hines said.

Hines was a responsible kid who still managed to test the limits of his father's strict schedule. Willie Hines was a former Marine, so when little Raymond had to clean something, he couldn't cut corners by simply wiping down the surface. The house followed a schedule and Willie — known for his generosity and preference for creating order — ran it to perfection. He rarely had to repeat his rules because they were easy to follow. His wife also was a person of repetition and took the family to the same Baptist church in Northeast D.C. every week.

Their youngest son grew up a child of habit. Raymond went to school, came home, did his homework and they went out to play. It was easy to prioritize his time because his parents instilled it. Years later, after Hines moved back into his parents' house and began working full-time, his father still ran a tight ship. "He's retired and I live at home so I have to get up around 5 a.m. to be at work every day," Hines said. "He gets up around 4:45 and you can hear him yelling, 'You ain't going to get up. Get ready for work.' I'm lying in bed thinking 'Why is he getting up this early?' He has a tight schedule and it carried through to me."

Like most of the neighborhood boys, Hines grew up playing sports. His first love was boxing — though Alva and Willie quickly nixed the idea of their son becoming a punching bag. In elementary school, Hines received a pass to the Boys & Girls Club and asked his parents about football. Though they were reluctant, they let him give it a shot. Hines was eight years old the first time he put on pads, and he was so small the helmet was cocked sideways on his head. But he quickly fell in love with the game.

Hines, though always small, was a good athlete from the start. He excelled as a sprinter and helped lead High Point High School to two state indoor track championships. His speed was his strength on the football field, where, as a tailback, he dodged and weaved his way to three straight 1,000-yard seasons. Hines possessed dazzling quickness. He was streamlined, strong and — thanks to a disciplined workout program — had nary an ounce of fat on his body. Seeing him shift gears was like watching a speedboat slice through the water.

Despite his willingness to work and his strong high school resume, Hines was passed over by many college teams. He was undersized, he did not have great hands and he was a below-average pass blocker. His offers came down to Fordham, JMU and Howard, and though Hines had urban roots, he chose Madison because it allowed him to leave home and live without the city's distractions.

Hines believed JMU gave him the best opportunity to earn a solid education and graduate on time. Yet he was not prepared for the rural college town and, at first, he wanted to come home almost every weekend. Hines missed the buzz of D.C. and it didn't help that after earning all-county honors at High Point, he couldn't crack the JMU starting lineup. He averaged 4.9 yards per carry as a freshman, rushing for 97 yards and a touchdown against Rhode Island in his most productive game of the season. But his success was sporadic. Hines bounced all over the depth chart. In 2003, with Banks and Fenner getting the ball on almost 65 percent of all running plays, Hines slipped to 3.2 yards per carry. He could not block or catch as well as Banks, nor could he hammer the ball between the tackles like the 220-pound Fenner. Hines was an unproven insurance policy entering 2003 spring practice. He had talent, but many believed he lacked the tangible traits to be a complete back.

Still, Hines always played well when he was given the opportunity. He played well that spring and his performance was enough to get back into the conversation — to the point that Matthews called the starting tailback job "a three-horse race" at the beginning of August training camp. Then the inconsistency resurfaced. Hines played poorly that August and watched as both Banks and Fenner leaped past him again. By the end of the month, he had slipped to fourth on the tailback chart, behind Banks, Fenner and 5-foot-7 freshman Antoinne Bolton. The poor showing bothered Hines, and more than once he questioned his own ability. "It was obvious his mind was not on football," Matthews said. "His body was here, but his mind was somewhere else."

...

HINES WAS thinking about something else, namely the future. His home had always produced people with vision. Willie Hines was a planner by nature. He constructed an entire basement-level living area for his family and in all the years he knew his father, Raymond Hines never remembered a repairman entering the property. Hines' sister, Ashley, graduated with honors from Florida A&M. Foresight was a common characteristic among the family. Shortly after graduating college, Hines took investing classes and began researching opportunities to launch a small business. He also became a student of the real estate market.

It was not surprising, then, that when Hines and his girlfriend, Jennifer Lassiter, began dating seriously, Hines thought about the future. The two began seeing each other in high school, and though Hines was three years older, they stayed together when he left for college. Though Hines never ran it across Lassiter, he sometimes thought about marriage. "I had a plan," Hines recalled. "If we were still together at a certain time I could see myself with her."

In the winter of 2004, after several years of dating, Lassiter learned she was pregnant. Hines was floored. He wasn't done with school and quickly began to process what it would be like to juggle classes, football and fatherhood. Lassiter's parents put her out of the house and she lived with Hines in Harrisonburg for a few months. Hines constantly worried about how he could manage his time during the pregnancy and after the baby was born. He was the type of person who wanted to examine and exhaust all options before he asked for help, but he also knew he was at a crossroads in his life. Hines wasn't getting much playing time and he often wondered if he was supposed to be playing football. The pregnancy, he believed, could be a sign that he was at JMU for another reason.

Hines went through a spiritual period that spring — an event that was in no doubt brought on through his familiarity with faith. He also began to focus on his primary responsibilities, the first of which was to ensure the health and safety of his pregnant girlfriend. Religion and structure — the two pillars Hines grew up with — helped clarify the moment. On April first, of all days, he told his parents about the pregnancy. At first, Alva thought her youngest son was playing an April Fool's Day joke, but Willie Hines saw right through it. They quickly offered to help and Lassiter moved into their house. "My parents are helpful people," Hines said. "I'm sure if I brought someone in off the street who could use some help they wouldn't question it. They would do whatever they could do. When [Jennifer] came and stayed with my parents it lifted a weight off my shoulders. I knew I had some type of help."

The world still wasn't all roses. Hines traveled back home when he could, but he spent the majority of the summer in Harrisonburg and found it hard to concentrate on a game when the real world was knocking at his door. The Madison coaching staff caught wind of the situation, yet Hines only told them enough to keep them informed. He opened the season with modest results against Lock Haven (seven carries for 39 yards) but touched the ball only eight times over the next three games. He often thought about God and purpose. Hines' belief in a higher power helped him understand his responsibility as a student and how that correlated to a successful future as a father.

On Sept. 16, Hines received a phone call from his mother, who told him Lassiter was about to go into labor. Hines didn't have a car at school, so two friends drove from Hyattsville and picked him up. "They got here around 3 a.m. [the next morning]," Hines recalled. "It was a dizzying experience. I remember calling one of the coaches and telling them I'd try to be at the game that weekend if I could."

Later that day, with Hines holding her hand at Prince George's Hospital, Lassiter gave birth to a healthy baby boy. They named him Marquis. After making sure his son and girlfriend were healthy and safe, Hines and his father got in the family car and drove through the remnants of a hurricane to Philadelphia for JMU's game against Villanova. It was textbook Hines, not wanting to abandon any of his responsibilities to family or team. Hines carried the ball only once in Madison's 17-0 win, but it was (several JMU personnel believed) as though the final weight had been removed from his slender, powerful shoulders. "He's a family-oriented guy and he didn't want to be the person who didn't take care of his child," Ulrick Edmonds said. "Those things weighed heavily on him. I think the things he did during the pregnancy showed his love was at home. It showed us we had a mature young man."

...

TWO WEEK after Marquis was born, Alvin Banks broke his leg in the midst of a 118-yard game against Hofstra. Banks was expected to miss at least six weeks. With redshirt freshman Antoinne Bolton still unproven, JMU — once loaded at the tailback position — was down to Maurice Fenner and Hines. Since Matthews preferred to employ a two-tailback system, Hines would get his shot. "I remember talking to Curt [Dudley] after the post-game show the night Alvin got hurt," Mike Schikman said. "We're thinking 'here comes another great JMU season in the dumpster' [because] Raymond had trouble holding onto the ball."

Fenner and Hines split playing time the next three weeks, averaging 165 yards per game in wins over Massachusetts, Maine and Richmond. Fenner shouldered most of the load, but Hines carried the ball 12 times in each game, providing a capable change of pace. He rushed for 123 yards and a touchdown in JMU's 28-7 win over UMass, highlighted by a 61-yard run late in the third quarter to set up Madison's first touchdown. As a secondary back, Hines gave opponents a different look. While Fenner ran over defenders, Hines usually slipped through them. But he also seemed capable of hammering the ball into the middle of the field and getting yards after contact. Justin Rascati said that while he never saw Hines as a third-string back, he was surprised at how well he transitioned into a prominent role. Edmonds remembered being impressed with Hines' intangibles. Hines, Edmonds believed, could not be measured the same way as Banks and Fenner because the tools used to evaluate players — speed, strength, agility — don't factor how quickly a person learns and evolves. Edmonds thought Hines — now in his fourth year with the program — had a tremendous ability to learn both by watching and through his own experience. This helped overcome his otherwise modest physical skills. "There was concern," Edmonds said. "He was probably closer to 155 [pounds] or so toward the middle of the season. Still, he was a fundamental guy and it was gratifying as a coach because he had success doing things the right way."

The 6-1 Dukes coasted over Virginia Military Institute on homecoming weekend, 41-10, getting big games from Hines (20 carries for 111 yards) and Bolton (11 for 103). But JMU also lost Fenner to a separated shoulder midway through the game. At the post-game press conference, Matthews placed his hands over his head in disbelief and told reporters that Fenner could be done for the season. Madison was at least one win away from securing a playoff spot and Banks still was a month away from returning. Delaware and William & Mary were coming to town, and while Hines and Bolton gashed VMI, the 0-9 Keydets weren't exactly setting the country aflame.

When asked what he would do about his tailback shortage, Matthews paused. Hines would start, he said. After that, he didn't know. The Dukes had talked about moving linebacker Akeem Jordan (a former tailback at Harrisonburg High School) into the offensive backfield. Madison also had safety Rondell Bradley, who rushed for 737 yards and six touchdowns on JMU's 2002 team. But Jordan and Bradley hadn't played the position in two years, and Matthews didn't think one week of practice was enough time for either to understand JMU's offense. "We were reaching at running back," Matthews said. "More than once as a staff we discussed what would happen if Raymond went down.

"We just looked up one day and he was all we had."

...

FOR A quiet guy, Hines wasn't short on confidence. It was an interesting contradiction considering he rarely spoke. Hines was about as far from brash as a person could be. It was surprising then, to learn that he was perhaps the only person unfazed by Madison's tailback shortage. To his coaches and teammates, Hines was capable of being the feature back until Banks and Fenner returned. But to Hines, this was his time to shine. "Ray's personality was always interesting because he was such a quiet guy but he wanted to play," Mike Barber said. "He really thought he could be the No. 1 guy and he believed it the whole year."

Barber thought Hines was overlooked because he wasn't built like a prototype JMU back (Banks and Fenner were fast, powerful, downhill runners). Hines had long viewed football as the great equalizer — a place where he could prove that size wasn't everything by outperforming bigger players. Hines didn't carry himself with the brazen confidence that attracted attention, but Barber believed he was good enough to be productive behind JMU's veteran offensive line. Pound-for-pound, Hines was JMU's strongest player. He was smart and fundamentally sound. He knew when to go for the big gain and he knew when it was best to lower his shoulder and fall down. Mentally, Edmonds thought Hines was the perfect player for the situation because he worked hard behind the scenes and performed well in the system as a role player. To Edmonds, Hines was the ultimate team guy waiting for his chance — a player who didn't measure well on paper, but had proven himself during the first half of the season.

Hines, after going through life-changing events off the field, wouldn't be overwhelmed by this transition. The concern, as Matthews said, was that Hines "weighed nothing" and the coaching staff didn't know if he could be productive early in games when opposing defenses were rested. Hines had gained most of his 839 career yards late in games as a backup. Now the Dukes needed to know if the wiry tailback could move the chains in the first quarter and prevent Justin Rascati from trying to win games with his right arm.

Offensively, the Delaware game was a disaster. Hines rushed 13 times for only 26 yards — 14 of them coming on one play — and Madison accumulated only 166 yards of total offense against the defending national champions. Thanks to three interceptions, a blocked punt, a blocked field goal, and Cortez Thompson's 87-yard punt return for a touchdown, the Dukes escaped with a 20-13 win. "That was a difficult game," Hines said. "It was a game that brought us closer as a team because we needed to pick each other up. It gave us confidence because we were able to win without playing well on offense, but it was a real frustrating day."

Madison was 8-1, and barring a collapse, the Dukes were heading to the playoffs. Still, their offense appeared cooked without Banks and Fenner. JMU had only four first downs in the second half against Delaware. Rascati, under constant pressure, was sacked twice. Matthews and Durden spent the next week searching for a way to jump-start the offense, eventually coming to the conclusion that there was nothing wrong with the game plan and Delaware simply was very good defensively. Adjustments would be necessary if they faced the Blue Hens again, but for the interim, the Dukes would hold the course.

The following Saturday, their faith was rewarded, as Hines torched William & Mary for 198 yards and a touchdown. The Dukes lost to the Tribe, 27-24, on a last-second field goal, but the offense was back. Madison cemented its postseason spot the following week with a 31-17 win over Towson. Hines, playing in front of his son for the first time, rushed 32 times for 142 yards and two touchdowns, ending the day by scooping Marquis in his arms as he celebrated with family and friends. Incredibly, the Madison attack adjusted to three different tailbacks during the season and barely missed a beat. By the end of the year, Banks, Fenner and Hines all would have at least three 100-yard games. "I wasn't surprised by [Ray's] performance," Edmonds later admitted. "I was astonished."

Hines vaulted the Dukes past Lehigh in the opening round of the playoffs, rushing 29 times for 191 yards and another touchdown in Madison's 14-13 win. He had closed November furiously, re-establishing JMU as a team that controlled the ball and the pace of the game. Hines caught passes out of the backfield, picked up blitzes and knifed through defenses with his elusive cuts. He had doubled his season rushing total in three weeks, passing both Banks and Fenner in the process. The performance, Matthews said, was nothing short of spectacular.

Madison marched into the NCAA quarterfinals as a 14-point underdog and used a relentless defense to hold Furman to 13 points. The Paladins — perhaps the most balanced team in the country — responded by shutting down JMU's running game, limiting Hines to 46 yards on 21 carries. After shouldering JMU's offense the previous four weeks, Hines was nearly on empty. But he got the tough yards the Dukes needed — the yards his body wasn't supposed to allow him to get — and scored both Madison touchdowns.

Down six and with the clock winding down on their season, Rascati used short passes to move the Dukes inside the Furman 10 with less than a minute left in regulation. A two-yard run by Hines, a four-yard run by Rascati and a one-yard plunge by Hines put JMU on the one with 33 seconds left. The Paladins burned a timeout to set up their defense. On the Madison sideline, the Dukes knew who they were going to. "During the timeout we made the decision to run to our right,"

Matthews recalled. "We thought they'd be blitzing so we ran a zone block. Coach [Curt] Newsome wanted to run the outside zone and that play involves either a handoff or a pitch. I turned to Raymond and I asked him if he wanted us to hand him the ball or pitch it to him."

Hines, sitting on 980 rushing yards for the season and playing with a painful ankle sprain, paused for a second. On the other end of Matthews' headset, Jeff Durden worked through the logistics of the play. "We chose the outside zone because we felt like they would pinch up the middle," Durden explained. "When you run the zone the running back's responsibility is to read the first down lineman. If you pitch it to him he has to look the ball in and then find his read. If you hand the ball off it's the quarterback's job to get him the ball."

Hines did not have great hands and caught only seven passes the whole year. He turned to Matthews. "And Raymond, who said about 100 words in four years here, whispered ever so strongly to me," Matthews recalled. "He leaned in and said, 'Coach, please hand me the ball, don't pitch it.'"

Matthews nodded his head in agreement and sent in the play. Rascati took the snap and handed the ball to Hines running to the right. The Furman defense collapsed into the middle of the field and Hines — on fourth down and with just 28 seconds left in the game — cut inside a block from fullback Chris Iorio and waltzed into the end zone. "They did exactly what we thought they'd do," Durden later said. "They pinched so hard [that] it was a walk in."

David Rabil's PAT split the uprights and the Dukes were off to the I-AA semifinals. They could not have known it at the time, but Hines was nearly done. He said he felt fine, but he practiced very little the next week and Matthews pushed both Banks and Fenner, hoping they would be ready to go before Hines ran out of gas. The two former starters did not respond well during the week and Matthews planned to go with Hines one more time. Over the course of his titanic effort in November, it was easy to think Hines was indestructible, yet a look at the numbers reflected the writing on the wall. Hines' 118 carries over a four-week stretch from Nov. 13 to Dec. 4 eclipsed his total carries from both his freshman and sophomore years combined. "When he got his shot he was a big reason why they got through the playoffs," Mike Barber said. "But he was basically run into the ground to get them to the William & Mary game."

Tired and weary, Hines dressed for the semifinal in Williamsburg and gave Madison an early lead with a 27-yard scoring run on the game's first possession. The touchdown pushed him over the 1,000-yard mark for the season and helped the Dukes storm out to a 21-0 first-quarter lead. But that was the final bullet from Raymond Hines. "Later in that half he came off the field and I could tell he was hurting," Edmonds said. "I thought it was the ankle so I asked him, 'How's your ankle?' and he said, 'It's good but I can't breathe. It hurts when I breathe.'"

Hines had felt pain in his chest after taking a hit during the game's first series and thought he had gotten the wind knocked out of him. He shrugged it off and finished the first half with 57 rushing yards on 11 carries but the pain persisted. The JMU medical staff gave Hines a quick evaluation and told him it could be a fractured rib. As the Dukes walked into the locker room (now leading 21-20 after a furious William & Mary comeback) Matthews knew his 1,000-yard back was spent. "We were out of tailbacks," Matthews recalled. "At William & Mary we were out. I'm not sure who we could have played. I haven't told too many people that, but at the half against William & Mary we were out."

"Raymond was done."

As team doctors evaluated Hines in the locker room, Matthews jumped on Banks and Fenner, dragging both players into the shower room for what he later called, "a revival meeting." The duo responded with a huge second-half performance. Fenner gained 106 of his game-high 117 yards in the final two quarters and Banks added a late touchdown run in a 48-34 win that sent the Dukes to Chattanooga. Though his blood was pumping and he wanted to play, Hines did not carry the ball in the second half. The Dukes traveled back to Harrisonburg that night and when Hines awoke the next morning in his Southview apartment, he could barely move. "My adrenaline was rushing the night before and I felt OK," Hines recalled. "I didn't feel it until the next morning. I couldn't get out of bed."

Hines had X-Rays taken that day and the examination revealed a cracked rib in his left cage. His season was over. It was remarkably ironic but Hines had come full-circle. On the biggest stages — back-to-back games on national television — he would slip into the background while Banks and Fenner again captured the spotlight. Hines had brought the Dukes within 30 minutes of the national title game, rushing for 1,038 yards and 10 touchdowns. Yet his season would end on the sideline, the same way it began.

…

HINES STOOD motionless on the Madison sideline and tried to imagine himself playing this game. That he was dressed in pads was both tactical and symbolic. Barber believed Matthews wanted to give Montana something to think about by dressing Hines — that Hines wanted to dress and "play" for the national championship and Matthews wanted Bobby Hauck to think Hines was available. At the same time, Curt Dudley thought letting Hines put on his pads and jersey was an appropriate gesture of thanks. "Ray represents a real feel-good portion of the story," Dudley said. "If you talk about the fabric of it all, the gauge of his thread is pretty huge."

The Dukes began to stabilize on defense. Montana's third offensive drive began with a nine-yard pass before JMU slammed the door shut and forced the Grizzlies to punt from midfield. After opening the game with a precise, relentless attack, Montana had regressed on its final two possessions of the opening quarter.

As the game flipped to commercial, *Daily News-Record* sports editor Chris Simmons glanced away from the television screen and turned his attention to a pile of papers on his desk. Simmons was in Harrisonburg managing the nightly workflow as Barber and staff writer Dustin Dopirak covered the game from Chattanooga. The DN-R did not have the staff to put together a larger section for the game. As

Simmons said, it was no different than any other late night at the office, with the first press run slated for 12:30 a.m. Simmons was in constant communication with Barber and Dopirak, but did not recall anything out of the ordinary as the night progressed.

Simmons was giving the game as much attention as he could afford. A good writer roots for a good story. He believed that if the Dukes won tonight it would make for a great story. Even if they lost a thriller it would be good. And JMU had come from behind often that season. "They had shown they could win a game regardless of how the first quarter went," Simmons said. And despite being dominated in the opening 15 minutes, the Dukes were down only 7-0 as Rascati and the offense took the field for their third drive of the game.

Simmons, with page proofs and notepads scattered across his desk, lifted his head and glanced back at the screen every few minutes, dividing his attention between the game and work. Back in Chattanooga, Maurice Fenner plunged into the line and gained four yards on the final play of the first quarter.

Part III: Elvis Has Left the Building

Chapter 8

CHRIS SIMMONS praised JMU's ability to win regardless of how it looked early in the game. But though they were at their best in the second half, the Dukes also had not trailed in the first quarter all season. Montana had Madison on its heels, and the Dukes, despite their confidence, had not competed so much as they had survived the first 15 minutes.

Still, the Madison defense had proven it could slow Montana. Craig Ochs was on his way to a 300-yard passing game, but the Grizzlies were beatable as long as the Dukes could come up with a few stops. The tempo of the game was there for the taking. If JMU could find a way to jump-start its offense, the Dukes could turn the track meet into a slugfest.

Maurice Fenner got the call on second down, this time hitting the right side of the line for four more yards and setting up third-and-short from the 22-yard line. For the first time all night the Dukes were in a manageable third-down situation. They went to Alvin Banks on the next play and Banks knifed through the middle to the 26 for a JMU first down. It had taken almost 16 minutes but the Dukes finally had moved the chains.

With a fresh set of downs, Jeff Durden sought to open the playbook. JMU came to the line with two tight ends. Rascati called for the snap, dropped back into the pocket and scanned the field for an open receiver.

Immediately, Rascati was pressured by Mike Murphy and forced out to the right. Slipping and stumbling on the unstable turf, Rascati floated the ball to Tom Ridley as he was being tackled. Ridley caught the pass in stride and rumbled for 14 yards before being knocked out of bounds near the 40. "Definitely not the prettiest play in the world," Rascati later joked. "But we needed to move the ball. I kind of just flipped it out to Tom and he did his thing."

A draw play and a 17-yard swing pass to Banks earned another first down and brought the Dukes into Montana territory for the first time. Surprisingly, of the 43 yards gained on the drive, 31 had come through the air. The previous week against William & Mary, Raymond Hines and Fenner torched the Tribe for 174 rushing yards, and they gained most of them running up the middle behind Leon Steinfeld and Matt Magerko. Montana's defense was nearly a replica of W&M's — small and agile — but the Grizzlies were blitzing and shifting linemen, turning their defensive front into a moving target. It was preventing the Dukes from blasting the Grizzlies off the line of scrimmage.

A draw to Banks and an incomplete pass set up a third-and-nine from the Montana 41 and forced Durden into calling an obvious pass play. Rascati brought the Dukes to the line, faked a handoff to Antoinne Bolton and looked for D.D. Boxley down the middle of the field. Boxley had been JMU's big-play receiver all season, averaging better than 14 yards per catch. Whenever the Dukes needed a completion, they looked for him. Now, in the face of a heavy rush, Rascati again found his favorite target, drilling a pass into Boxley's hands at 25 for another Madison first down.

A five-yard facemask penalty and a 10-yard gain for Fenner moved JMU to the 11. The Dukes had chewed up more than six minutes of clock on the drive and the change in pace was striking. Of the 16 teams who made the I-AA playoffs in 2004, the Grizzlies and Dukes provided perhaps the most intriguing matchup of opposites. While Montana's flashy offense would push opponents into a shootout, JMU hammered teams into the ground with numbing efficiency. And midway through the second quarter in Chattanooga, finesse and strength were in a power struggle over the tempo of the game.

Fenner gained four more yards on first down but an incomplete pass and a four-yard loss stopped the drive at the Montana 11. Less than nine minutes remained in the first half, and after putting together a 70-yard drive, the Dukes could not afford to come away empty-handed. The JMU special teams unit came onto the field. On the Madison sideline, David Rabil loosened up his right leg and jogged out for a 28-yard field goal attempt.

Rabil was a lanky collection of arms and legs — a soft-spoken kid who looked like an oversized teenager on a team of muscle. A sophomore from Franklin, Va., Rabil started kicking footballs after the local high school coach noticed the powerful right leg attached to his tall body. He was an all-state soccer player. Football was a secondary sport, but Rabil found he enjoyed it. "My friends said I should do it, why not?" he remembered. And Rabil enjoyed a modest high school kicking career, figuring it would be the last time he played the sport.

Rabil kicked for three seasons at Franklin. In the spring of 2003, while passing through the area on a recruiting visit, Curt Newsome stopped at the high school. Rabil had been accepted at James Madison earlier in the year and had submitted a recruiting letter to the football office. He and Newsome briefly spoke about Rabil coming to Madison as a walk-on. Rabil did not have eye-popping statistics. "I think I went 2-for-7 on field goals my entire high school career," he mused.

Football was something Rabil played to pass the time in a sleepy town. But he could kick the snot out of the ball. And since he already was attending JMU there was little risk in extending him an invite to preseason camp. Newsome told Rabil to sit tight. The call came two weeks before training camp. "They had a spot open up last minute," Rabil explained. "They said, 'you're going to be here in 10 days.' So I said, 'Heck, I guess I am.'"

Rabil appeared content to let the current carry him. He was a sharp student with a good sense of direction, but he appeared to lack any physical sign of worry. Nothing bothered him. His freshman year began in Hillside Hall, where all the football players lived for the first week of camp before most scattered to their assigned dorms and apartments. Rabil didn't have a football roommate and had no idea what he was getting himself into. Still, he kicked well in preseason and earned a spot on the team as the backup place kicker behind Burke George. When George began the 2003 season with four misses in his first six attempts, Mickey Matthews gave Rabil his shot.

Rabil, who kicked for a 22-man team in high school, made his first eight attempts — including a 48-yard missile against Rhode Island that would have been good from 50-plus. He possessed an average leg by collegiate standards (it would be his only successful field goal from longer than 40 yards in his career), yet the kick — coupled with a 38-yarder he made against Maine in nasty weather — demonstrated Rabil's resolve in tough situations. He finished the 2003 season with 10 field goals in 11 attempts, essentially locking up the starting job for 2004 and leading Matthews to call him a "mentally tough kid," a phrase he normally would not reserve for a kicker. "His laid-back personality worked so well on the field," Tony LeZotte recalled. "Kickers need to have a short memory and you don't want a nervous guy trying to make a pressure kick. David wasn't nervous about anything."

Rabil was popular on campus and had an equal number of friends on and off the team. He was the definition of casual and never seemed to fret. Sometimes he wore a bathrobe to class. It was just Rabil going with the flow. Kickers practice on different schedules; they rarely get hit and many are seen as outsiders. But LeZotte called Rabil an important figure in the Madison locker room. Rabil cracked jokes, played pranks and proved he was one of the guys. He also seemed oblivious to the idea that kickers were to be seen and not heard. He looked at himself as a member of the team, which — combined with his early success — helped him avoid the general disdain Matthews reserved for kickers.

Matthews seemed to believe that kickers and punters needed to toughen up. He spent one day a week grilling Rabil at practice as he attempted kicks. "I'm in your head Rabil," Matthews would say. "Everyone in this stadium thinks you're gonna miss this fuckin' kick." Rabil, more often than not, blocked this out. Matthews also was famous for lighting up players on the sideline to send a message, and kickers sometimes bore the brunt of his frustration. Madison punter Nick Englehart, a two-time all-conference honoree and former high school quarterback, was a proud competitor, and very confident in his ability. One day, Englehart shanked a punt at practice. "Hey God!" Matthews yelled. "You think you're God? God could have kicked that ball straight, long and with good hang-time!"

The love-hate dynamic between the two parties was obvious. Like a baseball closer who blows a save, a kicker who misses an important field goal causes an incredible amount of frustration. Matthews, like many coaches, was reluctant to kick for three if he thought he could run or pass for six. One former Madison player recalled that trust, even in successful kickers, was measured, and that Matthews longed to find a way to play football without having to rely on players who kicked for a living.

Rabil enjoyed a solid 2004 season, hitting 9 of 13 field goals and only missing one attempt from inside the 30-yard line in JMU's first 14 games. But he demonstrated a heart-stopping habit of walking the fine line between success and failure. Against West Virginia, Rabil shanked a 44-yard attempt midway through the second quarter that could have pulled the Dukes within four points of the Mountaineers. Later in the season against Delaware, he botched a 28-yard chip shot with JMU clinging to a 6-0 lead. Rabil, like most collegiate kickers, was subject to patches of inconsistency. He was accurate but far from automatic, and there remained a touch of tension in the Madison stands whenever he trotted onto the field — a mixture of fear, confidence and curiosity.

Here, that moment came in the form of No. 42 and the unstable turf at Max Finley Stadium. Though Rabil was composed and generally unfazed there was some tension as he tested the sod at the Montana 18-yard line. "You can't really whine about it because there's nothing you can do," Rabil later said. "[But now] I can say it was a disaster. It wasn't really a scary moment, but it was a curious moment. You could end up on stable turf or you could end up on a hell on earth."

Rabil lined up from the left hash mark. Englehart crouched at the 18, caught the snap and placed the ball on the ground. Rabil planted his left foot firmly on the turf, swung his right leg and heard the gratifying "thud" of a well-struck ball. His kick sliced to the right on an angled trajectory, then knuckled-over at the last second and smacked against the far goalpost. Rabil held his breath. The ball slammed off the inside of the post and ricocheted between the uprights. It wasn't pretty but the Dukes were on the board. "I've hit the uprights a few times," Rabil later said. "But those were the longest four seconds of my career."

...

RABIL WASN'T the only person breathing a sigh of relief. Across the field on the JMU sideline, the Dukes had a newfound confidence about their position. Madison had been overwhelmed in the first quarter, and yet with just under nine minutes left in the opening half the Dukes were within striking distance. Even more importantly, the butterflies of being in their first championship game seemed to have disappeared for good. Chalk it up to the bad turf, strong defense, Boxley's catch in traffic or just plain luck, but the Dukes seemingly had weathered the storm. "I could see we were feeling them out and gaining confidence," Raymond Hines recalled from the Madison sideline. "They were the big men on the block and their fans had signs that said, 'J-M-Who?' so it was like being the underdog there for a bit. [But] our coaches did an excellent job figuring out Montana, and as the game went along we knew we could hang with them."

Of course the Dukes still hadn't found a way to slow down Craig Ochs. Despite keeping the Grizzlies out of the end zone on the last two possessions, the JMU defense was giving up yards in bunches. As Montana lined up for its ensuing offensive possession, Ochs was 9-of-10 for 129 yards and the Grizzlies had run more than half of their 23 offensive plays in JMU territory.

The strength of the Madison defense was its ability to pressure the quarterback and shut down the run. In their opening-round playoff game, the Dukes sacked Lehigh quarterback Mark Borda 11 times. JMU entered the I-AA championship game with an NCAA single-season record 55 sacks. Matthews was of the philosophy that a good rush and good positioning in the secondary was the key to a strong pass defense. Yet Madison's defensive alignment (the eight-man front) put an incredible amount of pressure on the cornerback position because it took away the safety net of downfield help.

In previous seasons, safeties Tony LeZotte and Rodney McCarter would have spent more time in a Cover-2 formation, covering the top of the field on long pass plays. In the eight-man front, McCarter and LeZotte often were closer to the line of scrimmage and the cornerbacks (Clint Kent and Cortez Thompson) usually found themselves covering receivers one-on-one. Without much help over the top, Kent and Thompson had to be careful not to let receivers break tackles or get behind them.

The Dukes ranked in the nation's top 20 in scoring defense and run defense. They also gave up almost 240 passing yards per game — a number inflated because teams couldn't run the ball and often were trying to score quickly to catch up. "One thing Mickey understands very well is that a run-and-shoot offense will kill your defense," Mike Schikman said. "So he builds an offense that controls the clock and a defense that forces teams to throw the ball a lot. Giving up catches doesn't get you in trouble, it's yards-after-catch that hurt you."

In layman's terms, Matthews was content to let teams complete passes as long as his secondary kept long plays to a minimum. That Thompson and Kent could handle receivers alone enabled JMU to apply pressure up front. And because the Dukes could get to the quarterback, opposing teams could not exploit them down the field.

The defense relied on apt personnel in the secondary. Thompson and McCarter were seniors. Kent and strong safety Bruce Johnson were juniors. And LeZotte, though a freshman, was perhaps the best defensive back in Virginia. The unit, though not without flaw, was versatile — a trait the Dukes employed to their advantage both on defense and special teams.

Bruce Johnson, at 5-foot-8, was the shortest starter on the JMU defense and one of the smallest players at his position in the Atlantic 10. Johnson did not possess extraordinary talent and had the Dukes remained in a 4-3 defense that season he would have been the odd-man out in the secondary. He often was the target of opposing offenses — the player teams would single out to create matchup problems down the field. Yet he made big plays, often coming up with a key interception or quarterback sack to tip the balance of power. "We always looked out there and kept saying, 'we've got to have someone better,'" George Barlow said. "And we had some young guys behind him but none had his desire. His heart enabled him to play at a level beyond his body."

Perhaps. But more likely, it was Johnson's brain that kept him in the starting lineup. Though not exceptionally athletic, Madison's strong safety was incredibly bright and atoned for physical shortcomings with good technique. He had lettered four times in football at Lakeside High School in Lithonia, Ga., earning academic all-state honors and the *DeKalb Neighbor*'s Two-way Player of the Year award as a senior. In his first two seasons at JMU, Johnson was used in the secondary, on special teams and briefly as an offensive player. He lacked the size to play linebacker and the speed to play cornerback. But he was a good tackler, willing to play wherever he was needed, and took advantage of the eight-man front's need for smart, hybrid athletes who could play in the secondary and stop the run.

According to Matthews, Johnson — like many Madison upperclassmen — was a film junkie. Lacking the talent of others, Johnson gained an edge by breaking down opponents on game tape. He became adept at recognizing tendencies and uncovering ways to turn them in his favor, and usually found himself in the thick of things on the field. Much like a versatile sixth man in basketball, Johnson filled the stat sheet and his performance mirrored both his effort and preparation. He started every game in 2004 and finished the season with 45 tackles. Against Maine, Johnson had six stops and a quarterback sack. A week later, he had four tackles, a sack and a forced fumble against Richmond.

Johnson was best used as a run-stopper and often was key in blitz packages. He finished the year with 6.5 sacks —more than anyone else in the Madison secondary and tied for the second-highest total on the team. "When we went with the eight-man front Bruce was a guy in between a safety and a linebacker," Matthews explained. "He was our best blitzer and in small areas he was a tremendous defensive player."

Good positioning was the linchpin of Johnson's success. He forced three fumbles and recovered two. He intercepted a pass and blocked a kick. He was, Barlow said, a player who fully understood the game and his responsibilities. He might be burned on a jump ball, but Barlow knew Johnson would never miss an assignment because he wasn't prepared. "Bruce is pretty intelligent," Curt Dudley said. "Just like many other athletes who might sacrifice size, they find ways to be successful and Bruce did it from a mental standpoint. He knew to be in the right place at the right time."

Johnson's colleagues in the Madison secondary likewise often found themselves in the middle of the action. The defensive backs, LeZotte said, seemed to feed off each other. If Johnson forced a fumble, Clint Kent would recover it. If Rodney McCarter tipped a pass, Thompson would come down with the ball and LeZotte would throw a block during the return. "We were close," LeZotte said. "I've known those guys since Matt [LeZotte] came here. Our communication with each other was incredible."

Kent and Thompson were durable, proven cornerbacks who combined for 122 tackles and six interceptions in 2003. The decision to move to the eight-man front had a lot to do with the amount of faith Barlow and Matthews had in their veteran corners. Thompson and Kent were used to the Cover-2 formation and their ability to adjust to one-on-one coverage was critical to JMU's defensive scheme. "Going into that season Clint and I were asked to do a lot," Thompson remembered. "We had to rise to the challenge of playing out there on an island."

Kent had been a first-team all-state selection at Westside High School in Macon, Ga., where he set school records for most career interceptions in football and most career assists in basketball. A skilled playmaker with strong instincts, Kent led the Dukes with four interceptions in 2003, a number that McCarter believed could have been twice as high if Kent (then just a sophomore and in his first season as a starter) had been more experienced. Still, by 2004 Kent was one of Barlow's defensive generals. With a physical style of play and good cover skills, he had little trouble adjusting to the eight-man front and quickly became well versed in its parts.

Kent could not imagine life without football. He played with a blend of passion and discipline. By his own account, he was a quiet person who enjoyed his down time. But on the field, Kent was a showman — a high-energy player who created momentum. For a reserved person, Kent played with flair. After big plays, he danced and hopped around the field with the energy of a little kid. He grew up playing in front of big crowds and so Kent loved a good challenge, often performing his best when the stakes were highest. "As a player you should dream of being in the spotlight when the game is on the line," he said. "You should dream of making that big play."

From 2003-05, Kent's numbers were remarkably consistent. Every season he could be penciled in for 60-80 tackles, a handful of interceptions and at least a few plays he'd make due to a potent combination of instinct and intelligence. Kent valued preparation and thought it was important to develop a strong football I.Q. He often spent long hours studying receiver patterns to gain an edge on his opponent. His reliability and discipline often masked his greatest talent. Unlike other players with strong but unspectacular numbers, Kent's play was dynamic. While many players on that JMU defense enjoyed successful careers as methodical, no-nonsense performers, Kent was best known as a defensive playmaker. "He broke on passes so quickly it startled you," McCarter said.

In three years as a starter, Kent would have his hand in 19 turnovers. He finished his career tied for the most interceptions in school history (13). McCarter believed that last number could have been as high as 20 given Kent's feel for the game. Luck, Kent said, had little to do with his success; he attributed it more to skill and good study habits. But it also had a lot to do with his willingness to be proactive. Kent trusted his instincts when he recognized the play unfolding before him. He walked into every game believing he was going to make a play to help the Dukes win. More often then not, he was right. By 2004, Matthews had given up trying to explain Kent's ability to find the football, simply referring to him as "a great corner," and more than once remarking in his Texas twang that, "Clint Kent just makes plays."

Though his production rarely fluctuated, Kent was dynamite down the stretch in 2004. Of the nine turnovers he was involved in during the season, seven took place during the Dukes' late-season surge. And as other players broke down, Kent began to heat up. He intercepted a pass, recovered a fumble and made seven tackles in JMU's playoff-clinching win over Towson. Two weeks later against Furman, with the Dukes down 13-7 and the Paladins driving, Johnson and Sid Evans forced a fumble, and Kent fell on the ball at the JMU one-yard line to keep Madison within striking distance. And in their 48-34 win over William & Mary, Kent intercepted Lang Campbell's third pass of the game, dodged and weaved his way through traffic, and returned the pick 69 yards for a touchdown to put the Dukes up 21-0. He later called it one of his most memorable moments at JMU — another big play in a big game by a player who relished the chance to prove himself when the lights were brightest. "During that playoff run Clint was our best defensive player," Barlow said. "For me, in the last part of the season he was better than Tony. He came in and was a solid player for years, but during that stretch he want to another level."

Kent, it seemed, made big plays in almost every game and the challenge of playing on an island became a friendly competition between he and Thompson of who could have the best performance. "Those two really pushed each other, LeZotte said. A year older then Kent, Thompson was JMU's best pure pass defender. He had been a steady performer in the JMU secondary since his freshman season, totaling 125 tackles and collecting six interceptions from 2001-03 as a part-time starter. A speedy cover corner, Thompson understood football from almost every angle and was a useful utility man who could impact the game on special teams and defense. "We thought Cortez was a really good athlete," Barlow said. "He had done a bit of everything in high school and we thought he could help us in a lot of areas because of his versatility."

An all-state performer at Courtland High School in Fredericksburg, Va., Thompson was a running back, defensive back and punter for two state playoff teams. He was most effective on offense, but at 5-foot-9 and 165 pounds, had no illusions of playing Division I ball. Thompson verbally committed to attend Division III Bridgewater College in the spring of his senior year. He was on his way to a class trip at King's Dominion amusement park when JMU assistant coach Kyle Gillenwater intercepted him in front of the bus and asked him to come to Harrisonburg for a recruiting visit. JMU and Bridgewater were located less than five miles from each other and Thompson, without much knowledge of the JMU program or its coaching staff, told Gillenwater he'd consider the proposal.

Thompson visited Madison a few weeks later and met with Gillenwater, Barlow and Matthews. The coaches took him on a tour through campus and offered him a partial scholarship. "Coming from a small place that scholarship meant a lot and helped my folks pay for school," Thompson said. "I visited JMU again the first day of my last week of high school and everything looked great. I was sold."

Thompson signed with the Dukes. Like many of his classmates, he joined a team in transition. As true freshmen in 2001, Thompson, Rodney McCarter and Kwynn Walton — coupled with redshirt freshmen Trey

Townsend and Rondell Bradley — saw significant playing time for a team that finished 2-9 and lost seven games by a touchdown or less. Years later, Thompson and Townsend would refer to that first season as "difficult" and "unpleasant," yet both also credited their success as seniors to the growing pains they suffered as freshmen. "You build a lot of discipline from a season like that," Townsend said. "You hear how you're not good all the time and you learn what it takes to climb out of that stereotype."

Thompson was solid in his first three seasons, growing into an excellent pass defender and a capable kick returner. He made 49 tackles as a freshman, intercepted three passes as a sophomore and averaged 10.1 yards per punt return as a junior. He had perhaps his most complete game against Hofstra in 2003 when he made seven tackles, intercepted a pass and had kick returns of 24 and 33 yards, respectively, to set up Madison touchdown drives. "That was probably when he realized the impact he could make," Barlow said. "He's a pretty confident kid but that was one of those games that helped him get over the hump — maybe help him believe he really was a good corner and a standout special teams performer."

Thompson was a below-average tackler. This was cause for some concern at a position where a missed tackle could be the difference between 10 yards and 80. Barlow, Matthews and JMU defensive backs coach Chip West hammered Thompson to be more physical late in his career, even pulling him out of the starting lineup at times to show him that being a shut-down corner meant he had to be a better tackler. To Barlow, every defensive player was a run stopper, and he challenged Thompson to make himself tougher. Thompson struggled at times but also demonstrated a willingness to perform that kept him in the starting lineup for most of the 2004 season. It was, Barlow said, as though Thompson, after spending three years on mediocre teams, understood the urgency of the moment. Barlow believed that Thompson jumped to a higher level during his senior season and Thompson admitted the knowledge that this was his last chance pushed him to re-invent himself.

Although Thompson's final 2004 numbers (57 tackles and two interceptions) were not far removed from his previous totals, he was far more reliable in open space. "We needed him to help with the run as well as be a great pass defender," Barlow said. "He accepted that challenge, and while he didn't look great doing it, he became accountable."

Thompson had to make adjustments to fit into the eight-man front. Rodney McCarter simply needed to accept it. At 5-foot-10 and 190 pounds, McCarter was an athlete in the purest sense. He ran the 40-yard dash in 4.5 seconds and possessed a strong balance of size, speed and agility. Like Thompson, he had been an offensive player in high school, earning all-city honors as a running back at Bok Tech in Philadelphia. McCarter and Rondell Bradley (from nearby Levittown, Pa.) initially were thought of as foreigners on the Madison roster — a couple of tough Philly kids on a team full of Virginia boys. They were two of the first players brought in during the Matthews era outside of JMU's traditional recruiting zones.

McCarter grew up in Philly's south side, and was, by his own admission, a little rough around the edges when he came to Harrisonburg in the fall of 2001. He had developed a thick skin while growing up and it took him a while to understand the sociable atmosphere of the rural college. McCarter and Raymond Hines roomed together as freshmen didn't speak to each other for almost a month. Hines was quiet by nature and McCarter didn't understand why almost every stranger he passed on campus wanted to say hello. "I could walk past 300 people in Philadelphia and not talk to any of them," he explained. Walking around Madison's sprawling campus in the middle of the Shenandoah Valley, McCarter felt like an exchange student from another country. It wasn't bad. It was just different. "When [Rodney] came here I didn't think he would survive," Mike Schikman admitted. "He really had to work hard at his personal situation."

To fully understand that situation involved analyzing life in

McCarter's hometown. He grew up in relatively good areas and was instilled with strong values. But there weren't many players on the Madison roster who understood the pitfalls of the inner city like Rodney McCarter. He earned good grades in school and had uncanny discipline, but all around him, the world was full of turmoil, jealousy and wrong turns. "You deal with a lot," McCarter said. "A lot of people have negative attitudes about everybody else. They hope you don't make it. They get jealous because you can do something they can't."

McCarter's parents separated when he was 12 and Rodney moved with his mom and brother to New Jersey. He didn't play team sports, instead focusing his athletic ability on karate. He earned a brown belt by the time he reached middle school (uncle, Kevin Thompson, is a world-class martial arts master). In eighth grade, McCarter moved back to Philadelphia. He played football, earned solid grades and made plans to walk on a team when he got to college. He knew very little about the recruiting process and didn't send out highlight tapes or draft application letters. McCarter played with three of the best players in the city; two were NFL-size linemen and the third was a 6-foot-3 220-pound all-state receiver. None went to college. "Didn't have the grades," McCarter said. "They all washed up."

That was a phrase common to inner-city recruits. And the problem, McCarter said, usually came back to one of three things: grades, attitude and home life. A problem with either usually was enough to deter a coach from recruiting a player or prevent the player from accepting an offer. McCarter saw many great high school athletes fall short of college for these reasons. Some cared only about girls and money and let their grades slip below eligibility standards. Others had the right mental makeup but the wrong family situation. Some had kids or had to work to support family.

McCarter didn't have these problems. "When I came to JMU all I brought was a green duffel bag," he said. "No TV or anything like that." The lack of possessions carried metaphorical value. McCarter didn't come from luxury, but he also didn't bring any baggage.

Eddie Davis (Madison's offensive coordinator from 2001-03) found McCarter by accident. During a recruiting trip in New Jersey, Davis flipped on the TV in his hotel room and saw a local highlight of McCarter's Bok Tech game. Immediately interested, Davis recruited McCarter based on the highlight and invited him on a tour of campus. The Dukes ended up offering a half scholarship, believing McCarter would evolve into an athletic defensive back.

McCarter, however, would struggle with his new surroundings. He kept to himself, seemingly aware that the partial scholarship and abrupt change in scene did not guarantee emotional acceptance. McCarter rarely talked to people around campus and seemed to have trouble connecting. "I really didn't speak to anybody," he admitted. "I'm sure people walked around wondering, 'Why is this guy so mean?'" McCarter also lacked the job security of his Philadelphia predecessor. Bradley had been a first-team all-state running back in high school, earning a spot in the prestigious "Big 33 game" in 2000. He was a star when he came to JMU. He started almost immediately. McCarter would have a tougher path. He played through his first training camp convinced he wasn't good enough to compete for a starting job and more than once thought about transferring. As it turned out, McCarter was his worst critic and Davis assured him that he had a future at Madison. "He told me I was playing better than some of the full scholarship guys," McCarter said. "I really didn't believe him."

During that rocky freshman year, McCarter slowly began shedding armor. He and Hines became friends and McCarter warmed to the outgoing campus that served as a foil to his hometown. He declared a major in sociology and grew more comfortable with each semester. "By his second season Rodney was all purple and gold," Schikman said. And it was Davis, not McCarter who correctly observed his play. By the end of his freshman season, McCarter was starting in the Madison defensive backfield.

McCarter remained a work-in-progress because he lacked good technique. He led all JMU defensive backs with 103 tackles as a sophomore; a feat he later joked probably wasn't a good sign for his future as a cornerback — a position where more tackles means more receptions allowed. With Clint Kent waiting in the wings, McCarter believed his days at corner were numbered. Sure enough, the Dukes moved him to free safety in 2003, where he blossomed into one of the most feared rovers in the conference.

McCarter, Schikman recalled, hit with the force of a runaway freight train and would pop receivers so hard in the first quarter that they would be afraid to go over the middle for the rest of the game. "They would alligator-arm on routes," Schikman said. Although Matthews believes McCarter could have developed into JMU's best corner, the shift to free safety was one of the coach's shrewdest moves. McCarter, George Barlow said, had an insatiable thirst to compete. His drive was unparalleled and the safety position in the 4-3 scheme allowed him to play the physical, downhill brand of football he enjoyed most. "He was an unbelievable competitor," Matthews added. "[Rodney] would compete until there was no blood left in his system."

For three years the Madison coaching staff attempted to find the right home for McCarter. It seemed they finally nailed it. Given the freedom to roam the field and make big hits, McCarter made 94 tackles and forced three fumbles in 2003, earning third-team all-conference honors. Built like a safety, McCarter hit like a linebacker. His versatility gave him increased value, though it also likely prevented him from reaching his true potential. McCarter would play only that one season at free safety. He had offseason surgery on his thigh and missed all of spring practice in 2004. The Dukes were ready to red shirt him. "They were taking me off the magazine covers and everything," he said.

But McCarter rebounded and participated in summer sessions. By July he was back in the defensive backfield rotation. LeZotte had taken over the free safety position and McCarter was moved yet again, this time to a hybrid safety position created during the switch to the eight-man front.

The Madison coaches believed his physical play and hard hits would help JMU's run defense in the new defensive scheme. The Dukes gave up nearly 168 rushing yards per game in 2003 and Matthews wanted that number chopped in half. McCarter's new role, Matthews explained, blended elements of a safety, linebacker and cornerback. It sounded like the perfect fit for McCarter. It wasn't. "The position demands a lot of you physically," McCarter said. "And I'm a physical person, but switching from free safety to that position is hard because I wasn't in the action. All I had to do was contain and make sure nothing bounced to the outside. I was cut off."

Not that McCarter wasn't successful. He made an entire career as a square peg in a round hole. But the new position restricted what he could do. McCarter quickly discovered the difference between popping a running back in open field and charging a lineman on a blitz. "I learned quickly that I'm 5-9, 190," he said. "I can take a 220-pound running back but a 330-pound lineman is a whole different story. Dealing with Corey Davis, Harry Dunn, Magerko [in practice], that made things pretty clear for me."

McCarter's new responsibilities bored him and he often took it upon himself to make plays outside of his zone, trusting his instincts instead of the defensive formation. His teammates knew what he was doing and adjusted accordingly. Every Sunday, Barlow would grill McCarter during film session for making a tackle when he was supposed to be containing the play. And every week McCarter would keep doing it anyway. An unspoken agreement was formed within the secondary. McCarter would never put the Dukes in danger, but he was going to do his thing if he thought it could help — the playbook be damned.

Barlow, to his credit, never benched McCarter for his mild insubordination. In fact, the topic never came up. He too, recognized McCarter's thirst to win and believed McCarter's aggressive play — even his desire to bend the rules — gave the Dukes a swagger they lacked in previous seasons. Playing a position he hated, Rodney McCarter made 92 tackles in 2004 and the Dukes gave up a shade over 86 rushing yards per game. With Townsend and LeZotte making plays and McCarter pumping life into his teammates, the defense took on the characteristics of its leaders. "Rodney didn't get the fanfare that Tony and Clint got," Barlow said. "But he was the heart of that defense. If you carried the ball you knew he was going to try and knock your head off."

Like Thompson, McCarter was a key contributor on special teams. It was one area where his performance was not determined by his defensive position. He blocked kicks better than any player in school history. Again, his athleticism paved the way, and while McCarter's other feats were easily explainable, his freakish ability to get to the kicker required a crash course in simple physics.

McCarter lined up on the far edge of the Madison line with the kicker on his right side. His success, Matthews said, was attributed to getting a good jump by watching the center's hands (which quiver just before snapping the ball) and then bending off the corner blocker. The latter was where McCarter's athletic ability came into play. "It takes a 90-degree cut to come off that blocker and get to the kicker fast enough," Curt Dudley explained. "[Rodney] did it without losing any speed, which is something that can't be taught. If you were to take all these equations and put them on a bell curve he would be outside the curve. He was exceptional."

Most people need to slow down or change direction to cut that sharply but McCarter, Matthews said, actually accelerated off the side as he approached the ball and could blow past the lineman. He blocked three kicks as a sophomore, two as a junior and two more as a senior. The athleticism was half the battle. The other half was McCarter's cavalier attitude regarding his personal safety. Late in the 2004 season, *The Breeze*'s Matt Stoss wrote of McCarter's reign as Madison's kick-blocking king. "Like many things, kick blocking is dependent on … a sort of reckless confidence because getting kicked in the chest is a very real possibility," Stoss wrote.

McCarter even told Stoss that sometimes he closed his eyes just before impact and wouldn't see the ball, an admission that only added weight to his impressive ability. After enduring a rocky transition at school, McCarter's workman-like attitude made him one of the great success stories of the Matthews tenure. "Some kids can do it and some can't," Barlow said. "And by that I'm talking both physically and mentally. [Rodney] was a great athlete but he also had the desire to win and that's what took him to the next level. Most kids don't have the skill. Others have the ability but not the heart. Rodney had both."

...

WITH A four-point lead and the ball back in their hands at the 18-yard line, the Grizzlies began the ensuing drive looking to increase the game's pace to their liking. A nine-yard gain by Lex Hilliard on first down was followed by a 16-yard completion to Jefferson Heidelberger and then a three-yard completion to Justin Green that brought Montana to the 46. Ochs then found Tate Hancock on the far sideline for 22 more yards to the JMU 32-yard line. In less than two minutes, Montana had covered half the field. As Ochs and the Grizzlies again approached the line of scrimmage, the Dukes stood on the other side with their hands on their hips. The 55 sacks, the 33 turnovers and the aggressive play were nothing if the Dukes couldn't get to the quarterback. Playing on the tattered field, Madison's self-propelled defense was stuck in the mud. "The biggest problem was we couldn't rush the passer," Matthews recalled. "It's hard to cover them down the field when the quarterback is that good and he has all day to throw it."

Matthews, according to Gary Michael, had even gone as far as to call Ochs the difference-maker in the game. The Dukes were more athletic, had more speed and played with more power than the Grizzlies. In the week leading to the national title game, the JMU players and coaches were confidant that Montana did not have the athletes to chase the Dukes around the field. Certainly the Grizzlies did not have the size to stop Madison's ground game. But Montana had good receivers. More importantly, the Grizzlies had Ochs. And with seven minutes left before halftime, he was carving the Madison defense to pieces.

A two-yard run by Hilliard and a two-yard screen pass to Heidelberger set up third-and-six from the Madison 28. As Ochs brought the Grizzlies back to the line of scrimmage, Matthews glanced at the stadium game clock. Just over six minutes remained in the second quarter. A Montana first down would almost certainly shave two more minutes off the clock and would put the Grizzlies in prime position to add another touchdown before halftime. "Everyone talks about big plays," Tony LeZotte recalled. "But having someone drive on you wears you down. They just kept picking us apart down the field. The quarterback was on fire and the receivers did their homework. It was pretty scary there for a while."

Ochs set up in the shotgun with three wide receivers stacked to his left and Hilliard in the backfield. The Dukes, facing an obvious pass, dropped back into a Cover-2 defense. Ochs fielded the snap, backpedaled to the 37 and whipped a pass for the front corner of the end zone where Jon Talmage had a two-step lead on Cortez Thompson. As Ochs rotated his body to throw, LeZotte pivoted and began racing over from his free safety position to provide coverage help.

Years later, Matthews would recall that LeZotte was a bit out of position and likely allowed too much open space between he and Thompson. Still, Ochs put air under the ball and LeZotte looked ready to arrive in time. As Talmage ran down the sideline and the ball floated toward the end zone, LeZotte, still digging to break up the pass, stumbled on the turf. "I thought touchdown," he recalled. "And I remember it clear as day. It was right there. I remember slipping and my head went down when I slipped. When I picked my head up I saw he had beaten Cortez, and all I could think was touchdown."

Chapter 9

DESPITE JMU's ability to survive pivotal moments when its back was against the wall, Mickey Matthews didn't like using the word "destiny" when talking about his football team. In fact, he hated it. To him, the word was thrown around so much that it lacked significance. Fate did not determine the outcome of games — talent, execution and heart did.

But it was hard to dispute the evidence. During their 14-game trek to Chattanooga, the Dukes received more than their allotted share of fortunate breaks. Over the last month of the regular season and throughout the playoffs it seemed nearly every significant event on the field bounced in their favor. And if it didn't, the Dukes always found a way to survive. They were involved in seven games decided by 10 points or less in 2004 and they were 6-1 in those games. Some people attributed the success to JMU's experienced lineup. Others pointed to luck. It probably involved a both. And so if there existed a team of destiny in the 2004 playoffs, one would have to believe it was the Dukes.

The streak began in mid-October. In a game billed as one of the true barometers of the season, the 4-1 Dukes trailed Maine, 20-10, in Orono late in the third quarter. Maine, a playoff team in 2001 and 2002, had long been a thorn in Madison's side. The Dukes hadn't beaten the Black Bears since 2000 and JMU was 0-3 in Orono under

Matthews. Perhaps more than in any other I-AA conference, teams in the Atlantic 10 — located from northern New England to southern Virginia — enjoyed a climate-based home-field advantage when they hosted opponents from the opposite division. In 2007, JMU played three-time playoff participant New Hampshire and reigning Walter Payton Award winner Ricky Santos in an early September matinee at Bridgeforth Stadium. The game, tied at 17 at halftime, turned into a Madison rout in the fourth quarter, as Santos and the Wildcats wilted in the 95-degree Virginia heat. Likewise, the Dukes often struggled when traveling north. Mickey's bunch was 7-21 on the road in his first five seasons, including an abysmal 2-11 against teams from the North Division.

Maine involved particularly rough conditions. The facilities were below average and the games — though usually played in October — often were subject to cold conditions. The visiting locker room at Maine was located in the university's hockey arena. Mike Schikman remembered it having the insulation of a large tent. But in 2004, that arena was being renovated and the only available space was the locker room inside the faculty recreation center, which Matthews said, "was about the size of two broom closets." Matthews had his players dress at the team hotel instead. The Dukes held their pre-game and halftime meetings on the nearby baseball field. While Maine often struggled when it traveled to JMU, the Black Bears literally gave the Dukes fits in Orono and this trip was no exception.

With 2:32 left in the third quarter and the Dukes trailing by 10, JMU receiver Khary Sharpe caught a pass from Rascati but lost control of the ball as he was hit by defensive lineman Patrick McCrossan at the Madison 44. McCrossan fell on the fumble at the 41, and with a little more than a quarter to play, the Dukes were in danger of falling behind by three scores. The Black Bears drove to the JMU 28 before a holding penalty pushed them back near the original line of scrimmage. On the next play, sophomore linebacker Akeem Jordan intercepted a pass and returned it to the Maine 19. Four plays later, on the first play of the fourth quarter, Rascati raced into the end zone to pull the Dukes within three.

The 14-point swing kept Madison within striking distance. Years later, JMU equipment manager Pete Johnson remembered Rodney McCarter trying to spark the defense down the stretch. "He lit into them pretty good," Johnson recalled. "And Rodney doesn't do that much, but when he came out of his shell and spoke the defense turned it up."

Maine opened the fourth quarter by driving down the field and missing a field goal. Then the Dukes, heeding McCarter's words, clamped down. The Black Bears gained only one first down the rest of the way and the two teams traded punts for the majority of the fourth quarter. Up 20-17 with a little more than a minute left in the game, Maine elected to punt the ball on fourth down from the JMU 39, hoping to pin the Dukes deep inside their own territory. As Maine punter Mike Mellow lined up to kick the ball away, JMU freshman wide receiver L.C. Baker drifted back inside the 10-yard line to receive the punt.

Baker, a 5-foot-7-inch sparkplug from Richmond, had the type of raw speed that couldn't be taught, according to Durden. An all-region receiver and kick returner at Armstrong High School, he wowed Madison coaches with his big-play potential. Baker had been the primary punt returner for most of the year, averaging a shade less than 10 yards per return. He was electric when he touched the ball in open space, later earning the nicknames "Showtime" from his friends and "L.C. Baker the touchdown maker" from Schikman. But Baker also had moments of poor judgment, especially as a freshman. He often would field bouncing punts on the Bridgeforth Stadium turf, a maneuver that simultaneously would send the entire JMU student section into cardiac arrest. Somehow, though, his nerve-racking returns usually did not end in turnovers.

Mellow's punt did not have to be long, and the general rule of thumb for a returner was to stay away from a ball that bounced inside the 20-

yard line. Mellow's kick landed inside the 15 and bounced on the turf in front of Baker. It seemed the Dukes would be facing a long march down the field to avoid another loss to a northern opponent. But Baker, after eyeing the ball as it hopped across the 10, decided to pick it up. He slipped past tacklers and raced up the sideline to the Madison 45 before McCrossan and Ron Waller brought him down. "L.C.'s confidence level is through the roof," McCarter said. "He wanted to make a play all the time. Had he made a mistake I'm sure coach Matthews would have cussed him out. I think [L.C.] decided he was going to make a play. And if you know him than you expected that."

Thanks to Baker's gamble, the Dukes were near field goal range as they began the drive with 1:12 left in the game. A pass interference penalty, a 20-yard completion from Rascati to D.D. Boxley and a four-yard run brought Madison to the Maine 23. With less than a minute to go, Rascati walked the Dukes to the line, took the snap and lofted a pass to the corner of the end zone for Boxley.

As Rascati released the ball, Boxley became entangled with Maine defensive back Devon Goree. With his left arm pinned against Goree's shoulder pad, Boxley shielded himself away from the defender and corralled the pass with his right arm as he crossed the goal line. Boxley hugged the ball with one hand like a small child, Rascati raised both arms in the air and the Madison sideline erupted.

The Dukes would hang on for a 24-20 win. And though Rascati's clutch throw and Boxley's one-handed catch provided the decisive score, it was the other plays that stood out. The Dukes had never been quite so fortunate in a game where they made so many mistakes. The previous season, Madison had lost a road game to UMass, 31-26, when penalties killed a last-minute drive. Six weeks later, JMU threw away a win against New Hampshire by turning the ball over seven times in a 20-17 loss that killed its postseason chances. The Maine game should have followed the same script. Madison lost three fumbles. The Dukes gave up 166 rushing yards to Marcus Williams and let the Black Bears score on three of their four trips inside the red zone. "I remember the last minute of the game they were telling the Maine fans not to storm the field," Tom Ridley recalled.

Yet Sharpe's fumble, which in previous seasons would have buried the Dukes, instead galvanized the defense into getting the ball back. Baker's risky return, which in years past likely would have ended in a turnover, instead put the Dukes in position to go for the win. And the last-minute scoring drive, which always seemed to stall on the fridge of field goal range, instead was successful. "You need to understand the series of events that usually surrounded this team," Schikman said. "They never won these games. And so that became a great character win for the Dukes."

A week later, it was JMU's defense and running game that saved the day in a 26-20 win at Richmond. Up 9-0 in the closing seconds of the first half, the Dukes allowed a 41-yard Hail Mary touchdown pass from Richmond quarterback Stacy Tutt to receiver Arman Shields — an inexcusable score that had Matthews fuming as he walked into the locker room. Madison answered with a 24-yard David Rabil field goal and a 65-yard touchdown pass from Rascati to Ardon Brandford to open the second half. But the pesky Spiders took the ensuing kickoff and marched to the JMU six-yard line.

Now up 19-7, the Dukes were in danger of letting Richmond back into the game, but LeZotte made a touchdown-saving tackle on tailback David Freeman's third-down run, forcing the Spiders to settle for a field goal. Though Richmond eventually trimmed the margin to 19-17, they never took the lead, and Fenner's 46-yard touchdown run in the fourth quarter sealed the win. The Dukes again had walked the tightrope, allowing 310 passing yards and giving up a cheap touchdown in a rivalry game to a team that would win three times all season. Yet Madison escaped unscathed.

…

THE NO. 7 Dukes easily won their homecoming game against Virginia Military Institute the following weekend, setting up a Nov. 6 Atlantic 10 showdown with No. 6 Delaware. If the Maine game was a good barometer for the season, the Delaware game was a true test of the program. The defending national champion Blue Hens were 21-3 dating back to the start of the 2003 season and boasted two All-Americans in defensive back Sidney Haugabrook and defensive lineman Chris Mooney. Their top receivers, Justin Long and David Boler, would combine for more than 130 catches and almost 1,700 receiving yards in 2004. Though their quarterback, Sonny Riccio, was average, and their running game almost nonexistent, the Blue Hens were formidable. They were the class of the A-10, with more playoff appearances and championships than any other team in the conference, and they had dominated head-to-head meetings with the Dukes, winning each of their previous three games by an average of 19 points per game.

But this was a different Delaware team than the one that steamrolled to a championship the previous season. The 2003 Blue Hens overwhelmed teams with 1,600-yard tailback Germaine Bennett and quarterback Andy Hall — a Walter Payton Award finalist. They outscored teams by nearly 20 points per game and forced 40 turnovers. But in 2004 Bennett and Hall were gone, replaced by players who performed at rather pedestrian levels. Delaware was vulnerable. Injuries at tailback slowed the running game and the Hens were forced to implement a committee-based backfield, running just enough to keep teams honest. Delaware threw the ball 35 times a game, and Riccio, a transfer from Missouri, proved an underwhelming replacement for Hall, throwing 16 touchdowns and 14 interceptions.

Despite Delaware's run-and-gun offense, the likelihood of a shootout wasn't high heading into the 1:30 p.m. tilt at Bridgeforth Stadium. The Dukes didn't give up big plays, and they believed if Riccio threw the ball enough he'd make mistakes. And Delaware's defense was nearly as tough as Madison's. With Raymond Hines alone in the backfield, the Dukes couldn't pound the ball between the tackles all day. "I thought they had a great defensive football team," Matthews recalled. "And on offense they had veteran starters on the line but they had not shown any ability to run the ball in four or five weeks. Their quarterback was an average thrower and they were throwing the ball on every down anyway."

Sure enough, the game became a defensive struggle, though not the way Matthews anticipated. In an attempt to jump-start his running game, Delaware head coach K.C. Keeler had activated freshman tailback Omar Cuff two weeks earlier against William & Mary. The former walk-on saw limited action against the Tribe but performed well the next week in a 34-20 loss at Navy. Though he carried the ball only 13 times heading into the JMU game, Cuff was Keeler's secret weapon. He ran for 45 yards in the first quarter against the Dukes, effectively changing Delaware's offense overnight. Matthews, who had not seen any film of Cuff, was dumbfounded and kept glancing back at his assistants during the opening half. "Who the heck is this guy?" Matthews wondered.

Despite Cuff's hot start, the Dukes led 6-0 at the end of the first quarter. The Delaware game had been perhaps the most anticipated of the year — a late-season showdown between the defending national champions and the upstart challengers. Delaware, W&M and JMU had emerged from the pack as the class of the A-10 South. But while the Hens had pedigree and the Tribe had Lang Campbell, the Dukes, comparatively, were a bunch of no-names. This was a chance to prove Madison was a real player in the A-10 race, and in the week leading up to the game, the Dukes seemed to understand the significance of the moment. "That week defined our season," Cortez Thompson said. "At practice everyone was a little sharper — starters, special teams, even the scout team guys. Everyone poured everything they had into that game."

The Dukes needed every ounce of it. Delaware, with Cuff leading the way, kept piling up yards with a physical style of play that looked unlike anything they ran all season. Pete Johnson later called it the hardest-hitting game of the year from his vantage point. But though they allowed the Hens to move the ball at will, the Dukes kept Delaware out of the end zone. And Keeler, despite Cuff's brilliant play, kept falling back on old habits, letting Riccio sling passes across the field like a wild air cannon. Madison forced five turnovers on defense and special teams — two inside the Delaware 20. Still, JMU's offense was dysfunctional. The Dukes missed a field goal, fumbled twice and threw an interception on four consecutive drives midway through the game. Instead of a classic duel between two elite combatants, the contest was turning into an ugly brawl.

The teams were tied 13-13 midway through the fourth quarter when the Blue Hens went back to Cuff, handing him the ball 10 times on a 19-play drive that took more than nine minutes off the clock. Delaware marched to the JMU seven, where once again, the Madison defense regrouped, stopping the Hens two yards short of the end zone and forcing them to line up for a 19-yard field goal attempt. The Dukes had received career performances from many of their defensive starters. Thompson, Bruce Johnson and Trey Townsend all intercepted passes. Akeem Jordan blocked a Delaware punt that led to Madison's first score. LeZotte would finish with 19 tackles. Kwynn Walton would add 14 and Thompson another 10. Yet with 5:15 left in the game, Delaware was a short field goal away from taking the lead and forcing the Dukes to win with their offense. "Delaware really took it to the Dukes all day," Schikman recalled. "And you talk about big moments in a season, well this was one of them. The Dukes needed something."

Delaware place kicker Brad Shushman lined up for the field goal attempt. Shushman, a senior transfer from Louisville, was a two-year starter and entered the season as the most accurate kicker in school history. Yet on the Madison sideline, the Dukes were optimistic. Perhaps Jordan's block earlier in the day strengthened the faith they had in their special teams. Maybe the way they escaped with wins at Maine and Richmond reinforced their resolve. Not one JMU player had any evidence to demonstrate his attitude, but collectively, on a warm and virtually windless afternoon in Harrisonburg, the Dukes believed they controlled the moment.

The snap and spot were clean. But as Shushman approached the ball, a blurred purple figure came banking off the left side of the JMU line. A collective roar erupted from the Madison student section as Shushman planted his left foot and swung away, and then heard the "thud" of the ball hitting someone's forearm.

Rodney McCarter had done it again.

The blocked kick bounced on the turf before Thompson picked it up and returned it to the Madison 16. Incredibly, on four possessions inside the JMU five-yard line, Delaware had reached the end zone only once. Now, after an 89-yard drive, the Hens had been turned away completely — this time by another one of Madison's senior starters. "Collectively, we always thought we'd make something happen to win a game," Townsend explained. "We expected Rodney to block that kick. We watched him do it for four years."

McCarter's effort preserved the tie and the teams remained deadlocked with just over three minutes left in the game when JMU forced Delaware to punt from its own 46-yard line. The Dukes had been dominated and had not sustained one drive of considerable length all afternoon. Madison's running game was dead and Rascati — who would finish the game 9-of-21 for 103 yards — had completed only one pass since halftime. By the end of the game, JMU would tally a season-low 166 yards of total offense to Delaware's 466. Even the run defense — which had allowed only one player to gain more than 100 yards in a game all season — had been shredded by Cuff, who would finish the game with 162 yards on 34 carries. Had it not been for special teams and turnovers, the Dukes would have been blown out.

JMU lined up to return the pending Delaware punt. Across the field, Thompson rocked on the balls of his feet, awaiting the kick. Baker had fielded 22 punts in JMU's first eight games and was the primary returner, but he was breaking down under the physical strains of the long season. Though Baker fielded a punt earlier in the day, Matthews now decided to go with Thompson, who had fielded 28 punts in his career but just six all season and only three since mid-September.

Thompson lined up to return the kick. The Delaware line held off the Madison rush and Mike Weber sent a flat, spiraling kick that drove Thompson back to his own 13. "Very returnable," Curt Dudley said over the radio as Thompson camped under the punt. The Dukes were set for a return to the left side of the field, and despite catching the punt near the right hash mark, Thompson's first move was to the Madison sideline, knowing that was where his blockers were heading. "I didn't receive many punts that year," Thompson later said. "It's almost like one vs. 21 because everyone — even your teammates — are running right at you. It's like a big obstacle course."

Thompson zipped on an angled path to his left and crossed the 20. He scooted into a funnel of blockers before he shifted direction to avoid colliding with JMU safety Mike Wilkerson at the 25. The brief moment of hesitation caused two Blue Hens to fly past him and allowed Thompson to reach the Madison sideline as he approached the 30. By now, only seconds into the return, Thompson had circled past half the Delaware coverage team, and the Hens, trying to cut him off on the sideline, were running into a small convoy of blockers. Up in the JMU broadcast booth, Schikman began to see the wall developing along the sideline. Schikman was familiar with long punt returns dating back to former NFL great Gary Clark's days at Madison. As Thompson raced up field, he saw the makings of a big play.

"Thompson goes outside. Gets a block, to the 18, to the 30 … up to the 40."

At the 35, backup wide receiver Andrew Kern threw an off-balance block on Delaware linebacker Mark Moore, shoving Moore into Madison defensive back Adam Ford. Kern, a junior, would catch six passes his entire career and rarely played on offense. But he was a key player on special teams and recovered Jordan's blocked punt earlier in the game. Now he had thrown the block that got Thompson to midfield. Thompson, though blessed with great speed, was taking his time as he moved up the sideline, later saying that something told him to be patient and let his blockers lead the way.

Thompson's eyes were darting around as he neared the 50. There were blockers and defenders everywhere. He looked ahead and saw Clint Kent, bracing at the Madison 40 like an anchor leg at a track meet. Kent knew the Dukes were struggling to score points and decided right there that Thompson had to reach the end zone. "I took it in my hands to lead the way," he later said. Thompson shifted to the outside — running along Kent's left shoulder. The two cornerbacks tore across midfield into Delaware territory. Thompson had the same thoughts as Kent. "Gotta score. Gotta win the game," he would later tell Chris Simmons.

Kent and Thompson were at the Delaware 45 when Kent leveled the punter, Weber, with a shoulder to the chest. Thompson shifted to a higher gear. In the broadcast booth, Schikman's voice was doing the same thing.

"To the 45-yard line … has one man to beat — the kicker. Races down the sideline …"

Thompson had players all around him as he crossed the 40. One of them was Kent, who, instead of falling with Weber, had sidestepped past the punter after knocking him to the ground. Somehow, after throwing a block that slowed him down, Kent still was leading Thompson down the sideline. The pack crossed the 20 and Kent barreled into David Boler, giving Thompson a clear path to the end zone. "That will be the key to me when I replay it in my mind," Dudley later said. "Clint Kent threw *two* blocks. He could easily have taken out the first guy and just watched the rest, but he continued forward. I think he probably understood the sense of urgency."

Thompson now was the lead runner in an eight-man race to the goal line. Boler, completely off-balance, lunged as Thompson zipped past him. Andrew Kern raised his arms in the air and Kent somersaulted into the end zone as Thompson took the final steps into Madison folklore. As Thompson crossed the goal line, Schikman's escalating pitch reached critical mass.

"Down to the 20 … 10 … 5 … Touchdown! James Madison University. No flags. No flags."

The Bridgeforth Stadium crowd erupted as Thompson wheeled

around in the end zone to face his teammates. Kent, as was his normal reaction to big plays, danced all the way back to the sideline. Sensing the significance of the moment, it was almost as though the Dukes had willed the return to happen. Thompson later called it the best play of his career. The 87-yard run was the second-longest punt return in JMU history and with 3:04 left in the game, the Dukes led, 20-13. "Anything can happen on that play," Clayton Matthews later said. "And the thing is, no one stopped. When Cortez is on the 10-yard line there are guys at the 50 sprinting. You don't ever see that."

The defending champs, however, would counter. Thompson's return gave the Dukes the lead but it didn't give their defense any rest. Several JMU players — including Thompson and Kent — were back on the field two plays later as the Hens took over on their 27-yard line. As it had done all game, the Delaware offense moved down the field. Riccio completed 7 of his first 10 passes, and with 55 seconds left, a six-yard completion to Boler gave the Blue Hens a first down at the JMU three-yard line. Riccio spiked the football to stop the clock. The JMU defense had spent almost the entire fourth quarter on the field and the Dukes were gassed. "Thompson's return gave the whole stadium an extra boost," Jon McNamara said. "But by the time Delaware got down the field it looked like the Dukes were living off adrenaline."

Riccio fired incomplete passes on his next two attempts from the goal line. Of their 25 total plays inside the JMU 20, Delaware had given the ball to Cuff only four times. "I'm guessing here but sometimes when you take a redshirt off a kid you don't know what he'll do inside the red zone," said Mike Barber. "The red zone is where freshmen are more likely to cough-up the ball or not know the intricacies. Again, I'm just speculating, but that could have something to do with it."

The Dukes called a timeout with 41 seconds remaining. Earlier in the week, JMU spent extra time on red zone pass defense, believing the upcoming situation was likely to happen. After the game, Matthews would marvel that the outcome came down to a confrontation in the shadow of the partially constructed Athletic Performance Center. "Fact is we practiced the same scenario in the same end zone all week," he said.

The stadium was a palpable mix of anxiety and apprehension as Riccio walked the Blue Hens to the line on fourth-and-goal. A final roar from the crowd implored the Dukes for one more stop. "The fans were exhilarated to the point of exhaustion," McNamara recalled. Riccio deployed his receivers and sent his fullback in motion, then took the snap from shotgun and fired a pass to the right for Boler.

It never got there. On the most important defensive stop of the season, JMU's shortest defender was the biggest man on the field. Bruce Johnson — all 5-foot-8-inches of him — knocked the ball away.

Delaware ran an astounding 93 offensive plays and controlled the ball for almost two-thirds of the game. The Blue Hens had three cracks from the Madison three-yard line and still the Dukes found a way to win. Rascati took a knee and the panic-induced student section emptied onto the field. The champs were toast.

...

THE DELAWARE game would have a lasting impact on the rest of the season. As the Dukes advanced in the playoffs, the win over the Hens became more significant, the plays more dramatic and meaningful. Years later, Thompson's punt return would stand out as the most pivotal play of the season because of its timing, execution and improbability. The Monday after the Dukes defeated Delaware, Mickey Matthews and his assistants were grading game tape and found that every player on the punt team had done his job to near perfection. Clayton Matthews has a DVD of only that play and shows it to his players every year as proof of the perfect return. To date, Clayton and Mickey call it the most exciting football play they've ever seen. "In 30 years nothing comes close," the elder Matthews later said. "When I was at UTEP we beat Brigham Young in El Paso in 1985. A lot of people call it the greatest upset in college football history. We returned an interception 100 yards in that game. That play was big but Cortez's punt return was more exciting.

"I've been around some big ones, but I've never seen a play like that."

Thompson laughed when told this, downplaying the significance. Yet even he acknowledged that the whole story seemed too good to be true. Like all teams, the Dukes had nicknames for plays and formations to help cope with the mundane task of memorizing the playbook. Rascati had pass play he liked to run and the coaches began calling it "Derby," after the Kentucky horse race. In similar fashion, the Dukes — for reasons Thompson doesn't remember — referred to their punt return team as "Elvis." When asked why, Matthews smiled.

"We call it Elvis," he explained, "because it's the 'Return to Sender.'"

While Matthews would love to judge the play in the moment and for its execution, the return had far-reaching implications. The win over Delaware served as a springboard, providing Madison with the confidence to survive three road playoff games — two by a single point. Before that afternoon, big plays and fortunate breaks had been seen as aberrations of good luck. But after McCarter's block, Thompson's return and the goal-line stand, every moment the Dukes turned in their favor added to the belief that it was their time. In the years since their 1999 conference title, the Dukes had struggled to dispel the notion that they couldn't win. Now, the loser label was gone.

Geoff Polglase, who attended Madison in the early 1980s and currently is the university's associate athletics director for development and marketing, had a much larger view of the win over Delaware and Thompson's return. Polglase watched JMU baseball reach the College World Series, saw the football team beat Virginia and witnessed the basketball program's back-to-back-to-back NCAA trips while he was a student. His love affair with the school was deep, but also measured because it was his employer as well as his alma mater. For years, Polglase had worked to increase ticket sales, donations and national exposure for JMU athletics. And as Thompson raced up the sideline, Polglase, caught up in the moment and sensing the importance of the event, began to cry.

"I'm never going to apologize for being an emotional guy," he later explained. "You get those moments to really enhance your program. To me all those moments happened at once. When Cortez returned that kick you had the notion that we were going to win the game; and winning the game gets us to the playoffs; and getting to the playoffs turns the page for this team and this community."

…

POLGLASE WOUND up being correct in his assessment. The timing of the play, the magnitude of the game and the suspense of the moment turned Thompson's punt return into perhaps the most memorable play in the history of JMU football. But none of that would have mattered if the Dukes lost early in the playoffs. And that came close to happening. Long before they met the Grizzlies in Chattanooga, the Dukes nearly saw their season go down the toilet on a chilly November afternoon in Bethlehem, Penn.

JMU had drawn an at-large spot in the 16-team playoff field and was sent on the road to face the Patriot League champion Lehigh Mountain Hawks. Though the Dukes played in the nation's toughest I-AA conference, the Madison financial bid to host a playoff game was far short of what it needed to be — a fact Jeff Bourne later admitted. And so the Dukes, after being in the driver's seat for an automatic bid and at least two home games after their win over Delaware, instead were sent to the pastoral Lehigh Valley in round one. Though they publicly said they were happy to make the playoffs, many players and coaches quietly were miffed at going on the road to face the league champion from one of I-AA's weaker conferences.

This was discovery time for JMU. After a 9-2 regular season, Matthews would be back in 2005 and was in a strong position to ask for a new contract. But the Dukes hadn't won a playoff game in 10 years. Matthews had proven he could get the Dukes to the postseason, but his bargaining chip would be much larger if he could get JMU out of the first round.

The Dukes did little to justify their beliefs. They didn't play like a superior team and Matthews didn't scheme like a superior coach. Madison trailed, 10-7, late in the first half when Raymond Hines, coming off back-to-back 100-yard games, raced 44 yards to the Lehigh one-yard line. It appeared the Dukes, after playing poorly, would head into the locker room with the lead, but Rascati was stuffed for no-gain on first and second down and Hines was dropped for a two-yard loss on third-and-goal. Lehigh defensive lineman Josh Cooney was whistled for a personal foul after stopping Hines in the backfield however, and Madison was awarded a fresh set of downs back on the one-yard line.

Given new life, the Dukes again tried to pound the ball into the end zone with Rascati and Hines. Three times they ran the ball into the line. And three times they were stopped. Oddly enough, each of the six runs on the goal line went not to the left side (behind All-American tackle Corey Davis and All-American guard Matt Magerko) but to the right. "We had a lot of rushing yards that day but we didn't run well at all," Gary Michael said. "One thing I wondered was we kept talking about how good Magerko and Corey were but we kept running to the right side."

It did seem odd, though Matthews wholeheartedly believed he could get the yards behind veterans George Burns and Jamaal Crowder. On fourth-and-goal, the Dukes again ran their power play to the right. This time Hines bulldozed into the end zone. Hines, several people believed, saved Matthews and the offense with his 191-yard performance. The Dukes out-gained Lehigh by 180 yards on the ground but finished 9-of-22 on third- and fourth-down attempts. They had 11 sacks but racked up 91 penalty yards. They were the best team on the field but allowed the Mountain Hawks to hang around. "It worked," a reporter in the pressbox said in reference to the Hines touchdown. "But that doesn't mean it was smart."

JMU led, 14-10, at halftime. It still was a four-point game midway through the third quarter when Matthews, facing fourth-and-10 from his own 33, made another questionable decision, this time calling a fake punt inside his own territory. The Dukes practiced this play often — "every week," Matthews said — and punter Nick Englehart had played quarterback in high school. But the Dukes were locked in a tight playoff game on the road and Englehart, who led the A-10 in punting in 2003, hadn't thrown a pass all season. The Dukes ran the fake and Englehart's pass was intercepted at the 40. "This guy," someone in the pressbox said of Matthews, "is an idiot."

The Mountain Hawks converted the turnover into three points. From there, the defenses took over. The teams alternated punts into the fourth quarter. With six minutes left, the Dukes put together a small drive that stalled at the Lehigh 49 with 2:50 to go. Hines had been stuffed at the line on third-and-one and a punt seemed imminent. Englehart had pinned the Hawks inside their own 20-yard line three times in the game. But instead, Matthews burned a timeout, sent his offense back into the game and tried to pick up the first down. Comically, Hines — who was stopped for no-gain seven times that afternoon — was stonewalled again.

The Dukes attempted 16 fourth-down conversions during the regular season and were successful on 11 — a modest total with a high success rate. Yet they were 1-for-4 in that department in the opening round of the playoffs. It seemed Matthews, after playing things by the book all season, was walking the tightrope when he didn't need to. "The riverboat gambler," Schikman said. And even in hindsight, Matthews never wavered in his decision, saying coaches learn not to second-guess themselves. "You'll drive yourself crazy," he said. "You make a decision and you move on. If I could have looked into a crystal ball I wouldn't have gone for it."

But he did go for it. Perhaps he thought he could end the game without having to ask his defense for one more stop. Maybe his natural distrust in kickers convinced him to leave Englehart out of the equation. Whatever the case, the Dukes bailed him out by stopping Lehigh on downs and Madison ran out the clock. JMU had made a habit of overcoming its mistakes on the field all season. For one week at least, the Dukes overcame the mistakes from the sideline. At the postgame press conference, a confused Mike Barber asked Matthews about each questionable call and eventually, Matthews channeled Yogi Berra and found an answer well suited to the bizarre play-calling and his quotable personality. "Mike," he said. "If I knew it wasn't going to work I wouldn't have called it."

The response would up being one of the great quotes of the playoff run. But it did not reflect the battle Matthews waged within. "If we had punted and they had driven down the field and scored, I never would have forgiven myself," he later said in a candid moment. "You can't be afraid to take chances. You never get the credit you're due when you make a great call but you'll always get the criticism if you're wrong."

Indeed, Matthews came under fire. But because the Dukes won, it blew over by the middle of the week. Still, to this day, Madison personnel and reporters often point back to Lehigh as the game the Dukes (specifically Matthews) deserved to lose. "He had a great punter and a defense that played phenomenally," Barber recalled. "It looked like he had everything well in hand and then risked it all for a call that — to this day — baffles me. I remember thinking, 'I don't get it.' And I still don't get it [today]."

...

LUCK AND good fortune played an important role in Madison's road through the playoffs. The Dukes had been involved in nearly a dozen game-changing plays and almost all had worked in their favor. "I thought we dodged a bullet," Matthews later said of the Lehigh game. But he could have been talking about Maine or Delaware just as well. By the end of the season, Greg Kuehn's last-second field goal in the first William & Mary game remained the only blemish on Madison's "crunch-time" resume. "If you replay that season 100 times we don't win a lot of those games," Gary Michael said. "Look at the Maine game. If L.C. doesn't pick up that punt and put us in good position then we don't win. If we don't win the Maine game we don't go to the playoffs. If Cortez doesn't return that kick we don't beat Delaware and we don't go to the playoffs. Lehigh could have gone either way. We were a good team but we didn't dominate. We found a way."

Michael's comments were appropriate for this particular moment as the Dukes and Grizzlies battled beneath the lights in Chattanooga. JMU, through power, grit and a little luck, was finding a way. Rabil's wayward field goal ricocheted through the uprights. Montana's blistering offense was breaking down in the red zone. And the Dukes, despite being out-gunned in the first quarter, were in a one-possession game as Craig Ochs uncoiled a pass for Jon Talmage in the corner of the end zone.

LeZotte, still regaining his balance, watched as the ball passed over Cortez Thompson's head. There was no chance for him to break up the pass. Ochs had put the ball in the one spot where only his receiver could make the catch. The Grizzlies were about to take a 10-point lead. LeZotte lowered his head and sprinted for the corner.

He was still running when Talmage dropped the ball in the end zone.

"Even as he was falling out of bounds I thought it was a touchdown," LeZotte said. "It hit him right there. He had a chance. And then he missed it."

Ochs put both hands on his helmet in disbelief. Talmage buried his facemask in the turf. A sure-handed receiver, Talmage caught 49 passes during the regular season — nine for touchdowns — and averaged 15 yards per catch. He had been handcuffed by the pass and tried to make a leaping grab over his back shoulder like a kid holding a boom box to his ear. As he attempted to secure the ball and land in bounds, he lost control and was hit from behind by a charging Thompson. Talmage didn't drop many passes and he had picked an awful spot to drop one tonight. Another momentum-turning play had tipped in favor of the Dukes. "Certain teams seem to have the ability to either catch that ball when it matters or have the other team drop it," Mike Barber said. "JMU had that feeling all year. Montana's a good team. If they score there and go up, 14-3, do they run away with it? It's a very real possibility. But at the same time JMU was the team that could take the big shot and not get discouraged. They had an overconfidence, I thought, because they were good, but I don't think they were as good as they thought they were."

Faced now with fourth down, Bobby Hauck sent his kicking unit into the game for a 45-yard field goal attempt. Earlier in the night, Hauck had gambled from the same distance and faked the kick based on the turf. But now, the Grizzlies were in a street fight and Hauck needed the points to regain control.

The snap and spot were good. Dan Carpenter jogged forward, swung his right leg and sent the ball on its way. The kick sliced hard to the left and missed the uprights badly before striking a photographer in the back of the end zone. Carpenter yanked off his chinstrap, pulled out his mouthpiece and glanced back at the ground in frustration. It remained a four-point game.

Chapter 10

ALVIN BANKS and Maurice Fenner needed to get going. Montana's inability to produce points on three straight drives had left the door open for the Dukes. But to take advantage, JMU needed its running game. Since the beginning of the 2003 season, Banks and Fenner had played together in only 15 games, but of those, the Dukes were 9-0 when they combined to rush for more than 100 yards.

Of the two backs, Fenner was the quiet one. He and Banks were similar in very few ways. Both were sophomores and products of the Southeast portion of Virginia. They were part of the same recruiting class. They were powerful, downhill running backs, well suited for JMU's pro-style offense. But that's where the similarities ended.

Compared to the outgoing Banks, Fenner generally kept to himself. "Maurice just didn't say a lot," Mickey Matthews said. "He wasn't a very vocal guy." Fenner was polite and attentive, but he carried a nervous energy within, and never looked comfortable in a crowd. "I was open, but only around the people I knew," Fenner said. "The people who really knew me knew what I was like, but in my first year there I didn't speak much."

The quiet demeanor contrasted his talent. Fenner was a two-way star at Bayside High School in Virginia Beach and earned all-district linebacker honors in his final two seasons. Nicknamed "Juice" by a varsity coach who said Fenner reminded him of O.J. Simpson, Fenner split playing time in the offensive backfield. Madison coaches weren't sure where to play him. He was recruited as a linebacker by JMU coach Curt Newsome, but the Dukes also left the door open for Fenner to try his hand at tailback. That was fine with Fenner. He had grown up playing the position and wanted to run the ball in college, even if his ceiling was just as high as a defensive player. "Maurice was 6-2, 220 pounds and ran a 4.5 [40-yard dash]," Matthews said. "We weren't sure if he'd play linebacker or tailback. He didn't carry the ball a lot in high school. But the ability was there."

Fenner would become a full-time tailback at Madison. And he grew more comfortable with the position. After missing the first two games of the 2003 season, Fenner rushed for 633 yards in the final 10 and scored nine touchdowns — the latter a JMU freshman record. Fenner's massive frame made him an ideal short-yardage back, but he also had deceptive breakaway speed. Fenner wasn't a natural tailback like Banks. He ran toward contact — often bowling over smaller opponents. "[Alvin] was a slasher," Fenner said. "And I was more of a power guy."

Fenner could run through or past people and that made him difficult to defend, Ulrick Edmonds said. There was grace in Fenner's power. In open space, he shifted into high gear so smoothly it was hard to tell how fast he was moving. He played tailback with the power of a defensive player, using brute force to run over and away from defenders. There weren't many who could wrestle him to the ground alone. "When he dropped his pads on you and got low enough it wasn't pretty," Jeff Durden said. "Maurice was the hammer. There weren't too many safeties willing to come up and lay one on him."

Juice had his flaws. He was a below-average pass blocker and receiver. He ran with his pad level too high and had trouble holding onto the ball at times. "He was an up-and-down runner because he stood up," Mike Schikman said. "I always laughed and told him, 'you're going to get killed.' But he was so big and fast it didn't matter." Schikman had a point. Through his first two seasons, Fenner averaged 5.2 yards per carry. He scored three of his nine touchdowns in 2004 on big runs (25,

46 and 83 yards, respectively). Still, perhaps because he lacked Banks' showmanship, Fenner lagged behind his backfield partner when it came to popularity. Banks, at 5-10 and 215 pounds had a low center of gravity and technically was a superior back. He could run, cut, pick up a blitz and catch passes. He was extremely quotable and spirited. Fenner kept to himself. Though he was extremely confident, he never demonstrated it.

Fenner was faster, more explosive and — through their first two seasons — more durable than Banks. By the end of their sophomore seasons, Fenner would have Banks beat in career rushing yards (1,608 to 1,449) and touchdowns (18 to 12). But because he wasn't the headliner, he took a back seat to the man he shared the backfield with. It was fitting, actually, because Banks simply looked the part, as though he had been crafted to be a tailback, whereas Fenner appeared to be shoehorned into the role. "Alvin would move along the line looking for the gap to hit like you're taught to do," Schikman said. "Maurice would just run over people. And after he ran over them, he ran away from them. He hit the hole and he was gone."

Banks and Fenner — both 7-5-7 kids — were closer friends than most people thought. The two — along with wide receiver D.D. Boxley and cornerback Clint Kent — lived together in 2004 and 2005. Banks, Boxley, Kent and Madison coach Curt Newsome formed Fenner's inner circle, and according to Fenner, were a big reason why he graduated. The group looked out for him like family. Fenner, at times, struggled academically. He also had personal problems that affected his play. Sometimes he looked timid in the backfield and Matthews would wonder why his 220-pound power back was trying to be Barry Sanders. Fenner sometimes fumbled in big situations — the kiss of death for a Madison tailback — and Matthews wouldn't give him the ball the rest of the game. These situations, normally tough for any player to deal with, weighed heavily on Fenner.

Later in his career — after Kent graduated and Newsome took an assistant coaching job at Virginia Tech — Fenner began to weave his way in and out of Mickey's doghouse. He admittedly had a tough time holding things together. The JMU coaching staff kept many of his problems under wraps during his career, but later, Fenner was open about some of his off-field issues. He sat out a game in 2005 for personal reasons. In 2006, prior to an Oct. 7 game against Rhode Island, he missed several classes and was reprimanded (and benched) by Matthews. The following week, Fenner — upset, discouraged and unfocused — went out drinking on Thursday night and missed the team flight to New Hampshire the following morning. "It was a real bad decision and it really affected the rest of my life," Fenner later said. He was right. This became the final stone hurled through Mickey's glass house of trust. Fenner was suspended for two games and demoted to the scout team. He never again was an elite tailback.

Still, in his early years, with his support group whole, Fenner kept his academics and off-field issues in check. He opened the 2004 season with 165 yards on 16 carries against Lock Haven, including an 83-yard touchdown run midway through the second quarter. But Fenner, like all the Madison backs that season, was hit by the injury bug. He hurt his shoulder the following week against Villanova and missed the West Virginia game. Team trainers provided him with a brace, but also warned him the shoulder could pop out again.

Still, Fenner felt relatively healthy and rushed 24 times for 148 yards and three scores against Hofstra — a dominating performance that showcased JMU's ability to feature two elite backs (Banks added 118 yards on 19 carries). Teams were forced to prepare for both Banks and Fenner, which made life difficult, Durden believed. "You have to defend each of them differently, at least I would," he said. "The great thing was all three [Alvin, Maurice and Raymond] were different speeds and that made us hard to prepare for defensively."

Banks went down with a broken leg during that Hofstra game. Fenner kept rolling. He gained 85 yards and scored a touchdown a week later against UMass and was dominant in JMU's 26-20 win over Richmond, carrying the ball 21 times for 139 yards and busting loose for a 46-yard fourth quarter touchdown with the game still in doubt. By sharing the load in the backfield (Banks, Fenner and Hines all would finish the season with more than 100 carries) the Dukes were almost guaranteed to have a fresh back in the fourth quarter. Fenner, Matthews thought, was the most dangerous of the three in a two-tailback system because he was Madison's most physical runner. Late in games, Matthews loved having the luxury of handing the ball to his 220-pound battering ram against a tired defense.

Fenner had worked in a similar system in high school with success, once rushing for more than 100 yards on just 13 carries in Bayside's win over a top-ranked rival during his senior season. Everyone wanted to be the No. 1 guy, Fenner admitted, but no one had a problem with splitting the workload. "That's how it's been my whole career," he said. "And it's always worked." As defenses broke down, Fenner would bomb them for big gains. "He would knock you backwards," Durden said. "Maurice had great RPMs — he could really turn over. And you loved having a guy with his size late in the game when you needed to close out."

With 619 rushing yards under his belt by late October, Fenner looked poised for a 1,000-yard regular season. He scored an early touchdown against VMI, but then hurt his shoulder again midway through the game after falling awkwardly on the Bridgeforth Stadium AstroTurf. This was a full shoulder separation — an injury Fenner later admitted he had never experienced before. His options were limited. "The only way to fix it was surgery and I had to make a big decision during the season whether to play or not," Fenner later said. "I could have had surgery during the season but I decided I wanted to try and play through it."

Matthews was very concerned, later admitting that he thought Fenner's season was over whether he had surgery or not. Here were the Dukes, in the midst of their best season since 1999, with their best team in more than a decade, suddenly down to one healthy tailback. Fenner's injury thrust Hines into the spotlight, and Hines responded with an incredible performance — rushing for 603 yards in JMU's next five games. It was necessary. Fenner sat out the following week against Delaware, played sparingly against William & Mary and was a non-factor in wins over Towson, Lehigh and Furman.

Every time he tried to test the shoulder it responded poorly. Fenner was a power back who led with his upper body. He wasn't confident that he could be the same runner without worrying about his shoulder popping out every time he was hit. And the guessing game was driving him nuts. "I had to gain confidence that I could run the way I wanted to without worrying about my shoulder," he said. "It was one of those cases where the mental battle was tougher than the physical one."

By the time the Dukes arrived in Williamsburg, six weeks had passed. Team doctors assured Matthews that both Banks and Fenner were healthy, but both still were rounding into form. At halftime, while Hines slumped in a chair with a cracked rib, Matthews made his move. He brought his two former starters into the shower room for a powwow. The exact words used were never divulged, but Banks summed it up simply:

"He cussed at us. A lot."

Bullied back onto the field, Fenner's first carry of the second half was a bruising 29-yard run into the W&M secondary, capped by a hit on defensive back James Miller that landed Fenner a full-page photo in *Sports Illustrated*. The picture was classic Fenner: body angled forward and legs churning beneath him. He plowed into Miller and drove him backward before landing in a heap at the W&M 34-yard line. Even when tackled, Fenner dealt the hardest hit. "W&M was really the first game I played where I felt confident to run the way I wanted to without worrying about my shoulder," he later said. "When they called the play and I come through with that run I felt great."

Fenner gashed the Tribe for 106 yards on 14 carries in the second half and the Dukes scored four straight touchdowns in the third and fourth quarters to put the game away. Later told of his SI photo during championship week, Fenner laughed. "I didn't even believe it at first," he said. "I thought it was a joke." It wasn't. The publicity was as real as

Fenner's resurgence. Juice was back. Fenner had a full week of practice before Chattanooga and entered the national title game with 811 rushing yards despite playing less than eight full games. In an injury-plagued year, he averaged 5.6 yards per carry. A healthy Fenner was a productive Fenner, and Madison coaches were confident that, given enough reps, he could help the Dukes break Montana the way they broke W&M.

...

THE DUKES took the field following Dan Carpenter's missed field goal on their own 29-yard line with 5:21 left in the first half. Rascati called the cadence, took the snap and handed the ball to Fenner running off right tackle. Chris Iorio threw a key block and Fenner bulldozed up the field before Montana strong safety Van Cooper dragged him down by the facemask at the Madison 46. On the field, there was a noticeable turning of the tide. "During the season we would play harder during distress or when behind," Nic Tolley said. "We never got rattled. When we found our game plan [that night] we started to see some success."

Fenner's 17-yard run, combined with the 15-yard penalty, gave the Dukes the ball at the Montana 40. But Madison failed to capitalize on first and second down. A false start penalty, a two-yard run by Fenner and a four-yard scramble by Rascati left the Dukes with third-and-nine. "Montana has absolutely dominated first and second down tonight," Trevor Matich said in the ESPN booth. "The average to-go for James Madison has been third-and-seven."

The Grizzlies sent in substitutions, overloading the secondary with six defensive backs. Faced with third-and-long from the Montana 39, the Dukes had little choice but to throw the ball and Bobby Hauck knew it. For at least one pivotal play on the drive, he would make Rascati beat him through the air.

The Dukes came to the line with Iorio, Banks and L.C. Baker lined up off the line of scrimmage and D.D. Boxley as the lone receiver. Rascati sent Banks in motion to the near sideline and took the snap. Banks floated to the outside as Baker and Boxley raced toward the first down marker. Rascati's eyes were glued to Boxley the whole way. Boxley drove his defender downfield, slammed on the breaks and turned back toward his quarterback. Rascati pumped and drilled a pass into Boxley's hands at the 28 for a Madison first down.

For the second time in two drives, Montana forced Rascati into making a big third-down throw. And for the second time in two drives, Rascati found his go-to receiver. Boxley had caught a team-high 42 passes for 609 yards entering the national title game. Now, with time winding down in the first half, he had the Dukes on the fringe of field goal range.

...

IN THE first two years of JMU's rebuilding project, Mickey Matthews had a lot of problems with his offense. He lacked depth, senior leadership and explosive scorers. In 2001, the young Dukes scored 201 points in 11 games; in 2002 they scored 196 in 12. At most positions, Matthews was building from scratch.

Even in those early seasons, JMU was a running team. With a young quarterback and inexperienced receivers, the Dukes almost had to be. Madison lacked a legitimate deep threat at receiver who could stretch a defense (the Dukes, Matthews joked, led the country in receivers being tackled inside the five-yard line) and so JMU had to slug down the field. The more plays the Dukes ran the more chances they had to turn the ball over. "Every coach wants 'em big and fast but those guys go to Michigan," Matthews said of recruiting receivers. The Dukes certainly were not Michigan and so Matthews had to choose between size and speed.

Historically, dominant JMU skill players had been small and fast. Gary Clark was a standout receiver and punt returner at Madison and caught 699 passes in the NFL. Clark was 5-foot-9. Former A-10 offensive player of the year Curtis Keaton was 5-10. And Delvin Joyce, the school record-holder with 5,659 all-purpose yards, was 5-7. There were a few standout skill players who were bigger, notably Macey Brooks, a 6-5, 212-pound receiver who set the school's touchdown receptions record. But Brooks was the exception to the rule.

Still, early in his Madison tenure, Matthews opted for size over speed at the receiver position. He and his staff brought in Alan Harrison and Tahir Hinds, and both learned on the fly as true freshmen. Harrison and Hinds were solid players. They (along with Nic Tolley) represented the original wave of receiver Matthews developed: tall possession guys — physical receivers with good hands. They were not burners. Harrison's 123 career receptions, 1,907 yards and 14 touchdowns landed him in the top five in school history in each category. But Harrison was a good route runner, not necessarily a deep threat. Hinds, a 6-foot-3, 205-pound telephone pole, had range and was a big downfield target. He caught 60 passes in a career hampered by injuries and only one was longer than 40 yards. Tolley, like Harrison, was technically sound but not explosive.

They weren't the receivers who ran past defenders. And the Madison line hardly gave quarterbacks enough time to execute long pass plays, so the Dukes were never a threat to score until they got inside the red zone. But that all changed with Derone Lynell Boxley.

Matthews needed a burner to complement his possession receivers. Boxley, a 5-foot-9 speedster from King George, Va., ran the 100 meters in 10.8 seconds. He was a state champ in track and a standout basketball player in high school. He initially had visions of playing for a I-A school but most wanted him to walk on. Boxley, who knew Cortez Thompson from their high school playing days, accepted a scholarship to Madison instead. Curt Newsome, who recruited several of JMU's premier players during the early part of the decade, including Boxley, said if Boxley wasn't the fastest guy in the state he easily was in the top three. Boxley's 40-yard dash was once clocked at a blistering 4.36 seconds. It was speed Matthews coveted. "D.D. could flat run," he said. "You could just see how explosive he was out of the blocks."

Boxley was speed and hands. He was a first-team all-state receiver in high school and averaged nearly 22 yards per-catch at King George. In his senior season, he caught 34 passes for 867 yards and 16 touchdowns. Boxley was a player who could transform an offense without touching the ball. When he was on the field, teams always needed to give him due attention. "I had the mindset that I was going to help my team any way I could," Boxley said. "And the best way I could do that was by getting downfield."

Boxley suffered a significant muscle pull in his quad during the Virginia High School All-Star game the summer before he came to JMU. He and Hinds (who was recovering from a hip injury) sat out the 2002 season and were limited in 2003. They became friends in an encouraging, brotherly way. "When you're injured everything is repetitive," Boxley said. "Training room at 6 a.m., treatment three times a day and workouts to build your strength. Tahir and I pushed each other through it." Throughout the team, there existed a partnership that transcended recruiting classes because they were filled with players who were competitive and selfless at the same time, as though they realized they needed each other to succeed. "We were close from the jump," Hinds said. "There was a mutual respect because we both saw how we worked on the field and carried ourselves off it." Hinds was speaking about his friendship with Boxley, but he could have been talking about a number of his teammates from those first two seasons.

Boxley played just eight games in 2003 and at times looked like the injury still bothered him. But he also began to flash signs of his talent. In the third game of the season, the Dukes trailed Hofstra, 20-16, with less than a minute left in the game when Boxley got behind the Pride defense and caught a 32-yard pass from Matt LeZotte for the game-winning touchdown. Four weeks later, he and LeZotte connected on a 53-yarder against William & Mary. Boxley became Madison's breakout receiver, and the offense, Matthews said, was not the same without him in the lineup. The emergence of Boxley, Banks and Fenner, coupled with a big senior season from Harrison, transformed the Dukes' offense from lackluster to formidable. Madison scored 307 points in 2003 — nearly 10 points per game better than the previous season. "He was the one guy who had the extra gear to outrun the ball in the air," Matthews said of Boxley. "We used to laugh because he beat everyone. He even got behind Virginia Tech. We saw he was an exceptional deep threat. He just needed to stay healthy."

Boxley did get healthy in 2004. In preseason camp, he and Hinds — coupled with a more aggressive game plan from new offensive coordinator Jeff Durden — were poised to bring the A-10 air show to Harrisonburg. In the offseason, Boxley and Rascati had worked on their timing. "Whenever he wanted to throw he'd pick up the phone and call," Boxley said. "Instead of playing basketball or lifting we'd be running routes."

By August, Boxley finally had his extra gear back and Hinds, who averaged better than 17 yards per catch in 2003, was fully healthy for the first time in nearly two years. They had worked hard in the offseason with Madison strength coach Jim Durning and the results were obvious. Once fearful that his career might be over because of a recurring hip problem, Hinds blasted out of the gate, catching nine passes for 103 yards and a touchdown in games against Lock Haven and West Virginia. Against WVU, Hinds caught six balls for 71 yards while playing against All-Big East cornerback Anthony Mims and future NFL Pro Bowler Adam "Pacman" Jones. Hinds had come to JMU determined to become the best receiver in program history, and after his big day in Morgantown, he looked poised for a breakthrough season.

Instead, the game would be his last big performance of the year. Two weeks later Hinds fell awkwardly catching a screen pass against Massachusetts and tore tendons in his ankle. He missed four weeks and rushed back onto the field, thinking he could contribute even on a bum leg. Hinds spent the rest of the year fighting through pain and had arthroscopic surgery in the offseason. "I wanted to get back," he said. "In all likelihood I probably shouldn't have been out there. That was me being stubborn. I came back early and I wasn't ready."

Hinds caught only one pass the rest of the season and his injury — much like the ones to Banks and Fenner — could have cost the Dukes dearly. There were people who thought JMU's passing game would shrivel without the lanky, sure-handed Hinds in the lineup. Days after the UMass game, Hinds told Boxley it was his time to be the leader. The next weekend against Maine, Boxley was untouchable. "I felt so good that day," he recalled. "I had so much energy." Perhaps sparked by the challenge from his injured teammate, Boxley caught 11 passes for 108 yards and the game-winning touchdown against the Black Bears. He quickly grew into one of the conference's premier clutch receivers. It was another occurrence (along with Raymond Hines filling in at tailback) where the Dukes rallied after losing a critical piece of their offense.

Boxley and Rascati developed a strong rapport on the field. They took Boxley's raw speed and Rascati's natural accuracy and melded those traits into crisp routes and timely patterns. A trust was formed between quarterback and receiver. Boxley and Rascati executed plays with precision, and though the Dukes were a running team, they often connected for big plays in important moments.

What Rascati remembered most was that Boxley always was ready. Even though he might only get three or four looks per game, Boxley wanted the ball on every play and was prepared to get it. He emerged as Rascati's go-to target, catching a 35-yard pass against Richmond that set up JMU's first score, a 27-yard touchdown lob in the first William & Mary game and a 49-yard pass to set up the final touchdown against Towson. As the season progressed, when Rascati needed a completion and saw a defense in man-to-man coverage, he would look for Boxley; in zone coverage it would be Tolley over the middle. "He was the big-play receiver and he could give you separation when he was covered one-on-one," Durden said of Boxley. "Justin really appreciated [D.D. and Nic] when he was in a pinch."

Boxley seemed to play entire games in overdrive, like a roadster doing 105 in a residential neighborhood. He was not a defined route runner but he adjusted to the flight of the ball smoothly. Rascati would put air under the throw and watch Boxley track it down like a center fielder sprinting to catch a deep fly ball. His value was in his speed,

Durden believed, but Boxley's real talent was his ability to read the trajectory of a pass. He could get to nearly any throw.

Boxley was not outspoken or demonstrative but he played with flair. Late in his career he and fellow receiver Ardon Bransford would celebrate touchdown catches with flying chest bumps in the end zone. Hinds, known as "Cold Pizza" for his love of sports, roomed with Boxley on the road and believed he was a competitive entertainer at heart. Boxley and fellow receiver Mark Higgins were the team's best Madden video game players, and Boxley routinely torched Hinds when the two squared off. Hinds remembered beating Boxley once — in the hotel before the national title game — and gloating about it. Boxley was mad as hell and clobbered Hinds in the rematch, but Hinds never let him forget that one win.

His love of playing Madden, his competitive nature and encouraging, positive spirit made for a complex man. Boxley was a hard worker. When he stepped between the lines he was all business. But Hinds believed Boxley also understood that there was a time to relax. He had the right mentality, Hinds thought. Boxley could enjoy success and atone for mistakes without being consumed by them. "There is a very thin line that some athletes just don't understand," Hinds said. "D.D. was a great competitor but he knew he had to have fun. It's a game and he understood that."

Losing hit Boxley hard. He did not hide his emotions well. After the Dukes lost the first William & Mary game — and a chance to clinch the A-10 title — Boxley was one of the first players to arrive at the postgame press conference. The Dukes had won their first six A-10 games of the season but they no longer controlled their own destiny. Boxley slumped into a folding chair and stared at the ground before WHSV-TV sports anchor Joe Downs asked him how he felt. Boxley looked up, eyes glazed and frustrated, then quickly glanced back at the floor. Rascati or Townsend would have checked emotion at the door and given a quote about bouncing back the following week. Matthews would have paused for a few moments to diffuse his anger. Boxley, instead, swallowed his frustration and fired from the hip. "Man," he said without looking up. "It's hard to win every game in the Atlantic 10." Boxley was both accountable and honest. His response showed he could win and lose with class.

During the playoffs, Rascati seemed to rely more heavily on Boxley in big situations. Of the 27 passes he completed against Furman and W&M, 10 went to the burner from King George. In the third quarter against Furman, the JMU defense forced a turnover at the Madison one-yard line. Chris Iorio gained a yard on first down. Though they had possession, the Dukes were in dire need of a big play. On second-and-nine, Madison gambled with a deep throw on a play where the safe move was either another run or a short pass. Boxley got behind the Furman defense and Rascati lobbed a pass to the middle of the field for a 43-yard gain. It was a call that required icy confidence in both quarterback and receiver. "There was a period of time there for about eight games when Rascati and D.D. were like Peyton [Manning] and Marvin Harrison," Hinds said. "They couldn't do anything wrong. They were unstoppable."

Rascati and Boxley would hook up later on the game-winning drive. Facing second-and-22 from the JMU 14, Rascati completed back-to-back passes to Boxley for 16 and 11 yards to escape trouble. Ensuing passes to Tolley, L.C. Baker and Bransford would get the Dukes within striking distance, but Durden remembered Boxley's catches as the most pivotal. "The defining moment on that drive was the third down to D.D.," Durden said. "They blitzed and left that open pass in the middle. To get that [completion] really set us on our way."

Durden's praise for Boxley ran deep because he recognized — perhaps more than anyone — the importance of having a go-to receiver when dealing with a young quarterback. Rascati, for all his charisma and consistency, was a sophomore in a new system and Boxley (after Hinds went down) gave him the safety net of a clutch target. No play demonstrated this more than Boxley's outstretched catch the following week in Williamsburg. Madison had watched a 21-0 first-quarter lead disappear and the Dukes were reeling. Lang Campbell had completed 17 of 22 passes in the first half and JMU, down 26-21 with 11:37 left in the third quarter, was running out of magic.

With the crowd at Zable Stadium in frenzy, Fenner gained 29 yards to open the drive, rumbling over James Miller to the Tribe 34-yard line. As the Dukes moved to the huddle, Durden thought it was time to take a shot down the field. He told Rascati to run 62 Streak: a three-receiver pass play with Tolley and tight end Tom Ridley as targets over the middle and Boxley as a secondary option on a vertical sprint to the end zone. It was an out-of-character call for the Dukes and Durden believed it would catch the Tribe off-balance. In the huddle Rascati looked at Boxley. "I'm coming to you," he said.

The Dukes walked to the line. Rascati fielded the snap, took a short drop and quickly scanned the field. The W&M safeties were holding inside and Rascati knew he had one-on-one coverage up top. He lofted the ball for the corner. Across the field, Boxley ran for the pylon. It had rained all week in Williamsburg and the field was a muck-filled cow pasture. As Boxley sprinted for the end zone the ball seemed to sail on him. All year it seemed Rascati could not overthrow him, but now, on a damp night in Williamsburg, Boxley was losing ground. He strained forward, lunging and nearly losing his balance, and reached out as the pass crossed over his head. Boxley closed his fingertips around the ball and tucked it toward his chest. He crashed to the ground and hydroplaned across the wet turf through the back of the end zone. In the broadcast booth, Mike Schikman hesitated. "There was a three or four second pause," he later explained. "We had to wait and see if he actually caught it."

He did. Boxley later joked that it was the fastest 40 he ever ran and admitted that he was stretched to his limits. Years later, after watching a clip of the catch, he had no answers. "I don't know how I got there," he said. Neither did anyone else, but the Dukes led, 27-26, and in that moment the air seemed to go out of W&M. The Tribe erased a huge lead and battled back to take control, but D.D. Boxley had just knocked them out. Hinds knew it immediately. "That was history in the making," he said. "It was a game-changer. I'm a fan of the game even as I'm playing it. To see him pick it up the whole season and then watch him make that catch was truly incredible."

The Dukes never trailed again. In the years to come, Jeff Bourne would agree with Hinds' train of thought. Bourne believed the pitch-and-catch reflected the entire season for the Dukes — specifically Boxley. Eight of Boxley's final 12 catches in 2004 went for first downs, including his momentum-turning grab in Williamsburg. "I have a clip on my computer of that catch and I watch it every day," Bourne said. "That was talent; it was execution and most of all, it was synergy. If you could take that chemistry, put it in a jar and sell it … you'd make a fortune."

...

THE DUKES went back to the ground game after Boxley's third-down catch. A three-yard run by Fenner, a seven-yard swing pass to Baker and an eight-yard run by Banks brought JMU to the 10 with 2:18 remaining in the second quarter. After stunting and moving around the Madison offensive line for most of the first half, the Montana defense was cracking. JMU had dominated time of possession in the second quarter and the Madison front five was opening big running lanes. Montana could be successful if it continued to move, but when the Grizzlies planted themselves firmly in the path of the Madison line they were being blasted off the ball.

Banks gained a yard on second-and-two. A sneak by Rascati gave JMU first-and-goal at the eight with just under a minute left in the half. The Dukes were 25 feet from taking the lead.

Banks hammered into the line and picked up four yards on first-and-goal. Even on this remote section of the field, the turf at Finley Stadium was in shambles. Divots littered the area between the hash marks. Despite Montana's kicking problems, the unstable turf hadn't given either team an advantage. The Dukes were having trouble staying balanced and the Grizzlies looked out of rhythm. In a way, the field was taking both teams out of their element.

Fenner gained a yard on second down and the Dukes called their second timeout with 28 seconds remaining. JMU had done an extraordinary job controlling the clock, yet the goal line had been the toughest stretch of territory to conquer all season. It took four downs to get into the end zone against Lehigh and Furman. And though the Dukes were close, there was a feeling it might take four downs tonight.

On third-and-goal, the Dukes ran Fenner off right tackle behind George Burns and Jamaal Crowder. Fenner rolled past the line and reached the doorstep of the end zone before he was slammed to the turf by a swarm of Grizzlies at the one-yard line. For the third time in four postseason games, the Dukes faced a potential game-changing fourth-and-goal. Before Fenner got off the ground, Matthews and Durden were running through their options. Matthews, down at field level, didn't know where the ball was and thought about kicking the field goal. Durden, up in the coaches' booth, wanted to go for it. The offensive coordinator and the head coach were locked in a heated debate as the Dukes picked themselves off the ground.

The Grizzlies burned a timeout.

Chapter 11

THE DUKES has been here before. In late November it was Josh Cooney's penalty that allowed JMU to run seven plays from the Lehigh one-yard line. A week later, it was Raymond Hines, telling Matthews "hand me the ball, don't pitch it," in the quarterfinal against Furman. In the middle of both were Matthews and Durden — the head coach, who rose to his position as a man of defense, and the offensive coordinator, who had been on the job less than 10 months.

In a different time and place, Matthews might not have hired Durden. At their core, the two had different philosophies. Durden liked to air things out with a freewheeling attack that piled on points with big plays. At his JMU job interview, he described his offensive approach as "reckless," which raised a few eyebrows because Matthews preached a zone-running attack, emphasizing ball control and physical football. But Madison's vanilla offense wasn't winning. The Dukes averaged 20 points per game from 2001-2003 and were 13-22 over that stretch. Seeking a change, Matthews began searching for someone to jolt the JMU attack.

Durden, an all-conference defensive back at Georgetown College in Kentucky, bounced around the country as an assistant coach at his alma mater, West Georgia, California (Pa.), Morehead State and VMI. His 1997 Morehead State offense led the country in scoring. His 2002 and 2003 squads at VMI set team season records for points. Durden's teams had reputations for staying loose and using intricate designs to post big numbers. His play calling was difficult to predict and he carried a gunslinger's mentality — a blend of confidence and instinct. What impressed Matthews most was Durden's ability to produce points with minimum talent. Durden was bold, brash and knew his stuff. His relentless approach was exactly what Matthews was looking for — even if it meant deviating from a traditional offense down the road.

Matthews hired Durden midway through the offseason and the new coordinator went to work on JMU's attack. Known for opening things up with spread formations and motion, Durden, who doubled as Madison's quarterbacks coach, made careful evaluations of his players. Instead of bringing a system to JMU, he used the talent around him to build a plan based on personnel. It was common sense to Durden, who relied heavily on assistant head coach Curt Newsome for information. Newsome told Durden the Dukes were strong on the line and had depth at tailback. "I had every offensive coach write down our best 11 players," Durden said. "When I started looking at the lists most had the two tight ends, the center, both guards and tackles. And I had been hired to kind of spread things out but when you looked at the strengths of that football team you knew we'd be running the ball."

So the aerial assault would take a backseat to the ground game. No problem. Fact is, Durden wasn't just bringing Xs and Os to the table. His "reckless" style of play was a mentality. Durden wanted his offense to play loose and score points. If that meant running hog wild behind Matt Magerko and Corey Davis all day then so be it. JMU was a running team with a playmaker's mentality. The Dukes could wear down a defense with numbing efficiency or break it with a 40-yard play. Matthews loved the system because it kept Madison in control at all times. Durden liked it because it produced points and allowed him to sneak in a big play here and there. If a defense stacked up against the run, Durden didn't hesitate to pull the trigger. Against Richmond, with the Dukes up, 12-7, Durden noticed the Spiders routinely were biting on a screen pass, so he modified the pattern and told Ardon

Bransford to feign his blocking assignment and run a deep route down the sideline. Bransford faked, the Spiders bit and Rascati delivered a 65-yard touchdown pass. Boom. Instant offense.

Whether it was adding flavor or just the right mental makeup, Durden's impact on the offense was similar to George Barlow's on the defense. Both preached the need for a little swagger, a little more mojo, and they got it. The Dukes didn't need much more — three of their six losses in 2003 were by a touchdown or less — and if the right attitude could turn Madison into a winner than that was the first step. "You want to challenge players who might not have reached their potential so the ABCs of coaching really apply," Durden said. "Instill a winning attitude. Get their best and now be consistent. I'd like to think we were consistent in our game plans, consistent in our calls and consistent in our execution."

As his tenure progressed, Durden tweaked his offense based on personnel. When the talent around him favored speed over size, he worked to spread things out. In 2006, the Dukes had playmakers at wide receiver and a breakaway tailback (junior college transfer Eugene Holloman), and Durden's offense overwhelmed teams with its quick-strike potential, scoring 20 of its 42 offensive touchdowns on plays of 25 yards or more. In 2007, with running threat Rodney Landers at quarterback, Durden shifted to a spread option formation and the Dukes averaged 266 rushing yards per game. But in 2004, more often than not, he put the game in the hands of the front line. Durden was thorough when it came to evaluating talent and, in his first season, he found a way to meld his aggressive offense with JMU's monster running game.

At 39, Durden had the energy of a man half his age. He hit the gym often and kept in good shape. On the sideline at practice — wearing a T-shirt, mesh shorts and a visor — he had a boyish quality about him. When he answered a phone call from a familiar number all formality melted away. "Hey man! What's up?" he'd ask. Durden had a narrator's wit. He'd walk toward Curt Dudley and a reporter in the hallway and say, "time to meet the press," before stopping to say hello. Part of it was his drive and pure love of the game. "I never want to get a real job," he later joked. But another part of the energetic persona — especially in his first season — was he wanted to spread confidence to his players. The JMU offense had been bland for years and Durden wanted to shake that reputation. "Someone needed to believe we could score points," he said. "Sometimes you need to be a good salesman to get the thing going."

His energetic personality was well received. But Durden's criticism could be relentless if a player wasn't prepared. While Matthews had somewhat mellowed, Durden injected a little butt kicking into practice. The Dukes had talented players and Durden wouldn't stand for complacency. "If I have to be a hard-ass I'll do it," he once said. And if a quarterback wasn't making good reads, Durden would be all over him. "You've got to make better decisions," he'd say. "You are *killing* me, man."

Durden could immerse himself into an offense the same way a defense department analyst studied intelligence reports. He'd log long hours preparing game plans. It'd be 10 p.m. and Durden's office light would be on. He'd be rocking back-and-forth in his chair, JMU baseball cap turned backward and diagrams splattered across a whiteboard. With meetings and practices during the day, late night was the best time to process information. "I like having input but I don't want to bog [the staff] down with second-guessing," he said. "At the end of the day you want to take information and make decisions. I enjoy watching film by myself, taking the notes from earlier meetings and seeing how we can phase it into the game plan."

Like a chemist, Durden was forever experimenting on the whiteboard, tweaking the offense based on both available personnel and the upcoming opponent. The week of the William & Mary playoff game, a JMU sophomore was sneaking in a late workout at the campus gym around 9:30 p.m. As he walked to the recreation center, he saw Durden's office light was on. An hour or so later, on the way back, the light remained.

It later became known that Durden spent a good chunk of his first year sleeping on the floor of his office. His family was in Lexington — about an hour south — and his kids were in school. They, Matthews said, were ingrained in the local community and comfortable. Durden thought it silly to rent an apartment when he could make it home two or three times a week. He commuted from home on Tuesdays and Thursdays; he went to church on Sundays with his family and every other night he slept in his office. This went on for months — Durden was hired in March of 2004 and didn't move to Harrisonburg until the summer of 2005. Matthews had a hunch Durden was sleeping in his office and frowned on the practice. He came in early one morning during the '04 season to investigate. "I walked past his office and he was lying on the floor," Matthews said. "I put an end to that quickly."

Matthews offered Durden the guest bedroom at his house and Durden slept there a few nights a week during the season. Still, the idea of a good night's sleep was a relative concept. Matthews sometimes had to check to make sure his offensive coordinator came home — a bed check for his 39-year-old houseguest. "He's such a hard worker and there would be times when he'd come home after I went to bed and he'd be at the office when I woke up," Matthews laughed. "I'd have to ask Kay if Durden came home last night and she'd assure me she heard him come in the house. Jeff logged long hours at work, but I did make him quit sleeping in his office."

Or so he thought. Durden still managed to satisfy his work ethic and stole a night or two of rest on the floor. He followed orders, but when it came to his craft, Durden was a cowboy at heart. If his best work came late at night and ended with him sleeping at the office then that's what was going to happen. It helped that many of his players shared his passion. Rascati spent a lot of time preparing with Durden and the two were never afraid to speak their minds. Durden had a knack for checking a player's ego, especially during film sessions. Rascati, never short on confidence, watched more film with Durden than any other player, and he often received large helpings of humble pie when his coach thought he was getting a bit cocky. "You can cut 'em but you can't make 'em bleed," Durden later said. "If a good attitude and work ethic is how you got here then you shouldn't ditch it when you have success." Gary Michael remembered walking into the room during a film session and hearing Rascati blast an upcoming opponent. "Justin was watching tape of one of their defensive guys and he's going off," Michael recalled. "He keeps saying, 'This guy sucks. He's terrible. He just sucks.' And Jeff is trying to keep things in perspective but Justin keeps going on. Finally Durden starts jumping on Rascati to put him back in his place."

Fittingly, the players Durden pushed were the ones worth pushing, and they responded well. Rascati, even as a 20-year-old sophomore, had the study habits of an assistant coach. Matthews gave his players Sunday and Monday off during the season, and even though the coaching staff watched film of the previous game on Sunday night, the players weren't required to attend a screening until Tuesday. But Sunday night would roll around and Rascati would be watching film with his coaches. "A couple of guys would come every week," Durden said. "But he was religious about it."

Early in the 2004 season, Durden had a hard time putting his work into perspective. The Dukes opened the year against Division II Lock Haven and then had a bye week. Their second game was played in a driving rainstorm against Villanova and the third at Division I-A West Virginia. It wasn't until the Oct. 2 game against Hofstra that Durden was able to properly judge his offense against an opponent of common stature. "We really didn't know what we had," he later said. "We didn't want to give the farm away against Lock Haven because we were just better than them. We thought we had a lot to show against Villanova but the hurricane wiped that out. And against WVU we still had a quarterback competition going on."

The wait, however, was worth it. The Dukes were 5-for-5 inside the red zone and scored 31 points — a number they had reached only four times in 28 conference games from 2001-2003. Banks and

Fenner combined for 266 rushing yards and three touchdowns; Rascati completed 19 of 22 passes and the Dukes amassed 494 yards of total offense without turning the ball over.

It wasn't flashy — in fact, it was quite methodical — but it was relentless. Madison led, 21-14, early in the fourth quarter and faced fourth-and-four at the Hofstra 28-yard line. The way Fenner and Banks were going, everyone in the stadium expected a running play. Instead, Durden called for a play-action pass and Rascati hit Tom Ridley for a 19-yard gain. Two plays later, the Dukes were in the end zone. "Huge play," Durden later said, "not just for the game but our confidence on offense. That night we found out we had the tools. We could run; we had great blocking; we could throw and catch." The Dukes, Durden understood, weren't a traditional battering ram; they could be unpredictable.

JMU averaged 28.5 points per game in the regular season. But the offense sputtered in the first two rounds of the playoffs, scoring just 28 total points against Lehigh and Furman. Being bottom-line oriented, Durden believed a win was a win, but also recognized the reason for the lull: He didn't give Rascati enough wiggle room. Though the offense did not revolve around Rascati, he was the player who extended drives and made key decisions on the fly. In the first two rounds of the playoffs, Durden, knowing the postseason could unhinge even the coolest quarterbacks, wanted to take baby steps and protected Rascati from making an important play until it was necessary. "What Justin had to do all season was prove he could handle the situation," Durden explained. "When he succeeded we gave him a little more rope. In the playoffs everything starts all over and we were a little more conservative. It nearly cost us, but we won the games."

Of course, that only happened because Durden gave Rascati more room to operate when the stakes were highest — if nothing else, because the situation required it. And the stakes were never higher than Madison's second stop on the road to Chattanooga, when Rascati, Durden and the JMU offense mounted a drive to save the season, on a warm December night in South Carolina.

Chapter 12

THE CITY of Greenville, S.C. is nestled in the foothills of the Appalachian Mountains, amidst the rolling hills and knolls of the Palmetto state's northernmost region. It is a mid-sized city, located halfway between Charlotte and Atlanta, home to a minor league baseball team and located in the eastern heart of America's Bible belt. Eight miles northwest of downtown, and wedged between the Poinsett Highway and Duncan Chapel Road, sits the 750-acre campus of South Carolina's oldest private college, Furman University.

Since the inception of the Southern Conference in 1921, no football program has won more league titles than the Furman Paladins. A three-time NCAA title game participant and 1988 national champion, Furman is the most accomplished private school in the history of I-AA football. Its 16,000-seat stadium, with a small visitors' section and a massive home grandstand, was home to seven conference championship teams from 1981-1990. After a lull in the middle of the decade, the Paladins rebounded at the millennium, reaching the playoffs in all but one season from 1999-2006.

The 2004 Paladins were supposed to rewrite the record books. Furman had Ingle Martin, a transfer quarterback from Florida, leading an offense with size and speed. Martin, who had been part of a quarterback logjam in Gainesville that included Chris Leak and former JMU crush Pat Dosh, was a poised, confident redshirt junior and turned the Paladins from playoff qualifier into title contender. He threw for 22 touchdowns and 2,792 yards in 2004, pacing an offense that averaged 455 yards per game. Martin's top receivers, Isaac West and Brian Bratton, combined for 115 catches and 15 touchdowns. The Paladins did not have a workhorse in the offensive backfield; they had four. Cedrick Gipson, Brandon Mays and Daric Carter combined for 2,006 rushing yards. Bruising freshman Jerome Felton scored 10 touchdowns. Felton, Clint Kent thought, was one of the nation's best fullbacks. And Mays, who had battled a life-threatening inflammatory disease of the colon in 2002, had rebounded to lead Furman in carries and solidify the most balanced offensive attack in the country.

The Paladins also could play defense and held opponents to 16.6 points per game behind Southern Conference defensive player of the year William Freeman and the nation's best group of linebackers. Furman was relentless on both sides of the ball. The Paladins finished the 2004 regular season with a 9-2 record, losing on the road to Division I-A Pitt, 41-38, in overtime, and to rival Appalachian State, 30-29. But those games had been played early in the season. Furman was 6-0 since mid-October, undefeated at home and earned the No. 2 seed in the playoffs. In the first round, the Paladins throttled Jacksonville State, 49-7, as Martin threw for 282 yards and four touchdowns. When the smoke settled at the end of the opening weekend, Furman stood alone at the top.

In the week leading to their showdown with the Paladins, Mickey Matthews downplayed his team's chances, citing Furman's balance and tremendous home-field record. Though the Dukes barely squeaked by Lehigh, the grumbles around town were that Matthews simply was taking pressure off his players. JMU, after all, was no slouch, averaging nearly 370 yards of offense per game. And the Dukes had the nation's best pass rush. But Matthews, who had taken a talented Marshall team to Greenville in 1993 and lost, wasn't positioning and neither were his players. They knew the season could end in Greenville. "I don't think we thought we could beat them," Clayton Matthews later said. "That was the year for them. They were big, bad Furman."

Mike Barber, for one, agreed with the younger Matthews. The Dukes, he thought, were perhaps the most balanced A-10 team left in the playoffs, but they had the toughest draw. Delaware and William & Mary were playing each other, and while New Hampshire was going to Montana, Barber thought the Paladins were a better team than the Grizzlies. "Furman was as good as anyone that season," he later said. "I was so sure Furman was going to win that game that I booked my vacation for the following week. If there was anyone who thought JMU wasn't beating Furman, it was me."

Barber wasn't alone. The Paladins could do everything the Dukes could do. They had a transfer quarterback with pedigree and a stingy defense. They ran the ball effectively and controlled the clock. Furman won 80 percent of its home games. Head coach Bobby Lamb, a former standout Furman quarterback, was 24-11 since taking over at his alma mater. The Paladins had swept through the Southern Conference and rolled Jacksonville State. Their offense was perfectly balanced, their starting tailback was a walking medical miracle and they were 14-point favorites, according to Sports Network football director Matt Dougherty. The Dukes were going to Furman. And they were going to lose.

They would travel well, however. Since the Dukes weren't going to host a playoff game, the fans, instead, would go to them. About 1,000 made the trip to Lehigh for the first round game over Thanksgiving weekend. Madison originally intended to run two fan buses to Greenville, but higher demand increased that number to five. It was finals week in Harrisonburg, but many of the fans on those buses rationalized that it was the last time they would see the Dukes in action. Popular thought was that the convoy to Greenville would be a funeral procession on the way back. The coverage told the story: "Second-seeded Furman is the favorite for several reasons ..." Barber wrote in the Tuesday's DN-R. "Dukes face tall task at Furman," read the headline in Thursday's issue of *The Breeze*. And Matthews did his part to fuel the fire. "I think," he said, "we are the underdog."

Still there were people who thought the Dukes were an equal threat to the Paladins. Matthews, for one, believed points would be at a premium and both defenses would keep the game tight. Mike Schikman thought the key would be special teams. It was unseasonably warm during the day as the teams prepared for the 3:30 p.m. kickoff. Schikman, who had ties to the area stemming from his days as an announcer in nearby Spartanburg, was invited to help with the Furman pre-game radio show. Midway through the broadcast he was asked to disclose his key player of the game. "I said, 'Well I have a surprise key for you,'" Schikman recalled. "We had lost a bunch of games in the past because of bad snaps. And the difference between us and Villanova earlier that year was Josh Haymore because he could snap in the hurricane and the other guy couldn't."

Matthews had always told Schikman how essential Haymore (the team's long snapper) was to the Dukes. But in four years, Schikman never mentioned him with such importance. "No one ever talked about the snapper," Schikman said. "But here I was talking about him. I said, 'I think Josh Haymore is going to be a key in this game.' And no one knew who he was so I explained that he was the long snapper."

Schikman didn't know why he thought of Haymore at this juncture of the season. He also didn't know that the entire radio program was being pumped though the stadium loudspeakers. As Schikman was dissecting Madison's automatic long snapper, Haymore was warming up on the other side of the field. David Rabil and Nick Englehart heard Haymore's name over the public address system and started busting his chops. Haymore stood up and looked in their direction. "You ready Haymore?" Rabil yelled. "You gotta carry us today! You ready to roll?" Haymore again heard his name over the sound system and froze. "Oh God," he thought. "I hope I don't screw up."

Haymore was a bit nervous. Matthews was flat worried. He didn't know if his defense could stop Ingle Martin. And he wasn't sure how much petrol Raymond Hines had left in the tank. Hines had carried the ball 97 times over the previous three weeks and looked tired at practice. Meanwhile, Alvin Banks and Maurice Fenner appeared healthy but were not responding well to contact. Matthews couldn't get them out of the training room, and though they played sparingly, they were not enough to supplement Hines. "It was driving me crazy because I knew Raymond was a horse that needed to be put back in his stable," Matthews said. "I told my coaches we needed an open date for Raymond."

Instead the Dukes were facing the opposite — an upgraded version of themselves. "We were prepared for a very physical game," Kent recalled. "It was going to be smashmouth football." The Paladins also would be well prepared for the Dukes. Furman receivers coach Drew Cronic was a former Madison assistant and had coached many of the JMU seniors when they were freshmen. So the Paladins were balanced and somewhat familiar with their opponent. As kickoff approached and the teams met in their respective locker rooms, the late-afternoon sun splashed across the field and into the eyes of the visiting fans. Jon McNamara — still feeling the effects of the early-afternoon tailgate — was passing out purple and goal streamers when the Furman fans across the field began to pray. McNamara looked up. "I couldn't see a thing," he recalled. "But the sun was just about to settle behind the Furman stands and these people are all praying in unison. The Paladins come out of the locker room with those white helmets — the white knights of Furman. And here I am, in the middle of South Carolina, in a place I've never been before. I've been drinking and all I can think is 'not only are we facing a great team, not only are we underdogs, but now we have to play against God too.'"

McNamara, by his own admission, was exaggerating — though not by much. And Matthews, though truly worried about Hines, thought the Dukes were good enough to beat the Paladins. The teams traded possessions and punts through the first quarter. JMU's defense was relentless, sacking Martin twice in the first three possessions and nearly intercepting a screen pass deep in Furman territory. But Hines, as

Matthews feared, was sluggish, and the Dukes had trouble on offense, turning the ball over on their first two possessions, first on downs and then on an Alvin Banks fumble.

The game was scoreless early in the second quarter when the Dukes forced the Paladins to punt deep inside their own territory. In the week leading to the game, Matthews believed he found a flaw in Furman's punt formation. The Paladins often used a rugby-style kick where the punter catches the ball, sprints to his right and kicks while running to avoid the rush. From watching film of Furman's game against Georgia Southern, Matthews saw that when defenders broke through the front line, Furman's secondary blockers often let them pass through because the punter had already vacated the backfield. He instructed backup safety Isaiah Dottin-Carter to power through the front line and stay inside the secondary blocker, who was moving laterally across the field.

Dottin-Carter, a true sophomore, had emerged as a productive special teams performer. He, like Akeem Jordan and McCarter, had developed a knack for blocking kicks. The scheme was intricate. If the blocker forced his man to the outside, the Paladins would get the kick away. If the defender rushed through the wrong gap he would be in the backfield with the punter already past him. But if Dottin-Carter hit the right hole and cut inside the block, he could reach the punter before the kick. "We schemed it out at practice," Matthews said. "They ran the formation and Isaiah did the rest."

Furman punter Bo Moore fielded the snap and sprinted to his right. As Furman's backup quarterback, Moore was a threat to run and throw from this position and the pocket developed much like one during a rollout pass play. Dottin-Carter shot through the line and zipped inside the block of Furman tight end Brad Bell. He charged Moore, launched himself into the air and batted the kick to the ground, where is bounced and rolled out of bounds at the Furman eight-yard line. "The way they opened up when the line shifted gave us some room to charge," Demetrius Shambley remembered. "[Isaiah] got a big jump and made a play."

Suddenly, the Dukes were in business. Two plays later they were in the end zone as Hines barreled home on second-and-goal from the five. David Rabil's PAT zipped through the uprights and Madison, in a game that was shaping into a defensive struggle, had delivered the first salvo. "Mickey always talks about special teams," Schikman said. "You don't win championships because you have the best quarterback. You don't win championships because you have the Buck Buchanon Award winner on defense. If you have a great player in basketball you can put four stiffs around him and still win a lot of games. You can't do that in football. The Dukes shared the load on special teams so well and Isaiah's block was the perfect example."

The lead, however, was short-lived. Furman countered with a 14-play, 74-yard drive and tied it on a one-yard plunge by Felton. And the Dukes had no one to blame but themselves. On third-and-seven from the Madison 14, they forced a fumble in the backfield but couldn't recover. And when the Paladins came out for a chip-shot field goal, Madison jumped offsides twice, turning fourth-and-eight into first-and-goal. This wasn't the game most were expecting. The Paladins appeared vulnerable; the Dukes looked sloppy. "Too many mistakes," Matthews later said. And he was right. By the end of the game, JMU would be whistled for nine penalties and lose two fumbles.

It was 7-7 at halftime, but the Paladins had dominated the second quarter, running 21 plays to JMU's 12 and holding the ball for more than 10 minutes. The trend continued into the second half. The Dukes received the opening kickoff, but a Rascati fumble handed the ball back to Furman inside the Madison 20. Three plays later, Martin found Brian Bratton on a shovel pass and Bratton weaved into the end zone. The PAT was wide left but Furman led, 13-7. Slowly but surely, the Paladins were taking over, and though the Dukes were moving the football, they couldn't seem to string things together. "It was frustrating," D.D. Boxley said. "We knew we could do it, but we couldn't get rolling." Madison would take the ensuring possession down the field and had first down at the Furman 36, but back-to-back incomplete passes forced the Dukes to punt again. "They came at us a lot with field blitzes, which they hadn't done much," Jeff Durden said. "And that night we kept running the ball into the blitz. We moved the ball. We just weren't consistent."

Both teams had reached this point by running the football. But while Hines, Banks and Fenner were either banged up or recovering from injury, Furman's big four were producing. Mays and Carter were dual threats who could run and catch. Gipson was built low to the ground and was dangerous when he bounced to the outside. Felton, at six-foot and 260 pounds, was a sledgehammer. "You couldn't key on one guy," Kent later said. "They had a great quarterback who could run, a power fullback and a rotating system at running back. It made them hard to contain." And while the Dukes weren't letting any of them break the game open, the stubborn JMU defense was wearing down.

Englehart's punt pinned the Paladins inside the 10, but Furman moved down the field. A five-yard run by Felton, a 15-yarder by Gipson and a seven-yard gain by Gipson brought the Paladins to the 35. Six more runs — including a fourth-down sneak by Martin — had Furman on the Madison 47. The Dukes needed a stop. Instead Martin burned them with a 40-yard completion to little-used tight end John Rust. Suddenly, after poking and prodding down the field, the Paladins were inside the 10 with six minutes left in the third quarter. They had driven 91 yards in 10 plays. And with the ball on the JMU 7, the Paladins were 20 feet away from taking a two-touchdown lead and essentially putting the Dukes away for good.

Martin walked the Paladins to the line, called for the snap and pitched the ball to Gipson, running left behind Felton and tight end Willis Sudderth. Gipson cut inside a pair of blocks and breezed past an off-balance Tony LeZotte as he crossed the line of scrimmage. To the right, defensive end Sid Evans was racing over from the opposite side of the field. "I think with all of us, we realized that at any moment it could be your time to make a play," Evans later said. Gipson danced to the right and zipped past Bruce Johnson at the five, and Johnson swept an arm across Gipson as he passed by. A second later, Evans hit Gipson in the back and the ball popped loose, landing at the one-yard line.

Furman offensive tackle Stephen Schroeder flopped to the ground to recover the fumble. He was the closest player. But at the last moment, a running Clint Kent launched himself through the air and landed on top of the ball. "I was taking my pursuit angle and the ball just popped out in front of me," he explained. "I just dove for it." As Schroeder, Kent and Felton fought for possession, Kwynn Walton, Cortez Thompson and Shambley began pointing toward the opposite end of the field. The Dukes, Shambley recalled, had always spent extra time working on pursuit, and here, he thought Kent simply wanted it more. Officials bent over the pile and signaled JMU ball. To the left, a waiting Rodney McCarter spun around and punched a fist through the air. "I had it the whole way," Kent later said. "They tried to take it from me but I had it in my hands."

The Dukes were alive. Two plays later they were out of the woods, after Rascati and Boxley connected on a 43-yard pass to flip the field. As the game moved deeper into the evening, a rugged quality developed. What began as an ugly, mistake-filled game turned into a dramatic slugfest. Play was physical on both sides of the ball, Kent recalled. "Furman," Hines later said, "was the toughest team we went up against." The teams traded punts into the fourth quarter. With 9:21 left in the game, the Paladins picked up a first down behind runs from Mays and Felton. A 20-yard gain by Gipson moved Furman to the JMU 33, and after two short runs, a five-yard pass from Martin to Bratton set up fourth-and-three at the 26-yard line.

The fourth-down run against Lehigh and the fumble on the goal line earlier in this game were pivotal moments. But now, as Scott Beckler jogged out to attempt a 43-yard field goal, the Dukes were staring at the end of their season. With 5:15 left in the game, there wasn't enough time to score twice. JMU needed to stop Furman and get into the end zone, and at this point, the latter particularly seemed like a tall order. Beckler, a true freshman, had pushed a PAT wide left earlier in the game after a low snap interfered with his timing. But he was 5-for-6 on attempts outside the 40-yard line and had earned all-conference honors during the regular season. "Time was running out," Shambley remembered. "The thing I remember is their inside blockers were pretty soft. We knew we needed to make a play."

The Paladins set up shop. Across the line of scrimmage, the Dukes dug in. Shambley, Isai Bradshaw and Frank Cobbs anchored the middle of the Madison front. Behind them, Kwynn Walton stood with his arms at his side. McCarter lined up off the left edge. Ideally, JMU wanted to reach the ball before Beckler got the kick away, and that meant McCarter coming off the corner. But the Paladins had allowed only one blocked kick all season. If the Dukes couldn't get to Beckler from the edge, a strong push up the middle was their last shot. A 43-yard kick meant a flatter trajectory. Shambley, at 6-foot-4, had the best chance if the ball came out low.

The snap and spot were good. Beckler struck the ball just as McCarter was coming free off the edge. The kick was low — too low — and hugged the top of the Furman line. In the middle of the JMU front, Shambley wedged himself into the backfield. "The guard that was blocking [me and Frank] just fell backward," he later said. Shambley stuck his right hand in the air and felt the ball smack against it. He had been a part-time player his entire college career and spent most of the 2003 season battling injury problems, but with 5:11 left against Furman, Shambley gave the Dukes one last shot. "It was almost surreal," he recalled. "Each game it seemed someone new stepped up. That's just what we did all year."

Shambley jogged off the field pumping his fist in the air. "I'm not big on celebrating but I think we all knew it gave us a chance," he later said. And on the Madison sideline, the reaction was similar. The Dukes had done everything possible on defense and special teams. They blocked a punt and a field goal; they forced a fumble on the goal line and held Furman to 13 points. The game now rested in the hands of the

JMU offense. The Paladins had failed to bury the Dukes. Tom Ridley, a former high school quarterback, was holding court on the Madison sideline. Ridley wasn't an emotional guy, but like many of his senior teammates, he had a knack for finding the right words when they were needed. He gave a short speech before the final drive, reminding his teammates that they had some time to work with. "There were moments during that season where one of us seemed to have something to say," Ridley recalled. "That was one of those times for me." As Shambley crossed the sideline and Ridley gathered his teammates, a square-jawed Justin Rascati came into view. Usually loose and vocal, his face was without expression. Rascati was locked in.

Back-to-back penalties to start the drive pushed the Dukes back to the 14-yard line. In the huddle, Rascati thought it was time to speak. He told his teammates this was the moment they had worked for and that it wasn't time to go home. Meanwhile, Durden believed he finally had solved Furman's blitz packages. The Dukes had time to drive down the field and Durden wanted to get yards in chunks. He thought the big play was out of the question. It was time to give Rascati that extra rope.

The Dukes lined up with four receivers and Rascati in shotgun on second-and-22. Rascati took the snap, dropped back and sat in the pocket. Across the field, Boxley sprinted to the 35, slammed on the breaks and curled back to the ball. Rascati pumped and delivered a strike to Boxley at the 30. The 16-yard pass set up third-and-six. An 11-yard completion to Boxley on the next play gave the Dukes a first down at the 41 with 3:45 remaining. After struggling to throw the ball all game, the Dukes finally were finding space vacated by the Furman blitz. "From a play-calling standpoint we were a little more dialed in than we had been all night," Durden said. "Once we figured out that defense we found ways to get around it."

Rascati was stopped for no-gain on first-and-10. On second down he completed another pass, this time over the middle to a wide-open Nic Tolley, and Tolley swept across the field for 22 yards before being tackled at the Furman 37. On the sideline, Matthews was amazed at how much space Tolley had. "No one was there," he later said. "And when I checked the replay I saw they had a busted coverage. Half of their guys were playing zone and half were playing man-to-man."

It was another uncharacteristic Furman blunder. And now, the Dukes were building momentum. Rascati fired incomplete for Boxley on first down, but found L.C. Baker in the flat on second-and-10. Baker caught the pass in the backfield and turned on the jets, crossing the 30 and leaping over a block from Boxley before Cam Newton knocked him down at the Furman 22. "Coach Durden did a great job distributing the ball on that drive," Hines later said. "We just didn't want our season to end."

Less than two minutes remained as the Dukes broke the huddle. Hines was stuffed for no-gain on first-and-10. On second down, Rascati completed his fifth pass of the drive, this time to Ardon Bransford at the 15, and Bransford fought his way down to the eight-yard line to set up first-and-goal. Here, in the most pressure-packed situation of the season, Rascati and Durden were operating at another level. "That season was full of many game-changing events," Geoff Polglase later said. "But if there's a special moment, it's Rascati leading that drive at Furman."

Hines gained two yards on first down and was shoved out of bounds at the six. Rascati picked up four on second-and-goal and the Dukes burned their second timeout with 43 seconds left. In the JMU stands, fans were clutched arm-in-arm. Hines gained a yard on third down and the Paladins called timeout. Matthews met with his players on the sideline and asked Hines which side he wanted to run toward on fourth-and-goal. Hines wanted to run to the right, the same play they ran on fourth down against Lehigh.

The Dukes broke the huddle. Rascati handed the ball to Hines, who ran to the right and then — in what he later called his "Michael Jordan moment" — darted into the end zone behind blocks from Chris Iorio, George Burns and Jamaal Crowder to tie the game at 13.

JMU sports media photographer Cathy Kushner was snapping

photos of the Madison sideline as the play unfolded, and as Hines crossed the goal line, the Dukes erupted. In the middle of the crowd, bundled in an oxford grey sweatshirt, Clayton Matthews raised his right hand in celebration. To his left, Tolley dropped to his knees, raised his arms and pointed his index fingers skyward. Pete Johnson nearly jumped out of his body. Mickey Matthews drifted five feet over the sideline marker, clapped his hands and tried to compose himself. "I still think it's the moment of the year," Matthews said in 2007. "Let's be honest, it's the biggest play of that playoff run. You can't get bigger than that. [The photo] captured the entire emotional scene. It caught me because right after that I was looking for Rabil."

At that very moment, David Rabil already was on his way onto the field. He countered his nerves with outward confidence. The Madison special teams unit came into the game. Ridley, who had been pulled off field goal blocking duty during the William & Mary game because of a nagging injury, was approaching the JMU sideline when something instinctively told him to stay on the field. "Chuck Suppon had replaced me on special teams," Ridley said. "After we scored I just ran up to him and pushed him back toward the sideline. I have no idea why I did it."

Suppon took a step back, perhaps because he was just as shocked as Ridley. Years later Ridley still doesn't know why he pushed Suppon back to the sideline. He spun around and bolted back toward the huddle. As the Dukes lined up for the extra point, Rabil tested the ground. Ridley spun around from his place on the Madison line and looked back at his kicker. Rabil smiled. "If you're going to block one guy this season, block him now," he yelled above the noise. Ridley shook his head in disbelief and turned back to the line.

Rabil took a quick breath and signaled he was ready. Seven yards in front of him, Josh Haymore bent over the ball and looked through his legs into the backfield. Hours earlier, Rabil and Nick Englehart were ribbing Haymore for being Mike Schikman's "key player" of the game. Now, all three were in that boat together. Haymore snapped the ball to Englehart. Rabil jogged forward and swung his right leg at the ball, then hopped to jump over a Furman defender. The kick zipped through the uprights to give the Dukes a 14-13 lead. "Perfect snap, perfect hold," Rabil said. "And the second I made contact I knew we were winning the game."

Rabil was floating as he jogged off the field. Brandon Beach picked him up and gave him a hug. Bransford did the same. Haymore pounded the top of his helmet. In the Madison stands, there was bedlam, but Jon McNamara could barely watch. He remembered the Hail Mary pass the Dukes gave up against Richmond earlier in the season. He remembered the Furman fans praying for God's team. "That's all I was thinking about," he later said. "I was hoping [Furman] didn't get close enough to reach the end zone."

Brian Bratton returned Paul Wantuck's ensuing kickoff to the Furman 28-yard line. Martin fired incomplete on first down, but a hook-and-ladder completion to Daric Carter on second down put the Paladins on the 40 with enough time for two plays. McNamara held his breath as Martin fired two bombs for the goal line. The first was knocked away. When the second hit the ground in the Madison end zone, the Dukes piled across the field, their miracle victory complete. "It was our season," Leon Steinfeld later said of the game-winning drive. "That was the most memorable drive of my career."

And of the plays that made the drive possible: Dottin-Carter's blocked punt and Shambley's blocked field goal? "I still don't think people pay attention to how big we were on special teams that year," Tony LeZotte later said. "When Isaiah blocks that punt, it puts us in great field position and we go in and score. That was huge. And the blocked field goal? If he makes it, that field goal seals the game.

"Without those two plays we lose. Plain and simple."

It had taken two blocked kicks, a forced turnover at the goal line, a 74-yard drive with the clock winding down and a fourth-down plunge with less than a minute to go, but JMU was heading for a semifinal showdown with William & Mary. The road show would not be ending in Greenville. The battered Dukes, once an afterthought, were alive and well. "They've done it all year long," a drained Bobby Lamb told Mike Barber after the game. "They find a way to win in the fourth quarter. They found another way to win today."

...

BACK IN Chattanooga, the heated argument between Durden and Matthews was escalating. But the debate had nothing to do with the play call. It was about location. "The field was so bad you couldn't tell where the damn ball was," Matthews said. And while Durden had a better view, he also was farther away from the action. Both knew the Dukes had an advantage up front, but Matthews wanted to make sure JMU came away with points. Was the ball on the one-yard line or inside the one? "I didn't know," Matthews answered. "I don't even think Jeff knew. But he sounded pretty convincing on the headset." Durden kept telling Matthews the ball was inside the one. And finally, Matthews caved. They would run Fenner to the left behind Corey Davis. But as the Dukes rushed back onto the field, Matthews made a promise to his offensive coordinator. "Durden," he said. "Whether we make it or don't make it, if this ball isn't inside the one, you're fired when we get home."

The Dukes walked to the line of scrimmage and planted themselves in their jumbo package along the one-yard line. Six inches away, the Grizzlies dug into their goal line stand formation, feet anchored to the front of the end zone. Rascati barked the cadence, turned to his left and extended the ball to Fenner. The right side of the JMU line undercut the Montana defense. Matt Magerko pulled from his guard position and kicked out to the left. Chris Iorio plugged the gap vacated by Magerko and the Madison line surged forward.

The right side of the Montana defense began to buckle under the strength of the bigger JMU line as Fenner shot through the hole behind Iorio. Magerko blasted his defender off the ball and secured the corner. Five yards away, Rascati shuffled nervously and raised his hands in the air as Fenner powered toward the goal line.

Iorio and Montana linebacker Adam Hoge were in a stalemate at the one-yard line as Fenner approached them. Fenner drove straight into Iorio's back and momentarily was stonewalled. To his left, Montana cornerback Kevin Edwards was slipping free of Magerko's block. Fenner slid to his left into a small crevice between Hoge and Edwards and churned toward the end zone.

As he reached the goal line, Fenner lowered his head and barreled into Montana linebacker Nick Vella. To the right, Iorio fell to the ground inches inside the end zone. As Iorio rolled onto his back, a white jersey came crashing over him. Maurice Fenner was in.

On the far sideline, the fans in purple and gold erupted. For the first time all night, the Dukes had taken control and the Grizzlies had been powerless to stop them. Until now, the Madison faithful had been given little to cheer about, but Fenner's second effort had put the Dukes back in the national title game. They weren't just hanging around anymore, and they weren't simply the beneficiaries of a missed field goal and a dropped pass. Madison was alive and well. Streamers cascaded across the stadium grandstand and the JMU fans let out a collective roar that had been bottled up since the opening kickoff. "Everyone erupted," McNamara said. "I think that's when we started to believe. You could tell how much everyone wanted this."

David Rabil's PAT split the uprights. The Dukes were in front.

...

ON THE opposite sideline, Montana looked shell-shocked. Down 10-7 after all those yards? Down 10-7 against a team that couldn't do anything right in the first quarter? But the Dukes had rediscovered their offense and the scoreboard wasn't lying. Of the 13 plays on the JMU touchdown drive, 11 had been on the ground. Only 16 seconds remained in the first half.

Levander Segars patiently waited near his own goal line for the ensuing JMU kickoff. At 5-foot-8 and 180 pounds, Segars hardly looked formidable, but the speedy receiver owned most of Montana's all-time records for kickoff and punt returns. Matthews had no intention of letting Segars come anywhere near Paul Wantuck's kick, and Wantuck instead lofted a pop fly that was fair caught at the Montana 36 by Jaison Carringer. Though the move kept Segars from breaking a big return, it also gave Ochs good field position and failed to run any time off the clock.

The Grizzlies came to the line and Ochs dropped back in shotgun. Sixteen seconds was not enough time to reach the end zone without a long pass or a gadget play, but it was enough time to move 40 yards and kick a field goal. And 16 seconds for the Grizzlies was an eternity. Ochs fielded the snap and whistled a pass to Jon Talmage at the Montana 44, and Talmage scampered out of bounds, stopping the clock with 11 seconds remaining in the half. The hurry-up offense was built on quarterbacks who made quick decisions and accurate throws, and in 2004, Craig Ochs and the Grizzlies ran the best two-minute drill in I-AA football.

Montana again lined up in shotgun and Ochs dropped back to pass. He skipped and hopped in the backfield before Sid Evans flushed him from the pocket. As Ochs sprinted toward the Montana sideline, Jefferson Heidelberger broke free toward the same side of the field. Ochs swept around Evans, turned his body upfield and zinged a pass on the run. Heidelberger had a two-step lead on Tony LeZotte and caught the pass in stride as LeZotte dragged him out of bounds at the JMU six-yard line.

The stunning 50-yard completion gave the Grizzlies first-and-goal with one second left in the half and sent the Montana fans into frenzy. On the opposite sideline, the Dukes were stunned. After controlling the ball for more than 11 minutes in the second quarter, JMU was about to give momentum right back to Montana. So abrupt was the play and so glaring was the difference between the teams' reactions that no one seemed to notice the yellow flag in the offensive backfield. A holding penalty was called. The play was coming back.

Ochs popped his mouthpiece into the upper bars of his facemask and unbuckled his chinstrap. Another opportunity squandered. With one second left in the quarter and the ball back on the Montana 35, the Grizzlies were out of options. Ochs took the final snap of the first half, dropped to one knee and flipped the ball away. The Dukes, after a topsy-turvy first act, had won the opening half, and led by three as the teams entered the intermission.

Part IV: Welcome to Streamerville

Chapter 13

THE DIFFERENCE between Montana and JMU on the field was drastic. The difference in history was downright startling. The Grizzlies had been a national power for longer than the Dukes had existed. In Mickey Matthews, JMU hoped it had found the coach to lead the program to success. In Bobby Hauck, Montana simply was continuing its long line of dominance.

It was early in his coaching career but Hauck already was successful. That wasn't an easy task at Montana, where coach after coach was asked to uphold a tradition of excellence. Hauck was the fourth man in 10 years to lead Montana to the national championship game — a statistic so impressive it was hard to quantify. No matter how close a new coach is to a program's old regime, there is a change in philosophy, personnel and routine. Yet at Montana, where 33 men had preceded Hauck and where none spent more than 10 years as head coach, there was a seamless transition on the field. The Grizzlies were 133-31 since 1993 and an overwhelming 120-16 at home since the 1986 season. Despite staff turnover, Montana was a perplexing study in consistency. New coaches replaced old coaches; new recruits replaced graduates. The machine restocked and won football games. To average programs, consistent success was difficult. At Montana, it was status quo.

No one knew this better than Hauck. The Missoula native and Montana graduate was the tenth alumnus to coach the Grizzlies. When then-incumbent coach Joe Glenn left Montana to coach at the University of Wyoming after the 2002 season, he left a 39-6 record and two trips to Chattanooga in his old office. That was Hauck's immediate burden to uphold and the second-year coach had met expectations, piloting the Grizzlies to a 21-6 record and leading the program back to the national title game.

Hauck was candid when it came to his current status. He was asked earlier in the season if the Montana head coaching position was his dream job and he wasn't shy about saying no. Mentally, the idea of a new challenge energized him. The Grizzlies already were at the top of the I-AA world in most categories. Montana consistently drew the nation's largest crowds, averaging better than 22,000 fans per game for the last decade. While more than half of the country's I-AA schools played in glorified high school stadiums, the Grizzlies played in a state-of-the-art facility — a miniature version of a contemporary I-A stadium with seats so close to the field that players couldn't hear themselves think. In an interview before the national title game, Matthews said playing a game in Missoula was like playing a game at LSU's 92,000-seat Tiger Stadium. To other schools — JMU included — Montana was the gold standard. The program was strong from top to bottom and had all the necessary ingredients for success: top-notch facilities, winning seasons, devoted fans, large fund raising and brand equity. "They're incredibly established," Gary Michael said. "Every year you do the preseason rankings and it's, 'well, where are we going to put Montana?' They're one of the keystones of I-AA football."

For a program that was 70 years younger than Montana's, JMU wasn't in a bad place. Entering the 2004 season, Madison's all-time record was 180-158-3, but there had been several big seasons that, given a stronger program foundation, could have vaulted the Dukes forward. From opening day of the 1975 season to late September 1976, Challace McMillin's Dukes won 12 consecutive games, finished a season undefeated, earned a No. 1 national ranking and ended the stretch by playing in the first Division III game televised by a major network. In

1982, McMillin took a talented JMU team (including future NFL stars Charles Haley and Gary Clark) into Charlottesville and beat Virginia, 21-17. And in both 1991 and 1994, Rip Scherer piloted Madison to opening-round playoff wins.

But when the smoke cleared, each step forward was a small one, not a giant leap. The reasons varied. Madison's success at the Division III level didn't garner much attention given its low status on the national totem pole. The 1982 win over Virginia came against a 2-9 Cavaliers team and took place well before 24/7 sports news was commonplace. Had the game taken place in the late 1990s there certainly would have been more public knowledge on a regional level. It wouldn't rival Appalachian State's upset of Michigan in 2007, but McMillin's Dukes would have been a household name in the southeast.

Scherer's playoff teams, however, failed to launch the Dukes to elite status for different reasons. By the 1990s JMU was an established I-AA program, had sent a couple of players to the NFL with great success (Clark, Haley and place kicker Scott Norwood would combine to play in 10 Pro Bowls) and were playing in a state searching for a football power. In Charlottesville, George Welsh's Cavaliers consistently were winning seven-to-eight games a season but were outside the national championship picture. Down the interstate in Blacksburg, Frank Beamer's Virginia Tech Hokies were just starting to turn the corner. Scherer's 1991 team was solid, winning nine games and falling to Samford, 24-21, in the second round of the playoffs. His 1994 squad was better, outscoring opponents 388-224 and winning 10 games before bowing to a Matthews-coached Marshall team, 28-21, in overtime.

But JMU's athletics program lacked the means to showcase the Dukes beyond the Harrisonburg area. At a time when the dot.com boom was just beginning, there wasn't much media coverage for Scherer's 10-win team because, frankly, outside of major TV exposure and the newspapers, there wasn't any other medium to use. Madison also lacked a large-scale alumni fund raising system for its athletics programs. Without the tools to promote, the big seasons in 1991 and '94 flew under the radar. The Dukes simply were not a hot ticket because they lacked the resources to be relevant. "Rip's team had a home playoff game [in 1994] and the students had to pay to get in," Mike Schikman recalled. "That team was loaded with Kenny Sims, Mike Cawley, Macey Brooks and Ed Perry. The latter two were both NFL guys. I don't think they drew more than 7,000 people."

It's easy for college programs to lag behind without sufficient media exposure and marketing infrastructure, and the Dukes were in danger of falling into a hole. By the late 1990s, the program was stale. Bridgeforth Stadium had not changed in 25 years and JMU was settling into a large pool of modest teams with modest facilities and modest success. It was hardly the future many envisioned — especially after Madison's run of success in basketball in the 1980s and 90s. But support for those basketball teams did not translate to support for football. And the math was simple. No public knowledge meant no fans. Without fans — especially ones with deep pockets — there was no money. No money meant no operating room for facilities, which meant no upgrades, no growth and no recruiting edge.

The plateau was coming fast. At the beginning of the decade, the Madison administration recognized the need to improve their athletics infrastructure if the Dukes ever wanted to graduate from the middle of the pack. A chief member of the group charged with improving Madison athletics was Geoff Polglase, a 1985 JMU grad, who had worked for the alumni association and as special assistant to Linwood Rose in the 1990s. Polglase was an organized and patient man; he also was a passionate Madison supporter. From 2000-2004, he was in the middle of two important decisions that would change both JMU's athletics support capabilities and fan appeal. The first involved building alumni support by buffing up the Duke Club (Madison's athletics fund raising arm) and increasing campus involvement by working with associate director of athletics development Nick Langridge to establish the Student Duke Club. The second was the hiring of Brad Edmondson as assistant athletics director for marketing.

...

EDMONDSON WAS a spring chicken compared to some of his peers inside JMU Sports when he arrived in the winter of 2004. But the 29-year old had his sleeves rolled from the beginning. JMU needed a jump-start, specifically in its game-day atmosphere, which, according to former students, was nondescript. Edmondson, who previously worked in the athletics marketing department at Auburn, understood the need to establish tradition. "At Auburn, and around all the schools in the SEC, it's all about pageantry and the build-up to the start of the game," he explained. "It's truly amazing down there — almost like a theater production. That's what the fans come for."

Edmondson held an undergraduate degree in telecommunications and a Masters in athletics administration from Ball State. He loved sports, especially in the collegiate setting where students fueled the fire. At Auburn, where 15,000 undergraduates pile into Jordan-Hare Stadium every Saturday (about 18% of the average attendance) tradition and pageantry seep from the walls of the 70-year old structure. In 2001, after Auburn coach Tommy Tuberville called the home atmosphere "the jungle," Edmondson's boss, university assistant athletics director Marvin Julich, coined the phrase, "The Jungle at Jordan-Hare." Julich, Edmondson said, taught him the importance of 'tagging the atmosphere.' Fans embrace ideas that build identity for an organization. And given the chance to be active in the construction of that identity, students will run with almost anything.

A college football game plays to home-field advantage. At JMU, aside from the 300-plus piece marching band, that atmosphere did not exist. Though there was a structure in place for marketing and promotions, Edmondson essentially was given carte blanche for game events. The changes he implemented were immediately noticed. For years, the athletics department relied heavily on rented materials for home games, which was an expensive annual purchase. Edmondson approached Polglase with a plan to make an up-front investment, own the equipment and pay off the bill in two years. He and several other administrators also pushed to perform a little cosmetic work on Bridgeforth Stadium. Until 2004, the facility was two slabs of gray concrete sticking out of the ground. But with APC construction underway and a new scoreboard set to be installed, it was time for the stadium to change. Structural modifications were out of the question, but color wasn't. In the summer of 2004, the administration approved painting the inside stadium walls in purple and the railings in gold. Later, before the scoreboard was ordered, Polglase suggested that it too, be purple. It seemed like a small detail, but it turned a generic facility into something with brand value. "Amazing what a can of paint will do," Edmondson later joked. "It seemed so simple but it made a world of a difference. Add some color; make it JMU-related and suddenly you have a place that's unique."

There was, Edmondson said, a lot of thought that went into the changes. And that credit went primarily to Polglase, who kept the big machine moving forward. When the new scoreboard was ordered, Edmondson and Polglase knew they'd have to use it to its fullest capabilities. The old board was high school quality; the new one was 70-feet wide, 30-feet tall and sat 50-feet off the ground. It also came with a 220-square foot video screen, later dubbed "the medium-tron" because of its relative modest size. Still, it was a tremendous upgrade, but only if it could be used properly. That meant a new sound system (the old one was rumored to be a rental from a local little league), interactive video and replay. "We couldn't just have a scoreboard that had video capability," Polglase said. "We had to be able to run replay and interactive video elements from the beginning." So JMU contracted a Richmond-based production company to develop segments for game-day entertainment, including a pre-game video called "Watch Us Play" — a spin-off of "Walk This Way" — performed by a group of Madison students from the A Capella group, Exit 245. And Edmondson, by now knee-deep in re-structuring the pre-game program, began setting aside elements to use during the upcoming season.

Edmondson wanted to bring the pageantry and tradition of SEC football to Harrisonburg, which was impossible to do overnight. But he could help JMU build its game-day atmosphere. And he knew he had an ace in the hole with the marching band. Unlike the Madison football program, the Marching Royal Dukes were not a level below their peers at Virginia and Virginia Tech; if anything they were a level above. Nicknamed "Virginia's Finest," the MRDs performed at two presidential inaugurations and the 2001 Macy's Thanksgiving Day Parade. "The band," Matt LeZotte said, "rocks inside that stadium." Dr. Pat Rooney, the longtime band director and close friend of Mickey Matthews, would speak to the Madison football team at the beginning of every season about the traditions at JMU. It was important, Matthews thought, for his players to hear about this from a person with decades of experience at the university.

Rooney's MRDs were the big show in town. The running joke in bad football seasons was that fans came to the game to watch the marching band and tolerated the Dukes. Edmondson didn't know anything about that, but he knew how critical the band was. "The pre-game is all about them," he said. "The procession, the music, the pageantry — it all leads to them building the atmosphere for that team to come out of that tunnel. The halftime and post-game shows are great; but they're almost more important as a catalyst for everything else. They jump-start the fans."

With the marching band anchoring his program, Edmondson put together a 90-minute pre-game plan that coordinated cheerleaders, game-day personnel, dance squads, volunteers, video introductions, an inflatable Duke Dog, fog machines and both football teams into a schedule. Edmondson's game-day staff spent the entire summer putting it together and did full rehearsals at night the week before the Lock Haven game, sometimes running through countdowns at 2 a.m., while the rest of campus slept. The night of the home opener, as the Dukes waited on the concourse between the APC construction site and the student grandstand, Matt LeZotte felt his heart racing. As team captain, LeZotte would lead the Dukes onto the field. The atmosphere, he recalled, was unlike anything he had seen at Madison. "Before we came out I talked to a lot of the guys," he said. "I told them this was the start of everything we worked for." LeZotte was referring to the beginning of JMU's 2004 season, but his words rang true for the entire program. When the signal came for the Dukes to pile out of the paddock, LeZotte was pumping with so much adrenaline that he sprinted into the stadium with his arms raised to the sky, the perfect capper to an energizing introduction. At the end of the night, Curt Dudley named Edmondson and his staff co-players of the game during his radio broadcast.

The feeling, at least regarding the stadium atmosphere, was that the Dukes were entering a new era. The push, Edmondson explained, came from everywhere. The pre-game show, paint and scoreboard were university efforts, but Madison's success on the field and the positive response from fans caused the hype to spread through campus like a brush fire. "The perfect storm," Edmondson later said. And he worked hard to keep it that way. Every win changed the dynamic. When the school wanted to organize pep rallies before the Delaware and W&M games on short notice, Edmondson, Polglase, Dudley and dozens of volunteers made it happen. When students began to clamor for more freedom to tailgate before games, Edmondson and several progressive JMU administrators fought to loosen campus restrictions on drinking and parking. "There were a lot of moving parts in there," Student Duke Club president Ashley Sumner said. "Have you ever tried to turn around a pep rally in six days? It took a lot of people from both the administration and the student body to make it happen."

There was an incredible amount of synergy between the SDC, the Duke Club and the athletics administration, according to Sumner. And with program visibility on the rise and the football team winning, turnout went through the roof. "The students started to run with it," Polglase said. "We're the type of campus where our students will respond very favorably when you have success. And it's not just the team; it's the entire package, the idea that you're a part of it."

The final part was the most critical, because Polglase explained the whole point of being a fan. What he and Edmondson realized was that campus response was favorable not just because the Dukes were winning (though it didn't hurt) but because a large JMU-centric sports movement was the one thing missing from the current Madison experience. "[The students] were seeing their friends at Tech and Virginia," Edmondson said. "And the thought was, 'well why can't we have that here?' We actually used our student volunteers in the marketing department as focus groups for campus. When you create an atmosphere it becomes special. And when it's special for you as a student you'll come back as an alum. We kept coming back to the idea that we had to give the kids a chance."

...

BY THE middle of the fall semester, as the Dukes were in the midst of a six-game win streak that would vault them into the nation's top 10, the campus — never short on Madison apparel — was awash in purple. Cafeteria workers in the dining halls wore "GAME-DAY TOMORROW" shirts on Fridays. Orientation guides leading tours through campus would tell prospective students to check out the Saturday football game if they were in town through the weekend. In years past, the same guides would tell people not to bother with football because the Dukes were terrible. That message changed in 2004. "Going to football games became the social thing to do," Edmondson said.

Historically, Madison suffered from the same problem that plagued all un-established programs in unsuccessful seasons: declining attendance late in the year. In 2003, the Dukes averaged 9,982 fans in their first two home games. They averaged 7,581 in their final two. Weather is a huge factor when it comes to attendance in I-AA, but success during the season is critical. A major Division I-A program might see a five percent fluctuation in attendance based on weather and results. From 2001 to 2005, Penn State had three losing seasons and two winning seasons; its record was as bad as 3-9 and as good as 11-1, yet average attendance numbers for those seasons always fell between 102,800 and 107,500 — a change of less than five percent — a drop in the bucket regarding ticket sales and crowd size. But at JMU, the same drop in attendance (4,700 people) was almost 30 percent of the stadium capacity. A bad season for Madison generally meant the difference between averaging 12,500 and 9,500 fans per game — a 24 percent drop. Sustaining success would always be difficult given the modest size of I-AA stadiums. A 3,000-ticket hit is simply harder to take when the pot is shallow to begin with.

In 2004, however, the Dukes saw life from the other side. JMU averaged 12,358 fans per game in its first four home games (numbers inflated after the Homecoming and Family Weekend games drew 15,000-plus), but the Dukes actually increased average attendance in November, averaging 13,293 fans against Delaware and W&M. People would come to see a winner. A big difference was student turnout. According to Polglase, the university generally counted on 4,000 students at every home game. Bad weather and a bad team can drop that number under 2,000; good weather and a winning team can swell it to over 5,000. By the end of the 2004 season nearly half the stadium — 90 percent of the Godwin Hall stands and about 50 percent of the end zone seats — was filled with students or recent graduates. The high percentage of students per overall attendance turned Bridgeforth Stadium — especially the east stands — into hostile territory. Matthews, who had moved the Madison bench behind the west stands early in his tenure, now looked like a genius. "Initially I decided to move us to the other side because of the sunlight," he said. "You can't see anything from the east stands during a 6 o'clock game until the sun goes down. But I also thought it would be a huge advantage because our students would be behind our opponent. I know many coaches in this league have remarked when they play here that it was a stroke of genius to have the students behind the visiting team."

Bridgeforth had long been a tough place to play. The Dukes were 107-57 all-time at home entering the 2004 season and 20-9 under Matthews. But going on the road anywhere in college football is difficult and winning two-out-of-three at home is par for the course. The '04 season changed everything and Bridgeforth went from being a tough place to one of the nastiest stops in the conference. From 2004-2007, the Dukes were 20-3 at home. Teams — and their fans — dreaded the trip to Harrisonburg. JMU was a tough team and Durden's offense was nearly unstoppable at home. The stands were cramped; the fans were passionate; the students were loud, rowdy and drunk. "A lot of it is presence," said Sumner, whose SDC members took up almost two sections of seats at the 50-yard line. "You make a big statement when you have 1,000 people in purple screaming their heads off at mid-field. It's hard not to gravitate toward that. There are more pep rallies, promotions and tailgates. It all just caught on." And for every underclassman in the stands, there were two partying in the parking lot. "Tailgating is the big monstrosity now," Mike Schikman said in 2007. "You used to have a few diehards. Now, heck, forget about the 15,000 in the stadium because you've got another couple of thousand still tailgating during the game."

Madison fans have always had a tendency to tailgate longer and show up late, a common occurrence in many college football environments (sans the SEC). At pep rallies, Matthews would casually remind students that kickoff was at 1:00 and not 1:30. Still, dating back to the early days of the program, a large portion of JMU students generally float into the stadium at the end of the first quarter. And despite increased turnout, that trend continued. "Gary Clark used to complain to me about Homecoming crowds not getting into the stadium on time," Schikman recalled. "And it's funny because he came back for a Homecoming game a few years ago and he was supposed to be my halftime guest. He never showed. He was in the parking lot tailgating with everyone else."

...

MADISON'S NEWFOUND popularity was simple to explain: the Dukes were winning. As Matthews later said, "It's not hard to market a winner," though JMU proved in the past that it's very easy for a successful team to go unnoticed. But because of Edmondson, Polglase and JMU's athletics marketing department, fan support was going to a new level. There was a connection between this team and its fans unlike any other in program history. Edmondson's marketing theme for the academic year (One team. One community. One vision.) put the focus on the university coming together around its athletics program. For years, there had been a small group of diehard Madison fans who knew their teams, the players and the coaches. Everybody else cheered for the jersey, not the people who wore it. But in 2004, largely because of Edmondson's push to anchor football around senior leaders (Townsend, Matt LeZotte, Tom Ridley) and talented underclassmen (Rascati, Tony LeZotte, Alvin Banks) a larger portion of the fan base began to identify with the Dukes. A buzz was created. Sumner and the Student Duke Club executive board were in the middle of it. "We worked closely with the Duke Club, marketing and even the administration to create a unified student body," Sumner said. "When you have list servers for 1,000 students for eBlasts you're going to be a great addition to spread the word for a tailgate, pep rally or bus trip to an away game."

By the middle of the season, as the Dukes readied for consecutive road games at Maine and Richmond, the SDC already was running with the momentum from Madison's quick start. The organization of students was important to ensure sustained turnout, especially with three straight home games late in the season. The SDC was a liaison between the administration and the rest of campus — a vehicle for the athletics department to reach Madison students who wanted to be part of the growing movement to back JMU football. Sumner and her team worked closely with Duke Club advisers Matt Borman and Nick Langridge to promote JMU's on-field success. But they also took care of logistics, like bus trips and tailgates to away games. Sumner's approach was simple: volunteer to help with anything. "In years past our committee chairs within SDC were just carrying titles," she said. "But in 2004 they were very active." This approach took a lot of the groundwork off the hands of the administration and put the SDC at the forefront.

Another large push was viral in nature. While Rip Scherer's '94 team suffered from winning during the early part of the dot.com boom, the 2004 Dukes were successful during an interactive era. In an age of online message boards, diehard Madison fans — both students and alumni — congregated more on the Internet than in person. "It was funny because I would go to classes and ask students if they saw the posters or billboards and most would say no," Edmondson later said. "But if I asked them about e-mail we sent they would say yes."

Information among JMU fans was shared online more than anywhere else, with e-blasts and chat board messages being the top two sources. ESPN and major TV networks weren't covering I-AA football, so if you wanted the inside scoop on JMU sports, you went to the message boards. Same story if you had an idea to pump up fan involvement that needed to be spread quickly. Phil Cockrell, a 1985 Madison graduate, Duke Club member and longtime season ticket holder, used this forum to create a new JMU tradition during the 2004 season. Cockrell had experienced the Electric Zoo first-hand. In the mid-80s, when the men's basketball team was perhaps the most-feared mid-major in the country, Madison's home venues (first Godwin Hall and later the Convocation Center) were the toughest places on earth to find toilet paper on game day. That's because students would raid the bathrooms before tipoff and pocket all available two-ply before heading to their seats. When the Dukes scored their first basket of the evening, the fans would shower the floor with toilet paper, a unique tradition that later faded away when referees began issuing a technical foul against Madison for holding up the game.

Cockrell wanted to bring some excitement back to JMU sports. Both premier programs (men's basketball and football) had declined following the Lefty Driesell and Rip Scherer eras. Cockrell's initial idea involved car flags but it wasn't very successful. Before the 2004 season, he hatched another concept, one that involved bringing back an Electric Zoo tradition. Cockrell — through online message boards — began floating the idea of handing out purple and gold streamers before the game and throwing them into the air when the Dukes came out of the locker room. Since the Madison stands — separated from the field by an aisle, an eight-lane track and the sideline — were not close to the playing surface, Cockrell thought the idea was plausible. He had 1,000 streamers shipped to his house. Chris Nahlik — a Madison student and a diehard JMU fan — helped hand out the streamers in the student section. For the most part, according to Cockrell, the Student Duke Club was not involved. "They were told not to by the administration," he said. And so the movement — much like everything else at Madison — was a groundswell. "The coordination was where we came into play down the road," Sumner added. "And we did some promotion, too, but we all thought this would eventually sell itself."

On opening night against Lock Haven, Edmondson's timed and choreographed pre-game show was punctuated by an abrupt shower of streamers across the east stands. They were an instant hit among current students — who were looking to help create a unique atmosphere — and alumni — who yearned for a return of Madison's glory days. "Boy did they display well," Cockrell recalled. "Everybody at the game was asking about it and whether it would be done in the future. I said it would be up to JMU. The newspapers mentioned them in their articles about the game. I thought for sure it was a hit."

The initial conversation with Edmondson and Langridge the following Monday was positive, and Cockrell began spreading the word about the acceptance of a new tradition. He offered to donate the cost of the streamers for the first year. An hour later, Langridge and Edmondson called back. No more streamers, they said. The administration had responded with less enthusiasm. "Our initial meeting after the first streamer appearance wasn't very positive," Edmondson admitted. "A lot of people were worried about cleanup."

Insurance was the other issue. "Insurance?" Cockrell asked. "JMU had supported streamers in the past for basketball and there was never an insurance problem." Cockrell was baffled and let his supporters on the message boards know it. Edmondson, meanwhile, also was miffed at the situation. He sat in that meeting with the administration and nodded his head. The streamers could be a problem, he agreed. They could get out of hand. When the meeting was over he walked back to his office and paged one of his student interns. "This is the greatest thing ever," said Edmondson, who believed the fans were beginning to understand that they could create an atmosphere. Edmondson didn't care about cleanup. He wanted more fan involvement and now it was knocking at his door. The administration has to back this, he thought.

Later that afternoon, Cockrell received another call from Langridge and Edmondson. The streamers were back on the table. What caused the change is still up for debate. Maybe it was the positive press or a push from the alumni. Regardless, Cockrell's project was given a green light — albeit with a few rules. The administration still was concerned about people tripping on the stairs, so they asked Cockrell and the students to clear the aisles and cap the streamers at 2,000 per game. Additionally, they requested that the streamers be taken out of their individual wrapping to minimize cleanup.

Cockrell, for his part, was a tactical dreamer. He knew distribution would have to favor the student section and knew he had to keep streamers out of the hands of visiting fans. The streamers continued throughout the season, serving, many fans argued, as a symbol of JMU's resurgence in football.

The day the Dukes were sent to Lehigh in the opening round of the playoffs, Matthews and Cockrell were discussing the long road ahead. "Phil," Matthews said, "you make sure you bring those streamers up there Saturday." Initially, that path was blocked. No streamers at road playoff games. Cockrell spoke to Langridge. "Mickey told me to bring them," he said. Langridge told Cockrell to sit tight. An hour later, Jeff Bourne secured permission to bring 750 streamers to Lehigh. Cockrell had the streamers shipped to his hotel room and spent the night before the game unwrapping them with his son, Philip. Similar scenarios unfolded at Furman and W&M, and each time, the number increased. In Chattanooga, Cockrell reserved an extra hotel room to store 5,000 streamers and rented a Suburban to ship them to the game. By the end of the 2004 season, Edmondson and Sumner's initial thoughts were verified. The athletics department — once nervous about cleanup and insurance issues — embraced the new tradition. Madison's road to Chattanooga was paved with purple and gold tissue paper.

Edmondson's creativity, his partnership with the Duke Club and Madison's win streak brought in the students. The growth of the SDC and the game day takeover by its members ensured the influx would be proactive. And the work of alumni like Cockrell helped bridge the gap between current students and former ones. This partnership, born out of several moving parts converging at once, combined the resources of the Madison athletics program with a suddenly football-crazed campus and an alumni group looking to bring back the glory days of the Electric Zoo. It was, Edmondson later said, like catching lightning in a bottle.

The campus — never short on involvement — was making a massive push to back JMU sports. That fall, the JMU Duke Dog was selected as a finalist in the Capital One Mascot Challenge and the grassroots movement developed by campaign manager Mike Keown, a senior communications major, pulled the entire student body into frenzy. Madison was the fourth smallest school in the competition and was one of only two that didn't field a Division I-A football team. But Keown, who made campaign buttons, shot video promos, hung banners and coordinated public appearances, made sure that fan voting — which made up half of the overall score and was supposed to be a weak spot — was an area JMU would win. By the end of December, Duke Dog was 11-0 in a parity-dominated competition. So stunning was the Madison response that one of Edmondson's former colleagues at Auburn accused JMU of cheating. "They were in the competition too and couldn't figure out how our voting numbers were so strong," Edmondson later laughed. "But it was the little engine that could."

That little engine was derailed when Duke Dog lost the overall competition because its final score (half determined by fan voting and half by a panel of judges) was too low — a decision that created an immediate backlash and turned January into Edmondson's PR nightmare. But Keown's campaign had generated an incredible amount of momentum for the Madison athletics program. JMU might never earn a spot in the Capital One Mascot Challenge again, but between the football team and the school mascot, fans had two powerhouses to rally behind. Their causes were so similar the lines became blurred. Pulling for the team became pulling the mascot and vice versa. The fall of 2004, dominated nationally by John Kerry and George Bush and the Boston Red Sox, became the fall of football and Duke Dog in Harrisonburg.

At the end of the 2004-05 academic year, Polglase approached Edmondson regarding the program's new marketing theme. "One team. One Community. One Vision." had worked so well and Polglase wanted to know what was next. Edmondson was floored. There was nothing else. He started laughing. "I'm done," he told Polglase. "I can't do that again. I have no more themes."

...

POLGLASE AND Edmondson realized they were in a rare situation where action was not necessary to jump-start the big machine, but rather to feed it. It was a movement reminiscent of the one that took place in the mid-1980s when Lou Campinelli's basketball Dukes made three consecutive NCAA Tournament appearances. But Polglase was a student back then, Edmondson was in grade school and JMU lacked the infrastructure to capitalize on the momentum. Between 1982 and 1983, McMillin's Dukes defeated Virginia in football, Campinelli's team went to its second and third NCAA Tournaments (losing to Michael Jordan and North Carolina, 52-50, in one of them) and Brad Babcock's JMU baseball team became the first Virginia program to reach the College World Series. In 24 months, the university experienced arguably its greatest feats in each of its three major men's sports. But there wasn't a big alumni push, or a jump in donations, or a marketing strategy to move forward. The surge in popularity for JMU sports exclusively was a grassroots effort, passed down through word of mouth like a campfire story. And eventually, when the product on the field dipped, the support went with it.

JMU was a different university two decades before the run to

Chattanooga. There were many people close to the school who still referred to it as "Madison College" (the name change to James Madison University went into effect in the summer of 1977) and while the shift to a more diverse academic curriculum had been in place for decades, the university still was widely popular as a teacher's school. "You're looking at a totally different set of economic circumstances," Curt Dudley said in 2007. "Today you have roommates that go on to work for Lockheed Martin. If you sat down 30 years ago you had roommates that went on to work as teachers and coaches at public high schools. You had $100 contributors because they were in education. Not to slam educators, because we all know they aren't paid what they deserve, but now you have a bigger corporate alumni base so they have a lot more resources."

Dudley's assessment was spot on. Not only did JMU Sports lack the means to organize an alumni fund raising program in the early 1980s, the targeted alumni group wasn't capable of donating at a level to make it profitable. Both system and market weren't ready. "If [the success of the early 80s] happened now with what we have in place, it would have taken off," Polglase said. "We'd be a much different athletics program today if we had then what we have now."

What the Dukes currently have is a self-sustaining infrastructure, anchored by large-scale fund raising (the Duke Club), campus involvement (the Student Duke Club), and media marketing services. Shortly after the millennium, JMU began streaming online audio of football broadcasts. Now, after a Web site redesign in 2007, access to audio and video features, highlights and live broadcasts are part of a subscription package via the JMUSports.com feature, Madizone. In 2006, after Edmondson left to take a general manager position with Western Kentucky athletics marketing, Dudley shifted from assistant sports information director to JMU's director of multimedia communications, essentially strengthening Madison's media relations, sports marketing and communications departments. What followed was a boost in product — more interviews with coaches and players, more shows, more video, more coverage for press conferences and more access for fans. The increase in visibility was well received because the Dukes were a household name locally — even regionally. They were winning; they were relevant and they were taking advantage. In 2004, the Dukes played one regular season game on TV — the home game against William & Mary was televised on a FOX Sports regional network. By 2008 that number was up to five. JMU would never rival Virginia Tech or Virginia in size and scope — the I-A label and BCS money ensured that. But the Dukes could carve out a niche as a premier program in I-AA's toughest conference.

JMU was 36-13 in the four years after the national championship, keeping Matthews on the front page, his team in the spotlight and his program on the rise. And because the school could support growth, the money quickly followed. In 1999, Polglase and his staff began building an internal system for Duke Club members regarding donations and season tickets. The system — based on a points scale — ranked members in categories and afforded privileges — like parking permits and passes for hospitality tents — based on donation levels. A priority deadline was established (May 15) for season ticket and donation renewals. At first, because demand was low, the deadline was rather soft. That quickly changed after the national title. The most valuable thing, Edmondson said, is something you can't get. When the Dukes traveled to William & Mary in the 2004 playoffs they were allotted 2,000 tickets inside 12,259-seat Zable Stadium, and for the first time, the JMU ticket office had to turn people away.

JMU sold 2,272 season ticket packages in 2004, some of which were partial plans ordered during the season. In 2005, that number spiked to 3,640. In 2006 it passed the 4,000-ticket mark. And in 2008, JMU maxed-out, moving 4,335 season tickets by May 16 — 106 days before the start of the season. "We're light years ahead of where we were four years ago," Polglase said in 2008. "Our season ticket numbers in June of 2007 were where we were in August of 2006. It's jaw dropping. Ridiculous, actually. Winning creates anxiety and now our fans know that if they don't renew their tickets on time, they might not be there when the summer rolls around." In 2008, all tickets for a highly touted showdown between Madison and Appalachian State (aside from those allotted to students) were sold out six weeks before the game — something that rarely happened aside from Family Weekend and Homecoming. Seats were moving for as high as $150 each online. The game drew a Bridgeforth-record crowd of 17,163.

Being maxed-out, Polglase said, was a great problem to have. So was an increase in membership. For years, he explained, there had not been an emphasis on creating a culture of giving back. That became the Duke Club mission and it filtered down to the Student Duke Club, enabling the university to connect with potential donors while they were students, instead of waiting until they graduated. The Student Duke Club began with 123 members in 2000 and steadily increased to 708 in 2004 and 926 in 2005. But in 2006, thanks to campus awareness and consistent success in football, that number ballooned to 1,691. Sumner, who believed the 2004-05 academic year would be a turning point for the organization even before the Dukes began their season, had emphasized the need to retain members — and not just sign new ones — during her tenure as president. This meant increasing committee involvement. When JMU began to win, active participation was needed. It was the perfect forum to build numbers. "Look, there are a lot of perks to joining [the SDC]," Sumner said. "But now it's not just about the free T-shirt and the restaurant discounts. People who are involved tend to come back." In 2004 the Student Duke Club was named Duke Club Chapter of the Year. By 2008, the SDC was 2,000 members strong.

SDC's growth matched the growth of its parent organization. In 2004, according to Polglase, the Duke Club was raising about $465,000 a year and its annual increase consistently was between eight and 10 percent. In 2005, that number cleared $650,000, a 43-percent spike. By 2008, the Duke Club was raising $1-million a year. "[Back then] we weren't even engaged in discussions about when we could potentially raise a million dollars in unrestricted, cash Duke Club gifts," Polglase said. "All of a sudden, we were having that conversation daily."

By 2008, less than a decade after the university made a conscious decision to revamp its capabilities regarding athletics marketing and fund raising, JMU Sports had turned a 180 in terms of its ability to promote teams, fund programs and involve people. In football, the turnaround was dramatic. Winning and marketing led to an increase in ticket sales, donations and revenue. The jump in popularity made it easier to find willing donors with deep pockets for larger projects, like improvements to facilities, which (along with winning) enabled Matthews to sign better recruits and increase the end product. "When Mickey took the job I think he knew where it could go," Matt LeZotte said. "The facilities, apparel, sound system improvements all make it attractive for new students. That scoreboard — I'm not joking — recruits players."

By 2006, with the completion of the Athletic Performance Center and the installation of synthetic FieldTurf, JMU's football facilities had moved from the middle of the pack to among the best in I-AA. These upgrades, along with the new scoreboard, better video equipment and replay capabilities were not products of the 2004 title run, they merely coincided with it. "Coincidence is an interesting thing," Jeff Bourne said in March of 2005. "We laughed along the way in the playoffs and said, 'Wouldn't it be nice to open [the APC] and have people walk into the hall of fame area and stare at a national championship trophy?' And little did we know, that's what happened."

While the facilities upgrades worked with the title run to push JMU football to the next level, the timing wasn't planned. That would have been a bit too much to believe anyway. "We didn't put up the video scoreboard because we thought we were going to win a national championship," Dudley mused. And he was right. Madison simply was fortunate to have all its moving parts come together at once. The program also benefited from a resurgence in popularity for I-AA football. In the 10 years before JMU's title run, the emergence of the BCS and, perhaps more importantly, BCS money, caused an abrupt downturn in I-AA visibility. National network TV, newspapers, magazines and major sports Web sites, which at one time devoted a good deal of time and space to I-AA, opted to squeeze coverage and give more play to the big boys. This coincided with a number of top-flight I-AA schools — perhaps lured by the potential of big bowl money — making the jump to I-A, like Idaho, Marshall and Buffalo.

New powerhouses emerged in relative obscurity. Youngstown State won four championships in the 90s; Georgia Southern won back-to-back titles in 1999 and 2000. Both received little recognition until the coaches from those schools (Jim Tressel and Paul Johnson) received I-A jobs at Ohio State and Navy. But by 2003, ESPN, with little college football to air between Thanksgiving and Christmas, was broadcasting I-AA playoff games on its Gameplan package. In 2004, the Dukes played both William & Mary and Montana on ESPN2 in primetime. And in 2006, Madison's opening-round ESPN game at Youngstown was shown in high-definition.

The I-AA level received its biggest boost in 2007 when two-time national champion Appalachian State stunned Michigan, 34-32, on opening day in The Big House. The Mountaineers, America's new Cinderella and the visible face of I-AA football, would win their third straight national title that December. Division I football's lower class had its swagger back. Attendance at the national championship game increased every season from 2003-07, and while ASU had a stronghold on the national title, the overall level of I-AA football — and competition for recruits — was on the rise. The Dukes were right in the thick of it. In 2008, with attendance between 90 and 105 percent capacity for three straight seasons, JMU's push reached the wrecking ball, as the university announced plans to permanently enlarge Bridgeforth Stadium for the first time in three decades — not to make the jump to I-A, but to keep up with its new peers, namely Montana and Appalachian State. Once an afterthought in its own community, the program now was at the front of the I-AA arms race.

Chapter 14

PETE SLOAN'S second half kickoff bounced through the back of the end zone for a touchback and the James Madison offense began the third quarter on its own 20-yard line. Halftime adjustments by both teams would be on display on the opening drive, though the Dukes and Grizzlies likely were sticking to their original plans. "We're gonna dance with the one that brought us," Mickey Matthews had said in reference to his running game. And while Montana would try and turn the second half into a high-octane track meet, JMU would try to wear down the Grizzlies and keep the ball on the ground.

Justin Rascati opened the second half by handing the ball to Maurice Fenner, and the bruising tailback rumbled through the middle for 11 yards. After pounding the ball between the tackles on their second-quarter touchdown drive, the Dukes believed their ground game could not be stopped unless Montana overloaded against the run. That was a dangerous gamble given Rascati's accuracy, but one the Grizzlies might be forced to make. Montana had done nothing defensively in the first half to change perception. "We had a basketball game at Virginia Tech the day after we beat William & Mary," Gary Michael recalled. "Curt [Dudley] and Mike [Schikman] picked me up to drive down, so I got to watch the first part of Montana's semifinal game." Michael's observation: "These guys don't have the athletes to chase us on defense," he told Dudley and Schikman.

Madison came back to the line with Fenner in the backfield and three receivers. As Rascati crouched under center he saw the Grizzlies bring up a linebacker, leaving slot receiver Nic Tolley with an open running lane. Rascati fielded the snap, took a three-step drop and rifled a pass to Tolley, who stretched over the middle for a 13-yard gain. Tolley's eighth catch of the postseason gave the Dukes another first down, and with each passing minute, the JMU offense appeared to zero-in on the best way to attack Montana. Tolley had been a reliable target all season. When he and Rascati saw the blitz coming both instinctively checked to a quick pass. "We call that a sight adjust," Rascati said. "When we face a blitz we know to check to an alternate route designed to beat that blitz. He saw what I saw and knew how to beat that coverage."

Adjusting at the line was something Tolley and Rascati did with success during the 2004 season. Tolley, Rascati noted, was one of the smartest players on the field — almost like a second quarterback. Durden and former Madison offensive coordinator Eddie Davis had drilled their receivers to read coverage, and Tolley was JMU's best at finding open space. "Nic was one of the best receivers I've been around at reading the zone," Durden said. And Tolley atoned for physical shortcomings by being the most observant person on the field — even making it a point to know his teammates' responsibilities on every play.

Tolley was an overlooked linchpin of the JMU offense. The 6-foot-1 redshirt junior came to Madison as a skinny walk-on who lacked size and speed, but had good hands and athleticism. Tolley's father, Jeb, had lettered in gymnastics at Old Dominion in the 1970s and owned the largest gymnastics center in Virginia Beach. Nic grew up in the gym. He started competing at age six, and at 13 he finished second in the Region 7 all-around competition, which included the top gymnasts from New Jersey, Delaware, Pennsylvania, Maryland, West Virginia and Virginia.

Gymnastics, Tolley said, improved his strength and flexibility, and kept him injury-free. A background in activities that emphasized body control (gymnastics, ballet) had long been helpful to football players, especially receivers. Though slow for his position, Tolley was light on his feet and earned second-team all-district honors as a senior at Kempsville High School. Tolley was the poster-boy student-athlete. He had the top GPA on his high school team and later would be an Atlantic 10 academic honoree. After his senior year in football he ran winter and spring track for the first time, and his individual championships in the 110 and 300-meter hurdles helped lead Kempsville to the Beach District team title. "I had never jumped over a hurdle before," said Tolley, who began competing in the events halfway through his first season. "I asked my coach if he'd let me try it." That was Tolley, perhaps not the best athlete, but certainly a versatile one. "Deceivingly athletic," Matt LeZotte said. "You wouldn't understand it from looking at him but he was an incredible athlete."

Curt Newsome recruited Tolley and believed he could help the Dukes at receiver. He had a hard time selling Matthews on the idea. As a high school senior, Tolley weighed around 160 pounds and ran the 40-yard dash in a shade under 4.7 seconds. His team ran the Wing-T offense and he caught only 15 passes during his senior year. Tolley sent a few game tapes to Madison and Newsome's immediate response was to ask Tolley if he had anything better. Matthews and his staff were skeptical. Sure Tolley was athletic and had good hands. But could he take a hit? Did he have the speed and strength to get open? "[I think] coach Newsome had to convince coach Matthews to take a chance on me," Tolley said. "I think part [of it] was because I knew how to long snap and hold for field goals."

That probably didn't hurt. Tolley, after all, didn't add up on paper. "When Nic came here as a freshman he was this skinny kid," Matthews said. "He was just a guy. [But] I did think he could be one of those players who could get faster and stronger." The Dukes put Tolley on a rigorous lifting program during his redshirt season. Madison strength and conditioning coach Jim Durning, who played for Matthews at Marshall and worked with him on the Georgia coaching staff in the late 90s, was religious about the weight room — especially in the offseason.

Durning would put his players through daily workout sessions, often turning agility exercises into competitions to motivate the kids. The Dukes might have struggled in the early part of the decade on the field, but they never were out-conditioned, largely thanks to their strength program.

Durning, because of the size of the staff and the delegation of authority, had more direct contact with more players than any other Madison coach. While the Dukes sharpened their camaraderie on the field, they built the base in his weight room. "I think he was a big part of our synergy," Sid Evans said. "We weren't the biggest, fastest or strongest team, but we worked great together. He made us the best we could be." Durning was a constant presence, and over time, he helped the Dukes develop a mental edge. "The fourth quarter was Jim Durning time," said defensive tackle Brandon Beach, himself a future strength coach. "We thought we were physically more prepared than any team we played."

Tolley was a player who dramatically improved on Durning's watch. He'd push sleds, run cone drills, lift weights and do station workouts (agility drills designed to emphasize cardiovascular fitness) to build strength and quickness. In the years before the Athletic Performance Center, the Dukes did their lifting in a team weight room located beneath the east stands of Bridgeforth Stadium. It wasn't very spacious and players often had to share racks. Tolley frequently was stationed next to backup offensive guard Mike Jenkins — a hulking 6-foot-5, 290-pound brick wall, who looked like a cross between Vin Diesel and Mr. Clean. "Mike would have to steal some of my 45-pound plates when he squatted because he lifted so much," Tolley recalled.

Years three, four and five of the Matthews era were dominated by youth and the Dukes threw Tolley into the receiver rotation as a redshirt freshman. He played in 11 of JMU's 12 games in 2002, catching 16 passes for 191 yards. As a sophomore, those numbers doubled to 32 catches for 420 yards and three touchdowns. The more Tolley worked in the weight room, the faster he got. He bulked up from 165 to 190 pounds and shaved his 40 time to 4.59 seconds. Tolley thrived in Durning's program (after graduating he admitted he missed the early-morning workouts). Effort pulled him up to par with more talented players. "I definitely was not fast enough or strong enough [to be very successful]," Tolley admitted. "I had to use other assets to play. I always felt that if I slacked a little it would seem like a lot compared to other players."

Matthews thought Tolley's drive came from a need to prove to people that he could play at a level above his normal ability. He blocked well — a must for any JMU wideout — and made tough catches over the middle. He was Madison's best route runner. "No one was better going through the middle," D.D. Boxley said. "L.C., me and Ardon were young. Nic and Tahir were the leaders who showed us how it's done. Nic was the smart one. When we had a question he always put us in the right spot."

Tolley became known for the constant turf burns on his forearms — a painful result of diving and being tackled on Bridgeforth Stadium's unforgiving AstroTurf. Every day, Matt LeZotte watched him apply ointment to his arms. "Just wear sleeves, Nic," he'd joke. But Tolley didn't like wearing sleeves. "He was a competitive, hard-nosed player," LeZotte said. Rascati, who would play several years in arena leagues after graduating, called Tolley one of the toughest players he ever met. Hinds had better size and Boxley had better wheels, but neither carved out space in the middle of the field like Tolley. Years later, Boxley remembered that Tolley blocked more safeties than corners, a testament to his toughness. He seemed to relish the role. "We looked up one day and he was a real physical-looking guy," Matthews said. "Around August of his third year I realized Nic was our best receiver."

Tolley was a competition fanatic, which explained why he responded so well to Durning's workout routines and why he had a knack for winning — no matter how bizarre the forum. LeZotte joked that Tolley loved pancakes more than any person he ever met. During one late-night excursion to IHOP, Tolley and a few teammates asked their waitress what the restaurant record was for most eaten in a single sitting. Told it was 27, Tolley proceeded to eat 28. "The original buttermilk ones — full sized," he emphasized. Go figure. "Pancakes and turf burn," LeZotte deadpanned. And years later, he could not stop laughing about it.

...

TOLLEY ENJOYED another fine season in 2004, catching 36 passes for 395 yards. His value was in his reliability, but Rascati argued that Tolley's athleticism made him more than just a possession receiver. Many people deserved credit for the growth — namely Davis, Durden, wide receivers coach Tony Tallent and fellow receiver Alan Harrison. "He might laugh if he reads this, but Alan was my mentor," Tolley said. "He showed me that it's possible to be a star receiver even if you don't run a 4.4 40." This piece-meal education taught Tolley how to find open space, be physical at the line and use his body to separate the defender from the ball. Tolley's gymnastics background supplied the rest.

LeZotte and Rascati intentionally threw the ball higher to Tolley because it favored his athleticism. Tolley was graceful in motion; not shifty like an elusive tailback, but smooth like a dancer. He had an aerobic quality about him. "It was body control and balance," LeZotte said. "I remember him making a few tough catches, staying on his feet and picking up extra yards when any other receiver would have probably fallen down."

This control, combined with his knack for finding space, made Tolley a technically superior receiver — albeit one without 4.3 speed or a seven-foot wingspan. Tolley might never burn a cornerback deep (his longest collegiate reception was 29 yards) but he had the brains to read a defense, the discipline to run crisp routes and the body control to adjust on the fly. "A lot of his best catches were made on adjusted routes," LeZotte said. "Nic had a feel for space and understood scenarios."

In Madison's quarterfinal playoff game against Furman, with the Dukes trailing 13-7 late in the fourth quarter, Tolley lined up in the slot on first-and-10 from the JMU 41-yard line. Rascati had just completed back-to-back passes to Boxley, and Durden thought it was time to hit the Paladins over the middle. That meant Tolley or Tom Ridley — who had developed into Rascati's other reliable target on intermediate throws

— as the primary receiver. As the Dukes came to the line, Rascati and Tolley surveyed the Furman defense. The Paladins were in zone coverage and the zone routes called for Ridley to run up the field and occupy the outside linebacker, giving Tolley room to sweep underneath the defense for a quick pass. "I ran a drag to that side of the field," Tolley said. "When the strong-side linebacker went with Tom there was no one left to cover me." Tolley caught a short pass from Rascati and circled around defenders before being tackled at the Furman 37. The 22-yard catch showcased what the Dukes did best through the air: Read the defense, adjust the route and stretch the play.

There were those who believed Tolley was an overachiever. They had a hard time selling him and Matthews on that notion. "I think the best way to describe Nic was he was a late bloomer," Matthews said. "I don't think he overachieved because he was a heck of an athlete to begin with." Matthews wasn't dogging his player's work ethic. It's just that Tolley raised the bar for his head coach. Once a player proved he could do something once, Matthews expected it to happen with regularity. As far as he was concerned, Tolley's 84 career catches and 1,007 career receiving yards were not overachievements; they were reflections of his true capability. To Matthews — and teammates — Tolley simply maximized his potential. "He was really determined to prove he could play major college football," Matthews later said. "We were the beneficiaries." Yet Tolley didn't think he proved anything. Perhaps, teammates thought, self-motivation was the real source of his drive. Tolley convinced himself every day that he needed to earn his roster spot. Given his production, that mentality was a bit drastic. Nevertheless, it worked.

The drive carried into the classroom. Tolley arguably was — along with Matt Magerko — the smartest player on the JMU roster. He majored in business management, was named entrepreneurship student of the year and business management student of the year as a senior, and graduated magna cum laude. He was a bookworm and a realist. "I knew I wasn't going to the NFL," he said, "so I had high expectations of myself academically." Even as a senior, Tolley often stayed home to finish his work early instead of going out, a rarity for any college student. A good number of the Madison players underwent similar philosophy shifts during their careers. Priorities changed, Sid Evans said. Tolley, for one, was focused. Procrastination didn't really exist for him. "He was very disciplined," LeZotte said. "He and I had a few classes together and the reason I passed a lot of them was because he was around to help." LeZotte, an honors student in high school, likely was kidding, but he recognized that Tolley was a milestone-oriented player and student — that when Tolley completed a task, he often moved on to the next challenge.

This was an important concept for the Dukes, because Tolley, though a redshirt junior, was on track to graduate in four years and had been dropping hints that he might stop playing after the 2004 season. The debate would continue through the following spring. Tolley loved the camaraderie, the energy and the thrill of playing — heck, he even loved Durning's 6 a.m. workouts. But his grandfather passed away a few months after the national championship and Tolley was anxious to help with the family business. "He and I used to ride to school a good bit," said LeZotte, who lived with Tolley and was nearing the end of his own playing career. "We talked about taking the next step in our lives and a few times we had conversations [about him not coming back]."

Tolley wanted to wait until after the season to make his decision. But Matthews, who LeZotte believed had an uncanny knack for understanding his players, knew — given Tolley's approach and academic resume — that it was a possibility. "Nic was different," he said. And Matthews wouldn't be surprised either way. If Tolley came back in 2005 the Dukes would welcome him, but something told Matthews that the national title game would be Tolley's last in a Madison uniform. If it was, and if this catch against the Grizzlies was his last, it was a fitting final reception. Rascati had put a little extra on the throw. The pass was up and away from Tolley's body, causing him to stretch for the ball and maintain his balance as he glided into the secondary. He made it look easy.

Fenner gained two yards on first down from the 44, but a holding penalty on Magerko pushed JMU back 10 yards. Rascati countered with a 17-yard draw that crossed JMU into Montana territory. The halftime break didn't seem to be helping the Grizzlies, who, with the exception of the holding penalty, had given up 11, 13 and 17 yards on the first three plays of the second half.

The Dukes set up shop on second-and-three from the Montana 49. Rascati barked the cadence, turned to his right and handed the ball to Alvin Banks.

...

OF THE 63 scholarship players on the 2004 JMU roster, perhaps none entered to as much hype as the tailback from Hampton. That was the territory that came with high-impact players in high-profile positions. Like all other sports, the buzz generated by football fans was enormously devoted to the game's superstars. Alvin Banks certainly played the part.

Banks was a talented player from the state's unofficial athletic factory: Southeast Virginia — the 7-5-7. He appeared born to play football, and developed into an elite tailback under the watchful eye of Hampton High coach Mike Smith. Banks was on Hampton's 1998 state championship team and rushed for 1,302 yards as a senior in 2001. At 5-foot-10 and 215 pounds, Banks was "a heck of a player coming out of high school," according to Matthews. His footwork was good and his speed was solid; he had soft hands and he blocked well. Smith — the winningest high school football coach in state history — had a way of making his great players believe they were special. Banks certainly fit into that group. "He coached some of the best," Banks said of Smith. "You listened very carefully. The environment I grew up in produces some great athletes. In high school I felt like I was already playing against college-level talent."

Banks was self-assured — sometimes even brash — when it came to his ability. It wasn't limited to football. Confidence was not an issue for him. His mother was a teacher and his grades were solid. He excelled wherever he applied himself and had, what Schikman later called, a "winning personality." Matthews, trying to turn around the program, loved Banks' mental makeup. "Alvin was always talking," he said. The Dukes recruited him heavily. The second-team all-state honoree was perused by several schools during his junior and senior years at Hampton — including West Virginia — but ultimately was spurned. "They came to my school, watched my games and had me up for a few visits," Banks said of the Mountaineers. "And when signing day came there was no offer." It was discouraging for Banks. He committed to Madison — a steal according to Matthews — and set out to prove his worth.

Naturally gifted, Banks initially didn't appear to value preparation. He arrived in Harrisonburg overweight and out of shape. Matthews let him have it. "Initially we played him at fullback because he weighed about 230 pounds," Matthews said. "He looked like he didn't work out at all that summer." Matthews wouldn't stand for a player who wasn't prepared and Banks had to earn his way into the tailback rotation — a sobering experience for the heralded freshman. The Dukes sent him to the weight room. It was a wake-up call for Banks and he spent most of his freshman season working hard and letting his play do the talking.

Coming to camp out of shape gave Banks a one-way ticket to redshirt purgatory, and he sat out the 2002 season. Yet from his first college drills, he looked like a Division I tailback. "I remember he was very highly touted," Curt Dudley said. "There was a buzz about him." When Banks touched the ball, heads instinctively turned to watch as though a big play was imminent. Maurice Fenner was bigger and Raymond Hines shifted gears smoother, but even as a freshman, Banks was Madison's best all-around back. Dudley recalled talking with Matt LeZotte during one spring practice. "A.B.," LeZotte told him, "is the real deal."

Banks had the inside track at the starting job entering his redshirt freshman season, impressing Matthews enough to have the coach refer to him as the bell cow of the program. He also kept the brash statements in check, opting instead for modesty that endeared him to veteran teammates. Banks understood the hierarchy. Still, there was no doubt he and the Dukes thought his ceiling was high. "I think he's going to be a great player," Matthews said. "I don't think there's any doubt about that."

By August training camp, Banks was itching to play. His assurance, which began as a quiet evaluation of self-worth, slowly evolved into a cocky confidence as he grew comfortable. "I'm not looking for the 2- or 3-yard gains," he told Mike Barber in training camp. "I'm looking for the 30-yard runs every time I touch the ball." Banks could carry himself with humility all he wanted, but he would never hold back from who he was, even with a microphone in his face. His boldness was a big reason he was here. To lose that confidence would be to lose his edge. "I am," Banks later famously said, "an entertainer."

Initial impressions were validated in JMU's 2003 opener, when Banks torched Liberty for 157 yards and a touchdown. It was a pushover game for the Dukes, who beat the Flames, 48-6, but Banks did his part to entertain. He played to the crowd, added an electrifying 35-yard run in the first half, and the JMU students responded by serenading him with "Banks for Heisman" chants. "I kept telling Clint Kent how nervous I was before the game," Banks recalled. "Expectations were high but they kept giving me the ball. If I'm in front of a bunch of people I'm going to try and play perfect."

While the game was a tune-up, the performance was an unveiling. "During his freshman season I thought Alvin could be the greatest back in JMU history," Schikman said. To do that he would have to topple some big names — Warren Marshall and Curtis Keaton to name two — but on that warm August night in 2003, Banks was without limits.

A.B. would flash signs of brilliance throughout his first season, finishing with four 100-yard games and a JMU freshman record 895 rushing yards. But Banks was streaky. He looked jittery in a 21-carry, 53-yard effort against Virginia Tech in Week 2, bruised his ankle against

UMass in Week 5, missed the Villanova game, and was a non-factor against New Hampshire. By the end of the season, Matthews, who initially thought Banks could be the best tailback in the conference, reduced his young star's role. Maurice Fenner, much more consistent throughout the season, saw more playing time down the stretch, and Banks, despite rushing for more yards in a season than any JMU back since 1999, began to face criticism regarding his durability. "That became the big question," Barber said. "Alvin would run the ball, go down, limp off and he'd come back a few plays later. I don't know if that means he wasn't tough [because] he tried to play through things — but yeah, I think he had a lot to prove."

Facing criticism, even after a record-setting season, Banks talked about getting into better shape to help absorb hits. He stayed in Harrisonburg during the summer, improved his prep work and waited for the 2004 season to start. Banks likely was safe at the top of the tailback rotation anyway. Matthews could care less about the critics and he was perfectly content using Banks and Fenner in a two-tailback system. He later said the decision to reduce Banks' role was a personal challenge for him to be more physical. Banks took the challenge seriously. He had the second-most carries in the A-10 South in 2003, finished sixth in the conference in rushing yards and felt he had received very little acknowledgement for a strong rookie season. "Essentially he was out to prove something," Jeff Durden said. And Matthews kept Banks hungry, often calling him the best back and saying he had to be tougher in the same breath. "Alvin was the type of kid who seemed to show his skills more when he was pushed," Dudley said. "That's what I noticed at practice. Matthews would get on him like he gets on anyone and it would tick A.B. off and he would run for 150 yards that Saturday."

Detractors noted that Banks never looked like he was trying. Blessed (and perhaps cursed) by his talent, Banks appeared to be going half-speed even when he was working hard. "You know that 2+2=4," he explained. "The game just came naturally to me." But Banks looked more explosive and focused in 2004 training camp. He received an inadvertent boost from Durden, who wanted his tailbacks to be all-purpose players — receivers, blockers and runners. "I felt like it was built for me," Banks said. "Get me outside with those little DBs, get me in open space with a linebacker covering me."

Durden aimed to. Banks was challenged throughout camp by the faster, more explosive Fenner, but he was a better receiver and blocker. "As far as the total package, Alvin was ahead of [Raymond and Maurice]," Ulrick Edmonds recalled. Banks, according to Durden, was JMU's superback, and he played like one through the first month of the season. Pushed to be more physical, Banks gained 108 yards on 15 carries against Lock Haven and ran for 86 yards and a touchdown in the monsoon against No. 5 Villanova. "He wanted to prove to everybody he could be a healthy back," Durden said. "And he was delivering."

The Dukes traveled to Morgantown for a late-September meeting with Big East power West Virginia, a game Banks circled when the schedule was released that summer. These were not the Mountaineers of Steve Slayton and Pat White — that was a few years down the road — but WVU had Rasheed Marshall at quarterback, Chris Henry at receiver and Adam "Pacman" Jones in the secondary. The Mountaineers were coming off a New Year's Day bowl game and were ranked No. 6 in the country. Despite the daunting task, the Dukes expected to contend. "I actually saw the guy who recruited me," Banks said. "I wanted to play well and prove I belonged on that field."

Banks, for one, delivered. With Fenner nursing a shoulder injury, Banks rushed 30 times for 109 yards. Matthews later called it the best game of his career. It certainly demonstrated the difference between 2003 and 2004. Unlike his uneven performance against the Hokies, Banks was bruising in Morgantown. The Mountaineers were sluggish out of the gate and the teams were scoreless at the end of the first quarter, but a missed field goal by David Rabil and a pair of Madison fumbles quickly turned the game into a rout. Banks, winded from his performance, fielded post-game questions from a folding chair and gave even responses. He looked frustrated. Matthews certainly was. "We turned a 17-3 game into 45-10," he said. "I didn't know if we could beat them [but] we came over here to beat them. We came over here to take the game into the fourth quarter with a chance to win. Those two turnovers took us out of it."

Was Matthews posturing? After all, the Dukes hadn't scored against a I-A team since 1998 and hadn't beaten one since 1990. But the 35-point loss also wasn't a great indication of the game. The Dukes were pissed off for letting things get out of hand. They saw no victory in playing one good quarter of football. "People are just going to think we got blown out," a frustrated Tony LeZotte told reporters. LeZotte, just a freshman, was sending a message that the Dukes were embarrassed. They would not tolerate another performance like this one. Looking back, he and Matthews point to that afternoon in Morgantown as a critical moment of the season.

For some of the West Virginia fans, however, the Dukes — like Banks — already had proven themselves. When Dudley got back to his office that night he received an e-mail from a WVU fan. It read: "For a Division II team you guys are pretty good!" Dudley laughed. "I had to explain things a little bit," he said. "But I guess it's the thought that counts." The West Virginia players were more aware. Later that season, Mountaineers fullback Owen Schmitt placed a phone call to his high school friend and JMU student Reid Gadziala. "Your boys," Schmitt told him, "are going to win the national championship."

The Dukes rebounded the following week with an impressive 31-21 win over Hofstra. Banks, gaining confidence each day, rushed 19 times and caught four passes for 150 all-purpose yards — his most balanced performance of the season. He certainly was living up to Durden's "superback" nickname. What Banks could do better than any other JMU player was make people miss. Early in the third quarter, with the Dukes and Pride tied at 14, Banks took a handoff from Rascati on a power run to the right. "Everyone missed their block," Matthews recalled. "The tight end missed; the fullback missed; the tackle missed; the pulling guard missed. We did not block one person."

Banks gained 35 yards.

At 3-1 overall, the Dukes were beginning a five-week run to the top of the I-AA polls. Banks finished the season's first month with 421 rushing yards and the respect of his critics, who had no angle for complaint. A year earlier, Virginia Tech coach Frank Beamer told Matthews that he wished he had Banks on his roster. It was a flattering comment, and one that Banks was earning as his career progressed. Nearly three years after being spurned by West Virginia and 10 months after being passed over for conference rookie of the year honors, Alvin Banks had arrived. He woke up on Oct. 3 as the most productive tailback in the Atlantic 10, the focal point of the conference's best rushing attack, and with a nagging pain in his left leg that wouldn't go away.

...

THE FRACTURE affected a non-weight-bearing bone. That was the good news. The bad news was the injury likely would put Banks out of commission for five weeks. Somewhere during the first quarter against Hofstra, Banks felt something wrong. "I took a low hit and it felt like a pinch in the side of my leg," he recalled. "I tried to play through it. There wasn't any swelling or pain but something wasn't right."

Banks thought it was a break and X-Rays confirmed it. Matthews, who thought highly of Banks, felt sorry for him. Banks was the closest thing the Dukes had to a superstar. He generated a lot of buzz and carried himself with so much self-assurance that it was hard to remember that he was a 20-year-old kid. Banks generally handled his business and was fun to coach. Aside from nagging injuries, he was extremely low-maintenance. At the end of his career, Matthews met with Banks to talk about preparing for the NFL and it was one of the few times Banks had been in the head coach's office. Years later, Matthews only complained that he sometimes played with too much confidence. "And really, what's wrong with that?" Matthews said. "What was sad about his injury was he had just played his best game. I was on him so hard about being more consistent and he did that against West Virginia."

Ironically, after being called soft at the end of his freshman season, the toughness that Banks demonstrated in September resulted in an injury that would shelve him until Thanksgiving. "I saw [Alvin] that morning on crutches and he told me what the deal was," Dudley said. "And I thought it was one of those blows that can turn a good season into an average one."

Six games passed. Banks slid out of the conference's top 10 in every major rushing category. But the Dukes, behind their big offensive line, kept moving forward. Fenner ran for 288 yards and two touchdowns in wins against UMass, Maine and Richmond. When Fenner separated his shoulder against VMI, Raymond Hines replaced him and Fenner also was regulated to the bench. For five games stretching from early November to early December, the tandem that the Dukes planned to ride all season was non-existent. Hines, now shouldering the running game by himself, passed both Banks and Fenner with four 100-yard games in five weeks.

Banks and Fenner played sparingly in Madison's first two playoff games, combining for only 26 all-purpose yards in wins against Lehigh and Furman. Banks seemed particularly out of sync. He was hit hard once in each game and fumbled the ball both times. When Hines went down with cracked ribs in the national semifinal against William & Mary, a healthy Fenner came off the bench and rumbled for 117 yards in his place. Banks — still slowly rounding into form — saw limited action, carrying the ball eight times for 30 yards and adding a fourth-quarter touchdown run to put the game out of reach. "We ran a sweep to the right during that game and Alvin liked that play," Durden said. "He had a nice run and I think there was a good collision at the end of it. I think that's when he started to come back to form and trust his stuff again."

There likely was another reason. Banks loved the spotlight. He also loved playing in Williamsburg because it was close to home. Durden thought Banks wanted to play on national television and show everyone he was a healthy, dangerous tailback again. In the week leading to the national championship game, the swagger returned. For the first time in two months Banks was healthy — maybe not 100 percent, but certainly enough to make some noise. After all, he was the entertainer, a home run hitter who made people miss. The Dukes felt like they were back in September. Banks ran for 19 yards and caught two passes in the first half against Montana, and was pleased to see the leg holding up just fine.

As Banks lined up behind Rascati on second down, his big-play potential hovered over the field. It had been nearly three months since his last dominant performance and more than a year since his electric opening act against Liberty, but Banks still was a showstopper. There was no doubt he would play a large role in the second half, Matthews thought. It was just a question of when it would happen.

...

BANKS THRIVED when he got into the secondary, and the JMU offensive line was built to run-block. Matthews loved to line up his front five and bulldoze through teams. But the Madison line also was mobile, and so the Dukes could both overpower and outmaneuver opponents.

Banks took the handoff from Rascati and sprinted toward the middle of the field. To his left, Corey Davis cut down defensive end Mike Murphy and blitzing free safety Matt Lebsock. The block also caused blitzing linebacker Adam Hoge to alter his route and circle around the corner. Next door, Matt Magerko and Leon Steinfeld drove their defenders upfield. Banks shifted slightly to his left, aiming for the rapidly increasing hole in the middle of the Montana defense.

Banks crossed the line of scrimmage and saw nothing but open field. Later, a review of the game tape showed Steinfeld blasting through Montana defensive tackle John Cahill and then engaging linebacker Nick Vella. After Davis blocked Lebsock and forced Hoge to the outside, there wasn't a Montana player left in the middle of the field. Steinfeld and Davis had taken five defenders out of the play.

Banks stormed upfield and crossed the 40. At the 35 he cut back to his right against the grain of the Montana secondary. Ducking and weaving his way through traffic, Banks reached the Montana 21 before Shane MacIntyre slammed him to the ground. Banks popped to his feet and let out a short yell. D.D. Boxley nodded his head and smacked the side of Banks' helmet. The 28-yard gain was JMU's biggest offensive play of the night.

Fenner replaced Banks in the backfield and took the ensuing handoff from Rascati. He powered his way up the middle for 10 yards, dragging two tacklers with him until Tuff Harris finally brought him down at the 11. Five plays on the drive and each had gone for at least 10 yards. The Montana defense was losing its grip. "Montana is in trouble," Trevor Matich said. "They're in danger of getting worn down."

Durden was ready to punch one into the end zone. He called a play-action rollout on first-and-10 and gave Rascati the option to run or pass. Rascati took the snap, faked the handoff to Fenner and rolled toward the JMU sideline. He gave a half-pump at the 15 and veered on an angled path for the pylon. "Once I got outside the defensive end I knew I was running," he later said. Rascati wasn't one to slide or slip out of bounds; he'd rather pick up the extra yards and worry about his body later. "At the last second I realized I had a shot for the end zone," he recalled.

Tahir Hinds set a block on Montana cornerback Kevin Edwards at the goal line and Rascati charged forward. Hinds had been bothered during the second half of the season with a painful ankle injury, but he outweighed Edwards by 20 pounds. Rascati wrapped the ball with both hands, felt someone grab his legs and dove for the end zone. As Rascati neared the corner in mid-leap, Matt Lebsock dove at him from the left and the collision sent Edwards, Hinds, Rascati, Adam Hoge and Lebsock crashing to the ground. Hinds, Edwards and Lebsock landed out of bounds. Hoge wound up at the goal line. Rascati fell on top of the pylon, squeaking through for JMU's second touchdown of the night.

David Rabil's PAT hit the right post and ricocheted through the uprights — his second fortunate bounce of the evening. In a game of inches, the Dukes were benefiting from all the breaks, and with 11:55 to go in the third quarter, Madison led by 10.

Chapter 15

ON THE Montana sideline, Craig Ochs waited for his turn. After opening the game with immediate success, the Grizzlies had failed to score on their last four possessions, leaving the door open for JMU to settle itself. Now the Dukes were swinging like a heavyweight fighter eyeing a knockout. Montana had to answer. For the first time all night, the Grizzlies were in danger of being swept away.

Montana began its first drive of the second half on the 25 and Ochs started quickly. Back-to-back completions to Tate Hancock and Willie Walden gave the Grizzlies a first down at the 40. On the next play, a controversial pass interference penalty on JMU linebacker Kwynn Walton advanced Montana to 46. From the broadcast booth, Walton appeared to arrive just after the ball deflected off the hands of Levander Segars. Instant replay verified it, but the penalty stood. Mickey Matthews didn't need the replay to know what he saw. As the Grizzlies approached the line for their next play, a sideline camera cut to Matthews screaming at an official about the call.

The Grizzlies came to the line with four receivers and Lex Hilliard in the backfield. Ochs lined up in shotgun, faked a handoff to Hilliard and tried to run up the middle, but was met behind the line and dropped for a loss by Trey Townsend. As Ochs picked himself off the ground, JMU safety Mike Wilkerson smacked Townsend on the helmet in approval. Townsend hopped up, nodded his head and clapped his hands. After having moderate success running the ball on its first drive, Montana's ground game had been silent and Townsend was a big reason why. He had been all over the field in the first half and this latest tackle was his sixth of the game.

Townsend was part of Matthews' first recruiting class. An all-region Wing-T quarterback at Central-Lunenburg High School in Victoria, Va., Townsend was a member of two district championship teams. He was a star basketball player and an all-state hurdler, but his high school was small and he was not recruited heavily. Townsend had been offered an academic scholarship from Virginia Tech. He didn't think he'd play football in college, but a meeting with Matthews and Madison linebackers coach Kyle Gillenwater opened the door late in his senior year. Townsend was happy just to have a chance to get on the field again. He passed on the scholarship at VT and enrolled at JMU. The Dukes extended him an invite to training camp nine days before the preseason started.

A late edition to a veteran team, Townsend sat out the 2000 season and moved from defensive back to linebacker the following spring. He saw significant playing time on JMU's 2-9 team in 2001, a year he later called the most "unpleasant" of his career. "I've tried to think of a better word but I can't," he said. "The meetings were unpleasant; practice was unpleasant; being together was unpleasant. People just didn't smile as much and you didn't hear anything good coming from the media. It was a bad situation to be in."

Townsend was one of many holdovers from that 2001 team. And he wasn't exaggerating when he described his first season. The Dukes lost nine straight games from Sept. 8 to Nov. 17. But that team was the foundation for this one. They grew up together. And if there was a silver lining — especially for Townsend and Walton — it was that they were able to learn the college game at one of the only positions where the Dukes had ample veteran talent. Madison was loaded at linebacker in 2001 — a big reason why the Dukes allowed only 19 points per game. The group was anchored by national defensive player of the year Derrick

Lloyd, who registered 157 tackles, 7.5 sacks and five forced fumbles. Lloyd was the unanimous A-10 defensive player of the year and the most feared linebacker in I-AA football. "It felt like he had 20 tackles every game," Matthews later said. "[Derrick] was the best defensive player we'd ever had. He was a dominant football player."

Lloyd was a game-changer. He also was part of a long line of great JMU linebackers. The lineage dated back to the 1981 season when Clyde Hoy became first defensive player in program history to earn All-America honors. In total, seven Madison linebackers achieved this status from 1981 to 2001 and the Dukes had a linebacker on every All-American team from 1984 to 1988. In 2001, Townsend and Walton were backups to Lloyd, Derick Pack — a second team AP All-American in 1999 — and Dennard Melton — a future two-time all-conference honoree. Townsend and Walton combined for only 31 tackles that season, but watching Lloyd, Pack and Melton had an overwhelming impact on the two freshmen. "The biggest thing [Lloyd] showed me was the confidence to think you can make every play," Townsend said. "He seemed to make every tackle. Pack had a similar impact. They had the desire to make every hit."

Matthews believed Townsend and Melton were cut from the same mold. Both were superior athletes who the Dukes had to train to become linebackers. Melton, a team captain in 2003, was an easy-going guy and a player who preached the advantage of mental legwork. He made 161 tackles and recovered three fumbles in his senior season. Townsend recalled many games when his predecessor would react to plays as though he had been inside the offensive huddle. "It was like he knew the play before the ball was snapped," Townsend said. "He recognized formations and just reacted to them. Derrick Lloyd and Derick Pack told us there comes a time when the game slows down for you."

Townsend hoped hard work would slow the game for him the way it did for Lloyd, Pack and Melton. He was a good all-around athlete and had great hands. Townsend intercepted three passes, recovered two fumbles and totaled 199 tackles in his first three seasons. But he was undersized for the position. "Trey always knew where to be and he always had speed," Rodney McCarter said, "but he wasn't heavy enough to make the plays." Indeed, Townsend, at barely 210 pounds, was closer in weight to McCarter (a defensive back) than Melton. Still, he was very observant, "like a quarterback playing linebacker," Mike Barber once said.

Ironically, Townsend probably could have been a quarterback had Matthews given him the opportunity. Townsend was part of a huge recruiting class that included two-way star Rondell Bradley and Matt LeZotte, who Matthews pegged as the face of his new program. When Townsend arrived as a walk-on, Matthews knew little about him. "I knew his high school team ran the Wing-T," Matthews said. "I never asked him to throw the ball because he had quarterbacked an offense that always ran."

Matthews would kick himself for years over that assumption. LeZotte and Rascati developed into fine quarterbacks, but Townsend had a better arm than both of them. During a Thursday afternoon practice in 2003, backup quarterback Jayson Cooke stood near the 50-yard line and began throwing passes across the field. Townsend joined him. "Trey was throwing as far as Cooke, so Cooke started backing up," McCarter recalled. "They started throwing 60 yards, then 65, then from one knee. It became a bit of a competition."

Matthews couldn't believe it. "He could throw the ball 70 yards," he later said laughing. "I told my coaches I should have let him throw the ball because we probably would have left him at quarterback. Our linebacker had the strongest arm on the team." More than likely, however, Matthews simply missed this hidden talent because Townsend wasn't high on the Madison totem pole. LeZotte was a coveted recruit who Matthews had been eyeing since his days as an assistant at Georgia. Townsend was a recruited walk-on. Later asked if he could out-gun the Madison quarterbacks, Townsend laughed. "I had a pretty good arm but the accuracy wasn't where it needed to be," he said. Too bad. The Dukes, who later would employ a spread offense anchored around running quarterback Rodney Landers (3,468 yards rushing and 3,288 yards passing in his career) ironically could have tried it years earlier with Townsend under center.

Townsend, perhaps because of his age (he turned 22 the previous July) and his experience (five years in the program) was one of JMU's clear leaders. The Dukes had plenty of upperclassmen (including LeZotte and Leon Steinfeld) who took charge in the locker room, but Townsend was the closest thing the Dukes had to an ambassador. Bright, inquisitive and always alert, Townsend majored in finance, served as Madison's representative on the student-athlete advisory committee and was an A-10 academic honoree. His experience as a quarterback, his polished demeanor and his work ethic were evident. Townsend was a starter for most of his career and was a co-captain — along with LeZotte, Steinfeld and McCarter — in 2004.

Gillenwater called Townsend "steady" and that likely was the best way to describe him. Townsend was even-keeled, polite and knew his responsibility extended beyond the field and the classroom. He, along with LeZotte, was a go-to guy for the media. It wasn't surprising. Matthews referred to Townsend as JMU's "poster boy" and it wasn't clear if he was talking about the football team or the entire school. Townsend was so articulate and respected that Matthews was convinced he'd go into politics. "I've always thought Trey would be running for governor in a few years," Matthews said. "He's a physically handsome guy with a great family and a brilliant mind. You don't get to coach too many like him."

Townsend later dismissed the politics notion with a laugh. "I take it as a great compliment," he said, "but I don't see myself as a political type." Reagan himself couldn't have given a more courteous answer. But Townsend, whose father, Arthur, was elected as Lunenburg County sheriff in 2006, insisted that most of the Madison seniors were leaders in their own right. He used words like "responsibility" and "accountability" regarding his classmates. The Dukes clearly benefited from their experience. Twelve starters — including five of the nine spots on the offensive and defensive lines — were seniors. The Dukes, Townsend argued, didn't need rah-rah leaders because they knew what was expected. "We didn't have a lot of people who were spitting and yelling and getting in people's faces," defensive end Sid Evans added. "I think we were very positive for the most part."

After playing outside linebacker for most of his career, Townsend shifted to the middle in 2004 when JMU switched to the eight-man front. The transition caused him to revamp his style of play and focus on stopping the run. Akeem Jordan had the inside track at the starting job in training camp, but Townsend eventually earned it back. He became a rock for the JMU defense, starting every game and finishing the 2004 season with 102 tackles, three forced fumbles and 2.5 sacks. He tied for the team lead with five interceptions — a feat Matthews attributed to Townsend's good hands and experience as a high school quarterback. "He really understood offenses," Matthews later said. "Trey was an excellent pass defender."

Townsend's partner over the middle was more of a physical marvel. Kwynn Walton was a human bulldozer — big, fast and powerful. He could bench-press 405 pounds. He hit people with ferocious intensity and was a high-octane force on the field. On game day, the Dukes would huddle prior to kickoff in a team tradition that Townsend could only describe as "rowdy time." Walton led the charge. "In that sense, Kwynn was a spiritual leader for us," Townsend said. "He was a motivator." To complete the package, Walton wore a neck roll underneath his jersey that made his upper body look like something out of a science-fiction movie. He and Townsend were listed at nearly same height and weight in 2004, but while Townsend was impressive physically, Walton looked like Iron man in a football jersey. Facing him in tight space was a nightmare scenario for an offensive player.

Walton was an intimidating presence and thought the mental and physical battles were closely related, teammates said. "Kwynn wanted offenses to be scared of him," Townsend said. "He definitely wasn't looking to be buddies with anyone from the other team." For Walton, the preparation began early. He was a workout fanatic and seemed hell-bent on creating any possible physical and mental advantage. Matt LeZotte recalled that Walton was full of extra energy on game day, pumped up to the point of frenzy. "We'd be in the locker room before a game and Kwynn would be doing dips just to make his arms look bigger," LeZotte recalled. "He had huge arms as it was, but your arms and calves are the only muscles that show when you're wearing football pads, and he wanted his arms to be gigantic."

A Rochester, N.Y. native and former state player of the year, Walton began his playing career as a tailback, rushing for 2,112 yards as a junior at Aquinas High School. He played safety in 2000 at the Bridgton Academy in Maine before transferring to Madison in January of 2001 and shifting to linebacker. The position moves seemed logical given Walton's size, power and physical presence. Still, his career developed slowly. Walton bounced into and out of the starting lineup in his first three seasons. He generally progressed as a player, but it wasn't a steady ascent. Brilliant performances were offset by mediocre ones. Off the field habits were similar. Walton, Matthews recalled, had a discipline problem early in his Madison tenure. It wasn't anything defiant, but even an occasional lack of responsibility rocked the boat at Camp Mickey. "If we had a meeting at 9 a.m., he thought it was OK to walk in at 9:05," Matthews said. "We were always struggling with Kwynn. His behavior was a bit mischievous."

Blessed with incredible talent, Walton acted like he was above coaching and his play reflected this perception. "Kwynn was a hard head," McCarter said. "He didn't want to listen. He had all this strength but he didn't have control of it." Matthews briefly suspended Walton before the 2004 season. Somewhere during that time, sources close to the team believe that Walton grew up and started listening. "He progressed a lot," McCarter agreed. "He started putting speed with strength." The Dukes had very few issues with Walton the rest of the year. "He worked hard with the coaches and just blossomed," Matthews recalled.

Walton, like Townsend, rallied to earn a starting job in the final weeks of training camp, a commonality between two decidedly different players. Townsend rose above his lack of size and a position change. Walton overcame himself. He enjoyed his finest college season in 2004, finishing with 88 tackles and a team-high 7.5 sacks. He and Townsend — perhaps taking a cue from their predecessors — were everywhere on the field. Walton stuffed the run; Townsend did a bit of everything. "Trey was the all-around one and Kwynn was the downhill one," McCarter said. Years later, Tony LeZotte would credit them for his breakthrough freshman season. "You just look at the tape and the guys who were coming to block me were turning inside because Kwynn and Trey were so dangerous," LeZotte said. "Opponents had to pay special attention to them. They were physical and smart. Teams knew they would make plays if they weren't blocked."

Townsend and Walton were steady performers. But like most of the Dukes, they had turned things up late in the season. Walton registered a season-high 14 tackles against Delaware and had two sacks in Madison's playoff win over Lehigh. His play in 2004 earned first-team all-conference and third-team All-America honors. Townsend barely missed joining his teammate on the all-A-10 team (announced at the end of the regular season) and responded with what Matthews later called "our best defensive performance in the playoffs."

Townsend had been hiding a hamstring injury for most of the season. "I pulled it during the second game," he said. "I went through a lot of games just trying not to hurt it." He played the rest of the regular season at about 85%, but when the playoffs started, he said, there was no holding back. Snubbed by voters and pushed back to the second all-conference team, Townsend totaled 20 tackles and forced a fumble in playoff wins over Furman and William & Mary. "I wish they had made that all-conference team announcement in September," Matthews later quipped, "because [Trey] played his best football after that. He played like a house of fire."

...

OPPONENTS KNEW how important Walton and Townsend were to the Dukes. But the JMU defense — much like its offense — did not revolve around a core group of players. Instead, the '04 Dukes were an orchestra with interchangeable parts. Townsend and Walton were rocks in the middle, but talented sophomore Akeem Jordan was a capable backup. Sid Evans, Frank Cobbs, Brandon Beach and Isai Bradshaw saw the bulk of the playing time on the defensive line, but Chuck Suppon, Kevin Winston and Demetrius Shambley started games as well. The Dukes were so deep that Jordan — a future NFL starter — started only two games.

JMU blanketed its opponents in 2004 with the country's best pass rush. Seven Madison players had at least four sacks. The Dukes had 56 by the end of the season and forced 33 turnovers. This made life especially difficult for opposing quarterbacks. Some — like Lehigh's Mark Borda — avoided turning the ball over but took too many sacks. Others — like Delaware's Sonny Riccio — stayed off the turf but threw too many picks. Of the 14 quarterbacks who faced the Dukes in 2004 only two had successful starts. The first was Rasheed Marshall, who picked Madison apart in West Virginia's 45-10 win in Morgantown. The second was Lang Campbell.

The William & Mary quarterback knew about JMU's vaunted defense better than most. Campbell wasn't playing tonight because the Dukes sacked him twice and forced the Tribe into committing five turnovers a week earlier in Williamsburg. Townsend had been a primary catalyst, making 10 tackles and causing a fumble in Madison's 48-34 win. But Campbell was in Chattanooga for championship week anyway. He had been honored the night before, winning the Walter Payton award in a lopsided vote. In a year marked by great quarterbacks — including Ochs, Sam Houston State's Dustin Long, Eastern Washington's Eric Meyer and New Hampshire's Ricky Santos — Campbell was in a class by himself. He tossed only one interception during the regular season (a product of his quick release and accuracy) and threw for more than 3,000 yards. In a season where William & Mary finished with a school-record 11 wins, Campbell and the Tribe ran the gauntlet against perhaps I-AA's toughest schedule. Three of W&M's regular-season games were against A-10 heavyweights JMU, Delaware and New Hampshire — another was against Division I-A North Carolina. All were on the road. The Tribe had home-field advantage throughout the playoffs, but Lang's Legion certainly earned it.

Campbell led W&M to a 2-1 regular-season record against its fellow A-10 playoff teams, sneaking past New Hampshire in a rainy 9-7 win, falling to the Blue Hens, 31-28, and beating the Dukes, 27-24. He threw for 355 yards and four touchdowns against Delaware — a game in which the teams combined for 836 yards. Three weeks later, Campbell and the Tribe made the trip across the state to face the Dukes. It was a homecoming of sorts for Campbell, who starred for Handley High School in nearby Winchester. The Dukes, coming off their 20-13 win over the Blue Hens, were 8-1 overall and 6-0 in the conference. The Tribe entered at 7-2 and 5-1. The winner had the inside track at the A-10's automatic bid to the playoffs.

The teams staged a heavyweight fight worth remembering. Campbell was nearly flawless, completing 26 of 33 passes for 323 yards and a pair of touchdowns. But the JMU offense, which was so ineffective the week before against Delaware, was just as good. A second-quarter touchdown pass from Rascati to Boxley gave the Dukes a 10-3 halftime lead — part of a seesaw battle between the teams that included two lead changes and four ties. JMU would rush for 272 yards on the day (198 coming from Raymond Hines) but the Madison defense was porous. JMU had set out to prove that its defense could slow down Campbell. Instead the Dukes became another clip for his portfolio. "You talk about an annoying guy to play against," Tony LeZotte later said. "Lang was very smart and they tossed the ball all over the field. He knew exactly what to do in that offense."

Campbell drove the Tribe down the field with brutal efficiency. He broke free when he was cornered and completed passes when any other quarterback would have thrown the ball away. Down 17-10 and facing third-and-10 from the JMU 40, Campbell connected with Adam Bratton for a 35-yard gain. On the next play, he hooked up with John Pitts on a five-yard scoring strike to tie the game.

Knotted at 17 in the fourth quarter and facing third-and-one from their own 35, the Dukes tried to run Rascati up the middle on a quarterback sneak. Rascati plunged forward and extended the ball across the line of scrimmage, looking for extra yardage. It was, Matthews later said, a foolish mistake by a young quarterback. "You're never supposed to stick the ball out in traffic," he preached. Rascati knew this, of course, but he needed the yard. "I tried to make a play," he later said. "I had it and then it was gone."

Chris Ndubueze knocked the ball loose and it was recovered by W&M. Three plays later, the Tribe were in the end zone. "I thought that was the game," Matthews later said. But Rascati atoned on the next possession. He led the Dukes on an 11-play march down the field, picking apart the Tribe with precise passes. Antoinne Bolton, filling in for Hines, contributed a big 15-yard run on the drive. With less than a minute to go, the Dukes faced third-and-11 from the W&M 27-yard line. In the huddle, Rascati relayed the play to his teammates. Less than a minute remained in regulation and the Dukes needed a score.

Rascati took the snap and settled into the pocket. W&M was in a zone defense and the play was supposed to go to the left side of the field. Boxley, on the right sideline, was a decoy receiver. "I was supposed to run off my defender and take him out of the play," he recalled. But there was a breakdown in the Tribe defense. The corner didn't jam Boxley at the line and the safety stayed inside the hashmark. Given a clean release and an open lane down the sideline, Boxley went from decoy to open target. Rascati, facing pressure, rolled to his right and fired a pass to Boxley in the corner for a Madison touchdown. It was a broken play, perhaps as broken as a play can be for both teams, and certainly not the play the Dukes had in mind when they broke the huddle. But the game was tied again. "I got open down the field and I was hoping Justin would see me," Boxley later said. "That was all him [because] the play wasn't supposed to go there."

As the Dukes lined up for the ensuing kickoff, Rascati raced to the back of the Madison sideline and grabbed a headset. Throughout the season (and throughout his career) he proved that while he lacked the athleticism to take over a game, he certainly was capable of changing the outcome. Now he needed to talk with Durden. "We needed a game plan," Rascati said. "We were planning for overtime."

But overtime never happened. Campbell quickly marched the Tribe down the field. He completed all four of his passes and burned his three timeouts. "I was thinking, 'Just try to get into [kicker] Greg [Kuehn]'s range,'" Campbell said after the game. With five second left, W&M was on the Madison 29-yard line. Kuehn, soon to be named the A-10 special teams player of the year, had missed a 32-yarder earlier in the game and was facing a swirling 15-mph wind. The attempt would be from 46 yards out. "Anybody taking bets?" one reporter quipped as the Dukes burned a timeout. "I don't think he's got enough leg."

Kuehn lined up for the kick. Seconds before the snap the wind stopped blowing. "The flags weren't moving at all," Jon McNamara recalled. Kuehn fired a high kick that seemed to drift forever. Then it turned over and fell like a rock from the sky, landing a few yards beyond the crossbar. It was his longest field goal of the season.

Fans did not move from their seats. The Dukes stared as the Tribe celebrated. W&M tailback Jon Smith grabbed Kuehn by the jersey. "I told you [that] you were going to win it for us!" he yelled. The Dukes quietly walked across the field. Sid Evans dropped to one knee and lowered his head into his left hand, sweat glistening on his face. Matthews made his way to the Madison locker room. Finally, the stands began to empty.

After winning six straight games and climbing to the top of the conference, JMU was facing a must-win the following week at Towson. Kuehn had sent the Dukes packing. In the W&M locker room, Tribe coach Jimmye Laycock, a close friend of Matthews and the dean of A-10 football coaches, reportedly held a streamer in the air, dropped it on the floor and ground it with his shoe. The conference title, home-field advantage and the winning streak were over. The reaction among JMU fans — like the hysteria after the win over Delaware — was draining. Many of them (for the first time in years) had expected the Dukes to win. The reward for letting their guard down was a gut-wrenching loss that ended Madison's magic carpet ride. JMU had been flawless for more than a month, seemingly impervious to misfortune, but a fumble by Rascati and a last-second kick had the Dukes on the brink of elimination. "The W&M game was interesting because it was the first time people really cared," McNamara said. "You could see it in their faces." For McNamara, the loss galvanized the fans. Kuehn's kick did not break their faith. It reinforced it.

The Dukes, likewise, were confident. Kuehn and Campbell had knocked them down, but their heroics also masked a large chink in W&M's armor. The Dukes had moved the ball at will against the Tribe. For all its firepower on offense, W&M couldn't stop anyone. "We actually threw the ball too much in the fourth quarter," Matthews later observed. "I thought we coached poorly in the second half." Like their fans, the Dukes were coming to a resolution: If they could beat Campbell, they could beat W&M. The Tribe had a strong secondary and an explosive receiver in Dominique Thompson, but they were a one-man show, while the Dukes were an ensemble cast. The two teams would finish the regular season with the same record. They were nearly even — separated by a few inches and five seconds of clock — but they were decidedly different.

...

CAMPBELL WASN'T a gun-slinging quarterback so much as he was a precise one with a strong arm. But he also had a knack for the dramatic. He threw three interceptions in W&M's first playoff game and had to rally the Tribe for a 42-35 win over Hampton. In their second meeting against Delaware — this time in the NCAA quarterfinals — Campbell & Co. fell behind again. The Tribe trailed the Blue Hens, 31-

10, late in the game before mounting another comeback. Stephen Cason intercepted Sonny Riccio's first pass of the fourth quarter and returned it for a touchdown, trimming the Delaware lead to 31-17. Campbell then completed 10 of his next 12 passes, engineering an 8-play, 57-yard drive to cut the lead in half, and then a 12-play, 68-yard march to tie it, 31-31, with 1:56 left in regulation.

W&M eventually won, 44-38, in double overtime, when Riccio and the Blue Hens came up empty on four straight downs from the Tribe nine-yard line. By that point the hierarchy of the A-10's top teams was coming into focus. Upstart New Hampshire, after shocking perennial power Georgia Southern in the opening round, had fizzled at Montana. And Delaware, with Riccio under center, wasn't the same team that won the 2003 national championship. Despite playing a flawed game, W&M was moving on to its first I-AA semifinal. Three hours later, and more than 400 miles to the southwest, JMU capped its miracle comeback at Furman. The Dukes would have their second crack at Lang Campbell.

Admittedly, the Dukes were pleased to be facing the Tribe. It certainly beat the alternative. Despite defeating Delaware during the regular season and losing to W&M, Matthews thought his team had a better chance in Williamsburg than in Newark. He and Gary Michael spent some time before the Furman game talking about the draw. "We were talking about how terrible it would be to go to Delaware next weekend because Delaware was up 31-10 on William & Mary," Michael recalled. "[Mickey] wasn't taking anything away from Furman — he had tremendous respect for them. But the feeling was that if we could find a way to win we'd have a real tough time going to Delaware."

Midway through the second quarter, the Dukes heard about W&M's comeback. At that point, Michael said, Madison went from being a playoff team to a title contender. Going to Delaware, Matthews explained, would have been a nightmare scenario. "I thought they were better than us," he admitted. "I thought if Delaware had beaten W&M they would have won the whole thing." Matthews thought highly of Campbell but believed his team could out-muscle the Tribe. He didn't sugarcoat his reaction when the Dukes clinched their trip to Williamsburg. "We were thrilled," he said. And to a man, the Dukes agreed. Cortez Thompson said the chance to face Campbell again was an honor, but added that it gave the Dukes a chance to prove they were the better team. Separate interviews with Clayton Matthews and Madison equipment manager Pete Johnson yielded identical responses. "When we beat Furman," they said, "we knew we were beating William & Mary."

The first I-AA semifinal between two Virginia schools took place on a damp but mild December Friday. The week leading to the game unfolded like that of a showdown between rival high schools for a state championship. In Williamsburg, W&M students spray-painted the jersey number of Dominique Thompson on the campus statue of Thomas Jefferson. In Harrisonburg, JMU students scrambled to find tickets during final exam week. The Madison allotment was small and thousands of fans were resigned to watch the game on TV. Media members later wondered how large the crowd would have been if the game was played at a neutral site. Scott Stadium at the University of Virginia or University of Richmond Stadium would have been logical choices, and many believe the Dukes and Tribe could have drawn 30,000 people. Though there was no chance of moving the location, it was fun to speculate.

Rain had soaked most of the state by game day and the mass caravan from Madison was frantic. Campus closed for winter recess a few hours after the final testing session. Across JMU, students tossed clothes into suitcases and duffle bags. Most were going home, but about 2,000 were heading across the state for arguably the biggest football game in the history of the commonwealth. "Imagine if Virginia and Virginia Tech played each other for a spot in the national championship game," one reporter observed, "because that's exactly what this is like for people who follow JMU and W&M football."

Purple Madison flags and "Go Dukes" signs were visible on car windows during the three-hour drive toward the coast. Zable Stadium, intimate, old and tight, was a mad house as kickoff approached. Aside from the weather, the night had a celebrity feel to it. Governor Mark Warner and Senator George Allen were in attendance. They, along with a reported capacity crowd of 12,259 (likely closer to 14,000 with standing room), were witnessing history. This was a night for Virginia, a game between two schools with strong ties to the commonwealth. In one corner was W&M, the country's second-oldest college and the educator of Jefferson. In the other was JMU, named for Madison and centered in the heart of the historic Shenandoah Valley. And in the middle was Zable Stadium, a 69-year-old facility making history of its own. Zable didn't have lights, so temporary ones were wheeled in for the ESPN telecast. Night football had come to Colonial Williamsburg.

With a trip to Chattanooga on the line, the Dukes came out swinging. They needed just five plays on the opening drive to move deep into W&M territory. Play No. 6 was a handoff to Hines. Earlier on the drive, Hines had been hit in the chest on a nine-yard gain and felt the wind go out of him. "It was a little hard to breathe," he recalled. "I thought if I played through it, I would be fine." Hines took the handoff from Rascati and streaked untouched through the middle for a 27-yard touchdown run. He would carry the ball only eight times the rest of the season, but Hines had opened Superfight II with a bang. "That got us rolling," Matthews recalled. "I didn't think they could stop us enough to beat us."

For the first 15 minutes, Matthews was correct. The first quarter of the War in Williamsburg was a purple and gold fireworks show. Minutes after Hines' touchdown, Rondell Bradley, suspended from the team during the offseason after a brush with the law and later reinstated, delivered a jarring hit on W&M punt returner Jonathan Shaw and forced a turnover deep in Tribe territory. Bradley had been a vital part of Madison's rebuilding project and had been a returning starter until he was convicted on misdemeanor charges of assault and battery and property damage in late August. He returned to the team mid-season, mostly on special teams. Years earlier in Williamsburg, Mike Schikman recalled, Bradley had single-handedly shut down Tribe receiver Rich Musinski, W&M's all-time leader in receptions and receiving yards, holding the future All-American to three catches. Back on the same field, Bradley now triggered a barrage. Nick Englehart's punt was high and Bradley crushed Shaw just as the ball was arriving. Isai Bradshaw fell on the fumble at the W&M 25 and the Dukes were back in business.

Three-yard runs by Fenner and Boxley moved JMU to the 19. Rascati followed by hitting Casime Harris in the back of the end zone for a 14-0 lead. On the next possession, Clint Kent intercepted Campbell and returned the errant pass 69 yards for another touchdown. Less than 11 minutes had lapsed in Williamsburg and the Dukes led by three scores. The Madison faithful, overly hyped at the start of the rematch, now were in frenzy. "YOU-CAN'T-STOP-US!" they chanted as the first quarter came to an end. But Matthews knew it was far from over. "They had the best player in the country," he said. "I knew they were going to score points. I thought it would go back and forth all night."

It certainly did. The Tribe tipped the scales all the way back in the next 15 minutes. A Kuehn field goal and two Campbell scoring drives made it 21-17. With Hines banged up and Fenner ineffective, the Dukes were struggling on offense. "Some of us got a little over-excited," Demetrius Shambley said after the game. "We thought the game over in the first quarter, so we really let up in the second."

The game had the abrupt flow of an old wooden rollercoaster — fast-paced, and with dramatic changes in direction. Less than a minute before halftime, Englehart again sent a high punt toward Shaw. This time Shaw called for a fair catch and Bradley ran into him. "The same play that went perfectly in the first quarter went completely wrong in the second," Jon McNamara said. The penalty moved W&M from its 26-yard line to the 41. Campbell promptly drove the Tribe into JMU territory and Kuehn zipped another field goal through the uprights as time ran out in the first half. The three-score lead was down to a single point.

The halftime conversation, Matthews later said, was extremely one-sided. Matthews had been confident that the Dukes would stop the Tribe. But the field, muddy and slippery, bogged down the JMU pass rush and Madison had let W&M back in the game. Though they had turned two Tribe turnovers into 14 points, the Dukes certainly were not in control when the second half started.

The frustration was palpable. Zable, for all its history and aesthetics, had perhaps the most outdated pressbox in the country. Like the one at Madison, it sat low regarding the field, but it also obstructed the view of coaches in the upstairs booths. Durden, who had called games at Zable before, slowly was losing his mind. "I kept yelling at some guy who had a big, gold No. 1 finger waving back and forth in front of me," he recalled. "I couldn't see a thing." Pushed to his limit, Durden climbed out of the pressbox, went into the stands and found the fan. "Dude, you have to put that down. You are killing me!" he yelled. The fan, a Madison student, wheeled around. "Coach Durden!" he screamed. "It's me! I'm from JMU!" Durden shook his head. Obstructed by his own fan. What else could possibly go wrong?

Durden was having a rough night. Next door, Mike Schikman and Curt Dudley were entertaining politicians while calling the game. Governor Warner had joined them in the booth during the first half and the guards cleared people away, giving Schikman and Dudley a clear line of sight. "The best view we've ever had in Williamsburg," Schikman cracked. Warner left after halftime and Senator Allen was slated to join the broadcast in the third quarter. Meanwhile, Campbell and the Tribe continued to roll, taking the second half kickoff and marching down the field for the go-ahead touchdown. A two-point conversion attempt failed, but with 11:37 remaining in the third, W&M led, 26-21. Matthews, despite his fire-breathing halftime speech, later had a Zen-like view of the game. "I knew they'd score," he said. "I just thought that through four quarters they couldn't stop us enough and somewhere along the line we would stop them. I didn't feel any differently before the game, during the game or after the game."

For Matthews, it was a rare sign of inner stoicism. Still, the Dukes were on the wrong end of a 26-0 scoring blitz. "We definitely lost control of the game for a second," Townsend later said. He was off, but not by much. It took the Dukes 37 seconds to take the lead back. A good kickoff return by Ardon Bransford put the Dukes on their 37. Fenner followed with a bulldozing run through the middle and Boxley capped it with his outstretched touchdown catch. In the JMU broadcast booth, Allen had just settled into his seat. "He joined us just before the drive started," Schikman said. "[So] I made him stay with us the rest of the game."

Turnovers and pressure told the rest of the story. On the ensuing W&M drive, Townsend forced a fumble and Kent recovered, leading to a touchdown run for fullback Chris Iorio and a 34-26 Madison lead. On the next Tribe offensive play, Brandon Beach sacked Campbell and forced another fumble, this time recovered by Shambley at the W&M 18. Three plays later, on third-and-five, Rascati dropped back in the pocket, started to scramble and then tossed a pass on the run to a wide-open Antoinne Bolton, who twisted in the air as he caught the ball for another score. The rout was on.

The Dukes would outscore the Tribe 20-6 in the third quarter, on their way to a 48-34 win. Despite the glaring storylines of the JMU running game and the W&M air attack, the difference was possession. The Dukes took care of the football; the Tribe did not. Campbell, playing in his final college game, finished 30-of-39 for 315 yards and three touchdowns, but he was undone by two fumbles and outplayed by the methodical Rascati, who was 11-of-14 for 143 yards and three scores of his own. In total, Madison forced five turnovers and scored 28 points off them. "I don't know how you explain it," Matthews later said. "They hadn't turned the ball over all year." W&M was good enough to beat JMU when Campbell was hot, good enough to win even when Hines ran wild, but they couldn't overcome that many turnovers. The Dukes, Mike Barber wrote that night, had taken William & Mary's best shot, and then delivered one of their own.

...

TOWNSEND'S SIXTH tackle of the national title game brought up second-and-13. With the running game nonexistent, Ochs went back to the air, slipping a pass underneath to Lex Hilliard for 11 yards. On third-and-two he drilled a pass to Segars at the marker. Segars absorbed a vicious hit from Tony LeZotte and his forward progress gave Montana another first down.

Ochs was operating with precision. He swung a pass outside to Hancock on the next play and Hancock slipped his way through the JMU defense for 16 yards to the Madison 28. On the next play, Ochs rolled out of the pocket, bought himself extra time and floated a pass to Segars for 11 more yards. For the first time since the opening drive, Montana was beginning to exert its own muscle and the Dukes were scrambling to keep up. JMU, McCarter recalled, had emphasized keeping Montana in third-and-long situations, but sloppy play was making that impossible. "We were missing a lot of tackles," he said. "We knew they were going to catch the ball, but we had to make the hits and knock them off their rhythm."

The Grizzlies were on the JMU 17. Ochs again lined up in shotgun, this time with Talmage, Hancock and Segars stacked toward the far sideline. Ochs called for the snap and zipped a screen pass to Segars. Talmage moved outside and put a block on Cortez Thompson; Hancock stepped forward and cut down Tony LeZotte. Segars sprinted for the alley between his two teammates, hurdled both Madison defenders and turned on the burners.

From across the field, McCarter saw the play developing. The Dukes, he later recalled, were in Cover-2 and he was responsible for the back side of the field, opposite to where the ball was thrown. Thompson was supposed to contain the alley along the sideline and force Segars to run at LeZotte. But the Grizzlies had out-schemed the Dukes on this play. "There are three receivers and only two defenders out there to handle this," Rod Gilmore later said. Thompson couldn't contain and LeZotte couldn't make the tackle. They were cut off.

McCarter saw that Segars had a shot at the corner and he had the best chance to catch him. He drove hard, tearing toward the pylon on a collision course with the Montana receiver. McCarter would be arriving at a 90-degree angle with Segars. If he won the race to the corner he had a good chance of saving a touchdown.

Segars was flying and McCarter appeared to be losing the race to the corner. "I was surprised at how fast he was," McCarter said. "He didn't look that fast on film." McCarter launched himself in the air, a final attempt to make up for lost time. As the two players neared the goal line, McCarter was completely horizontal. Segars shrunk himself and lowered his right shoulder to absorb the hit, causing McCarter to partially pass over him. "I wasn't sure if he got in," McCarter said years later. "I just dove for it." As McCarter clipped past Segars, his forward progress took him into the pylon and out of bounds. Segars spun to the ground and slid across the goal line for Montana's second touchdown.

Dan Carpenter's kick sliced through the uprights. The JMU lead was down to three.

...

ASIDE FROM the turf, which by now looked like the infield at the Kentucky Derby, people had to be pleased with the 2004 national championship game. The 16,771 fans marked the highest title-game attendance since 2000, and with JMU clinging to a 17-14 lead midway through the third quarter, the two teams — though different in style — were evenly matched. It was a welcome contrast to the previous year, when Delaware annihilated Colgate, 40-0. And although the field was an embarrassment, it hadn't significantly lowered the quality of play. Penalties were at a minimum, and as Ardon Bransford awaited Pete Sloan's kickoff, neither team had turned the ball over.

Bransford had bounced around the Madison roster. The Harrisburg, Pa. native rushed for 1,888 yards and 25 touchdowns as a senior at Central Dauphin High School. Not surprisingly, he began his JMU career as a tailback, but the Dukes were loaded at the position. Bransford switched to corner and then was converted into a receiver before the

2004 season. He caught 20 passes for 295 yards and three touchdowns, and carved out a spot as JMU's most reliable kick returner. Bransford gathered Sloan's end-over-end kick at the two and returned it to the Madison 26. In a tight game, field position was crucial and, so far, both teams had managed to stay away from the shadow of their respective end zones.

The Dukes began the drive by handing the ball to Alvin Banks and Banks carried to the 29 before Nick Vella and Dustin Dloughy brought him down. After rushing for 19 yards in the first half, Banks now had 50 for the game, and with each carry he appeared to be gaining confidence.

Madison came back to the line on second down with Rascati in shotgun and Banks to his right. Rascati took the snap and moved toward the far sideline. Dloughy cut him off from the corner and Rascati pitched the ball to Banks. It was the first option play JMU ran all night.

Rascati's pitch was ahead of Banks and the JMU tailback had to fully extend his right arm to catch the toss. As Banks brought his left hand around the ball to corral the pitch, he lost control. The ball slid up his forearm and fell toward the ground. It hit Banks in the shin and rolled up the field. Banks stumbled forward but he was too late. The ball rolled to the 29 where Nick Vella slid and recovered it. In the broadcast booth, ESPN announcer Rod Gilmore thought this could be a window of opportunity for the Grizzlies. "That pitch was a little in front of him and he couldn't one-hand it," Gilmore said, "and now you have a short field for Montana."

On the Madison sideline, the large personnel exchange was underway. The Dukes lost 20 fumbles in 2004 — more than Delaware and W&M combined — and had just seven more takeaways than giveaways. Conversely, Montana was plus-23 in the turnover department for the season. If the Dukes had a statistical weakness it was their inability to hold onto the football. "That was frustrating," Durden later said. "If he catches that then he's gone." Likewise, Matthews couldn't fault the play, just the execution. "We run the option every week at practice because it's a check against the blitz," he said. "It was the correct check. He just dropped the ball."

With a chance to regain the lead, Ochs and the Montana offense came back onto the field. The machine started quickly. Ochs connected with Jon Talmage and the big wide receiver broke three tackles before Walton dragged him down at the JMU eight. The Grizzlies were knocking on the door and the Dukes — after playing brilliantly from the beginning of the second quarter until now — were about to watch their lead evaporate.

Ochs was flushed from the pocket on first-and-goal by Kevin Winston and threw the ball away. On second-and-goal, the Grizzlies came to the line with Ochs under center and three receivers. Ochs called for the snap, took a five-step drop and looked over the middle for Willie Walden.

It's difficult for a 275-pound tight end to be slight of hand, but as Ochs dropped back to pass, Walden took a few steps forward, stopped and turned around at the five-yard-line. Ochs looked directly at Walden and the moment of hesitation caused Tony LeZotte and Kwynn Walton to bite. As the two All-Americans broke for the apparent pass, Walden pivoted and split them down the middle. Ochs waited and then lofted the ball down the field. The pass floated just over Townsend's outstretched hand and Walden caught it as he slid through the back of the end zone for a touchdown. "[Ochs] was the one guy who concerned Mickey all along," Dudley later said. "The quarterback was the X-factor and right there he became Triple-X."

JMU had taken firm control of the game at the start of the second half. Now, Montana had answered impressively. The Grizzlies erased a 10-point deficit with two lightning-quick drives, successfully tipping the game's tempo back in their favor. Carpenter banged home the PAT. The Grizzlies led, 21-17.

Part V: Baby Bulls

Chapter 16

THE DIFFERENCE between the 2003 and 2004 Dukes was obvious at face value. One team was mediocre; the other was playing in the national championship game. Still, a closer examination countered the notion that the '04 team was dramatically different from its predecessor. Both offenses were built around a strong running game. Both teams had playmakers. The rosters were remarkably similar. In fact, Tony LeZotte and Rascati were the only impact starters missing from the 2003 roster. Yet neither represented the greatest upgrade between the two teams. That distinction went to Leon Steinfeld, a burly fifth-year senior and one of many offensive holdovers from Project Ground Floor.

Steinfeld, like his classmate, Trey Townsend, was a walk-on player when he arrived in Harrisonburg in the summer of 2000. He came from a military family and grew up in Virginia, North Carolina, Colorado and Japan. His most recent stop had been New Orleans, and so that was listed as Steinfeld's hometown on his player biography. His family ties to Madison (uncle Woody Bergeria was a JMU Hall of Fame defensive end) were as strong as any place he had lived. Despite earning all-state honors as a high school senior, Steinfeld did not give much thought to playing football in college — or attending college, for that matter. And so, when it was time to pick a school, Steinfeld applied only to Madison and only because of football. "I had been to a few JMU games as a kid," he said, "so I sent film to see if they were interested."

The Dukes were interested enough to invite Steinfeld to camp, and he played as a reserve defensive lineman during the 2000 season. In 2001, as a true sophomore, he shifted to the offensive line, first at guard and later at center, where he anchored a young group that included George Burns, Jamaal Crowder and Mike Jenkins. These four players, coupled later with Harry Dunn, Matt Magerko and Corey Davis, became Matt LeZotte's main bodyguards.

Steinfeld, even as an underclassman, was an outspoken leader and clubhouse cut-up, a player who instinctively knew when to be serious and when to have fun. This trait was vital in the development and preservation of the Dukes' collective psyche, because as far as statistics go, the Madison linemen were overwhelmed. "We had five guys who didn't know each other," Steinfeld said. "I think a big reason why Matt got hit so often was we weren't good. We were worried about each other and that's how a quarterback gets hit. Matt suffered because of that."

The Dukes surrendered 70 sacks in 35 games from 2001-03. By comparison, the 2005-07 teams allowed 30 sacks over the same number of games. LeZotte, relatively mobile early in his career, bore the brunt of the mismatch. He never played a full season. "Matt was battered behind a young offensive line for three years," Mike Schikman said. "And the O-line loved him to death. They knew they were the reason he had been beaten up so badly. And they felt horrible about it."

With a bunch of kids on the line and a quarterback running for his life, the Dukes began the arduous process of growing up in the trenches. "A lot of those guys played before they were ready," Mickey Matthews admitted. "We called it the 'dark ages.'" Curt Newsome, Matthews' top assistant and the offensive line coach, deserved most of the credit for pulling the linemen out of futility. Newsome preached a tough, hard-nosed brand of football. The Dukes, he believed, could not afford to give an inch because their youth was an inherent disadvantage.

The JMU line, even in those early years, adhered to Newsome's warning. They played a physical (sometimes chippy) brand of football, and several later were accused of being dirty players. But they surrendered nothing. Newsome, according to Magerko, was a second father for many of the offensive linemen. He was personable and preferred to keep his game plans simple. "His philosophy was to be physical," Magerko said. "We were taught to wear down the opponent and take over the game."

Magerko's words suggested that the Dukes were in the hands of a straight shooter. There was a survivalists' mindset. "Take no prisoners," Steinfeld later said. "Coach Newsome turned us into players who took nothing. All of us had so much pride and we didn't want to give up. We played hard together."

This especially was true along the offensive line, where Matthews aimed to turn his fledgling program into a contender. JMU went three seasons (2000-02) without having a back come close to reaching 1,000 rushing yards. This had little to do with the Madison passing game. The Dukes were a running team; they just weren't very good at it. But Matthews kept preaching development along the line. "There were a couple of people who realized that Mickey had been building a monster," Schikman said. "He was old school in that sense. Run for dough, pass for show." The strategy eventually paid off. In 2003, Banks and Fenner combined for 1,528 yards and 17 touchdowns. And from 2004-08, the JMU line paved the way for five 1,000-yard rushers.

...

NEWSOME, THROUGH genuine affection and an open-door policy, had no trouble building trust with his players. The tough part was getting them to trust each other. Time and talent took care of most of that problem. Crowder, a 6-foot-3, 300-pounder from Temple Hills, Md., spent most of his college career at tackle, where his good footwork made him a solid run and pass blocker. He was the laid-back member of the group. Crowder was a poetry lover and one day would publish his own collection of works. Writing, even more than football, was his passion. He majored in English and helped mentor the generation of players who followed him into the program.

Crowder took Davis under his wing in 2003. "I was out with him when I came on my recruiting visit," Davis recalled. "We liked the same music (mainly R&B). Jamaal handled his business. He was smart, got good grades; he was good in the weight room, too. Jamaal was the cool guy."

Crowder and Steinfeld were consistent starters in 2001. Burns, a heady, hard worker, entered the rotation the following year. He paired with Magerko, a transfer from Virginia, to give the Dukes two rocks at offensive guard. A fellow 300-pounder, the 6-foot-2 Burns was a gritty competitor. "The meanest, toughest person I ever played with," Steinfeld said. Burns was a technician. He was not blessed with great athleticism or a height advantage, but he had good instincts. In later years, Burns and Crowder would be the forgotten men of the 2004 offensive line, lost behind Steinfeld's leadership, Magerko's drive and Davis' talent. But they were vital. Schikman later referred to Burns as "the single-most underrated lineman in JMU history," and as a player who, if his talent had matched his heart, could have made a run at the NFL.

Burns was a complex character. His teammates believed he was a little crazy. "He was off the wall," Magerko said. Burns had a sarcasm that was tough to read. Davis admitted that he rarely knew when his fellow lineman was being serious or kidding, that Burns "was totally out of control in every way possible." This, however, wasn't obvious to the casual observer, because Burns could be downright generous, even to complete strangers. A pair of freshman students once walked into D-Hall and unwisely filled their lunch trays with food without first finding a place to sit. They wondered aimlessly through the packed cafeteria until Burns offered two seats at the end of the table he and his teammates were sitting at.

Still, Burns was best known for his daily antics. Pressed for examples of his teammate's finest work, Magerko could only pause. "There's probably nothing I can say that should be printed," he laughed. Steinfeld however, was willing to offer a few G-rated anecdotes. "Someone once dared George to eat a brisket with mayo and wash it down with half-

and-half," he laughed. "They said he'd never do it. George just looked at him with this grin. He finished the whole thing."

Burns held the starting job at right guard from 2002-04, starting 35 games over that stretch. Magerko — a brains and brawns combination who would graduate magna cum laude — manned the other guard position. Like Steinfeld (6-foot-1, 295 pounds), the 6-foot, 280-pound Magerko was considered undersized at a position where Burns was the prototype. But those who believed Magerko did not have the size to be successful underestimated his intelligence, athleticism and stubborn will.

Magerko had been a two-time state wrestling champion at Northumberland High School in Farnham, Va.; he also lettered in football and track, and was a second-team all-state soccer player. Wrestling was his passion sport. On the mat, Magerko was in total control. He wrestled at Virginia for a year before transferring, later saying he didn't fit in on the team or at the school. JMU was his only option. "I had played in an All-Star Game with Clayton and a few of the guys," he remembered. "I thought I had a pretty good connection with them."

So Magerko packed his bags and trekked west. He broke into the starting lineup midway through the 2002 season, displaying a rare combination of speed, balance and power. Magerko turned a weakness into a strength. His squat build and relatively light frame made him susceptible to power rushers and bigger defensive tackles. But in JMU's power and zone blocking schemes, Magerko became a weapon. Bigger linemen struggle in open field; Magerko thrived. He could chip a defender into Steinfeld and then blast forward to engage a linebacker. "You never expected Matt to be able to match up with those bigger defensive linemen every week," Schikman observed. "But he was so smart — maybe the brightest football player I've ever known. Offensive linemen are never given enough credit. In general they're the smartest players on the field because they have to know everyone's assignments. I think Matt's intelligence made him a great player."

His teammates, meanwhile, preferred to focus on his drive. Magerko was a mule, "a fighter who didn't know how to lose," Steinfeld said. He was accountable. Above all else, there was an unspoken competition among the linemen. "We didn't want anyone to beat us," Magerko explained. "And you certainly didn't want to be the guy who lost it for the group." Magerko believed camaraderie was necessary. He spoke gently and properly, and was rather benign off the field. But between the hashmarks, where he and his teammates relied on each other, Magerko was ultra competitive. "Determined," Davis said, "is a good word to describe him." Magerko and several teammates started growing their hair out during the 2003 season. They repeated the process in 2004, and as the Dukes began winning, it became a sign of good luck. "We didn't want to jinx it," said Magerko, who also grew a Fu Manchu mustache. This look gave him an intimidating boulder-like presence, like that of a Roman warrior on the field of battle.

This would be the core of the line for the rebuilding years under Matthews. Dunn and Jenkins rounded out the original mix, both starting in stints between 2001 and 2003. Jenkins, a physical freak, was 6-foot-5, 290 pounds and looked like a bodybuilder. "Mike was a man-child," Steinfeld said. Jenkins was a transfer from Kent State, had lettered in football, basketball and lacrosse in high school, and was one of the more recognizable Dukes around campus. He shaved his head, wore earrings and spent most of the offseason in the gym. A few Madison students referred to him as "Vin D-Hall."

Dunn, meanwhile, was 6-foot-7 and 325 pounds, a three-sport captain at Surrattsville High School in Clinton, Md. and one of the largest men ever to play for the Dukes. Asked to describe Dunn in one word, Davis didn't hesitate. "Goofy," he said. "Harry was a character." Former *Breeze* assistant sports editor Meagan Mihalko remembered Dunn as one of the nicest players on the team, a gentle giant who majored in health sciences and wanted to pursue a career in public health education. This did not deter Davis. "Yeah, he was nice," he acknowledged. "But he was a goofy kid." Mihalko recalled that Dunn and Davis once tried to bum a ride from the practice field back to the locker room. She took one look at the twin 300-pounders and decided it wasn't going to happen. "I didn't think they'd both fit in my car," she laughed.

It was funny that Davis would describe Dunn as a goofy kid because that adjective sometimes also applied to Davis. A highly spirited talent, Davis blended nicely into the linemen rotation. The group had a distinct, collective vibe. They were cool, laid-back, and, at times, appeared nonchalant. Observers easily could have mistaken them for being lazy. But they handled their business. Davis could have been the poster child for this group, not because he was its leader — that distinction went to Steinfeld and Magerko — but because he reflected its public image. He was a relaxed presence. He was 6-foot-4 and 335 pounds, but had a soft voice that carried the tone and laughter of a child. Perhaps the strongest indication of Davis' personality was his love of music. Davis could not stop singing. He'd sing on the way to class, in the weight room, at practice and during games. "Corey," Magerko later quipped, "thought he was auditioning for American Idol."

The Madison locker room generally was split regarding game-day preparation. In one camp were guys like Steinfeld and Rascati, who preferred to keep things loose before games. The other group included Tony LeZotte and Walton, high-intensity guys who were ready to bust out of their jerseys by kickoff. Matt LeZotte's locker was next to his brother's and he remembered Tony transforming before games. Hours before kickoff, the LeZotte's would do a light workout and throw the ball around at the stadium. When they entered the locker room, Matt would go through some of his mental preparation — snap counts, defensive schemes, blitz reads. After a few minutes he'd glance at Tony. "He'd be listening to music," Matt said, "and he'd go from relaxed to a focused zone. His eyes would change." At that moment, Matt said, he was thankful that Tony LeZotte was on his side.

Davis, meanwhile, was a member of the first group, often relaxing and cracking jokes prior to kickoff. This, at times, even extended into the game itself. Davis, especially in opening quarters, was loose, sometimes jawing with defensive linemen in a form of playful banter. He once was hit hard at the end of a play and shoved the defender in retaliation. The defender got in Davis' face and the two quickly were separated. As they walked away, Davis tapped him on the back of the helmet and ran back to the huddle, laughing. "What I loved the most about playing here was that all the linemen and the guys I came in with — Marvin [Brown], Akeem [Jordan], D.C. (Isaiah Dottin-Carter) — were about having fun," Davis said. "Football was what we loved to do."

Yet Davis had a mean streak, often triggered by seemingly innocent events like a post-play shove. Something would snap. "He'd be singing and laughing and having a good time until someone made him mad," Magerko said. "Then he'd transform." When that happened, Davis went from an over-sized teddy bear to a force of nature — driving, shoving and smacking defenders all over the field. Davis' intensity, Mike Barber noted, was relentless once it started, like an 18-wheeler rolling downhill. He blocked to the whistle, and sometimes past it, rarely leaving a play to chance. In 2005, he and Magerko had a play where they were responsible for the same defender. "We just kept hitting him back and forth between us until the ref threw a flag," Davis said. "He didn't whistle us for unnecessary roughness. He said it was 'excessive blocking.' I had never heard that in my life!"

This was a glimpse into the physical nature of Corey Davis, who had Dunn's size, Burns' mean streak and Magerko's athleticism. He was, without a doubt, the most talented Madison lineman. Newsome had been eyeing him as a potential recruit when Davis was in 10th grade. Back then, Davis was a defensive lineman at Kecoughtan High School in Hampton. He hated offense. "I just wanted to play defense forever and hit people," he said. One night during Davis' junior year, the Kecoughtan offense was struggling and Davis was frustrated. "I came off the field and said something like, 'man I hate offense,'" he recalled. One of Davis' coaches turned to him. "Oh you hate offense?" he yelled.

"Well you're not playing defense the rest of the game. I'm putting you on offense."

From that day forward Davis was an offensive lineman. He found he could hit people just as often and that his physical play was vital to his quarterback's effectiveness. Newsome and the Dukes offered him a scholarship early in the official recruiting process. But Davis had other options and did not immediately accept. He and Kecoughtan defensive back Allyn Bacchus looked to be heading to Virginia until their offers fell through on the same day. That afternoon, both were contacted by Michigan State, which had just hired former Louisville coach John L. Smith. "They told us they were interested," Davis said. "And two days later a guy flies all the way from Michigan to tell us it wasn't going to happen."

Spurned by two mid-level BCS programs, Davis and Bacchus fell back on old offers. Bacchus went to Villanova, Davis to JMU. Both played as true freshmen and were four-year starters. Bacchus would finish his career with 374 tackles. Davis, meanwhile, was considered the final piece to the puzzle on the Madison offensive line, a gifted young player to add to a veteran rotation that was beginning to find its feet. "Corey definitely was mature for his age," Steinfeld said. "The way he played early in his career, it was like he had been there all along."

Matthews was adamant about Davis' potential. He had a great work ethic and the agility of a man half his size. Like many of the Dukes, Davis played pickup basketball in the offseason. It wasn't his sport, but everyone played, and a game of hoops was a good way to get away from football. Instead of planting himself in the low post, Davis often ran the floor with guys like Rascati and L.C. Baker. Still, this wasn't the most startling display of his athleticism. A more accurate one was described during a conversation between Matthews and Schikman during Davis' freshman year. "Mickey sold me on Corey Davis early," Schikman said. "He came up to me and said, 'Mike, this kid is so damn big. And would you believe it, he plays on the damn high school tennis team.'"

Unlike some of his famous "Mickey-isms," this statement was 100%

factual. Davis and a friend had been dragged into a casual doubles match during his sophomore year of high school. There, the varsity coach glanced over and recruited both to fill out his men's team roster. Davis possessed remarkable quickness. He played doubles for three years and cracked the top singles rotation as a senior. And he enjoyed it, though it was clear Davis was a football player who played tennis, not the other way around. "My coach always joked when I did crazy things on the court," Davis said. "I was doing up-downs and then hitting the ball."

Mihalko, a former varsity tennis player at Oakton High School, covered Davis extensively during her editorial stint at *The Breeze* and decided to pursue the angle, even attempting to arrange a one-set match between them as part of a feature she wrote on Davis and Dunn in 2005. That match never took place — though both parties say they wished it had. At Madison, Davis often was challenged by friends and teammates to a few sets. More often than not, Davis surprised them. "People always wanna play me because they underestimate me," he said. "But my boys know. I'd take Marvin and Akeem every now and then and go play. They know what's up."

This was Davis in the raw — lively, entertaining and youthful. After his playing career was over, he'd come back to football games and stand in the front row of the student section (instead of using a guest pass for the home team sideline). Davis would greet old friends, cheer with the rest of the JMU faithful and wave a rally towel in the air. He was, in this sense, a big kid, totally at ease with himself and his friendships, which often were filled with boyhood antics. Davis and his roommates (Brown, Jordan and Dottin-Carter) had a rowdy form of camaraderie, often messing around and wrestling in their rooms. Brown, a fullback, and Jordan and Dottin-Carter, both linebackers, were instigators more often than Davis. One of them would walk into the room and slap someone on the back of the head. Then all hell would break loose. But when Davis was the victim, he often funneled it away. "I'm saving that one for practice," he'd say. No one wanted to mess with Davis at practice, not when a shove or a push could send the 335-pounder into ass-kicking mode. Davis, as a result, would torment the tormentor, a friendly reminder that the room and the field were connected. "I'd get to practice and start talking up how I'm gonna get D.C. or Akeem back for smacking me," he laughed. "I'd be like, 'Oh man, I'm gonna get you now.'"

...

INJURIES AND bad timing prevented all the linemen from playing together consistently until 2004, but Magerko, Steinfeld, Crowder, Burns, Dunn, Jenkins and Davis shouldered the load in combination. The big guys constantly were around each other, lumped together by their athleticism, their camaraderie and, yes, their position. Linebackers hung out with linebackers; receivers hung out with receivers and the linemen hung out together. Dinner trips, parties and workouts were orchestrated endeavors. The pack mentality dominated. Davis later remembered Burns as the leader of this approach. The Madison coaches encouraged the linemen to stay together. "That was the thing," Davis said. "It was 'stay in a pack', don't break the pack,' all the time. George always liked to have fun with that and rip on it. We'd have an early morning workout and he'd be jabbering the whole time 'C'mon guys, c'mon, stay in a pack.'"

But Burns and the Dukes believed in this mentality. Davis, who joined the group as a true freshman in 2003, experienced only an aftertaste of the chaos from previous years. Steinfeld said that was the lone positive thing that came out of the 2001 season. Forced to play at an early age, the Dukes had gelled by the time Davis arrived. They were closer to a well-oiled machine than five separate parts on the field. And off the field, they had developed a strong bond. "You're with each other all the time," Steinfeld explained. "I think all of us combined to have an outgoing personality."

Steinfeld likely was the catalyst on that front, often going from locker room leader to ringleader in a matter of minutes. He was serious about football, but also believed there was no reason to cause stress when it wasn't needed. "He was a vet," Davis said. "He knew when to joke and he knew when a guy was feeling uncomfortable how to make him feel good. He knew how to get people to open up." Magerko was Steinfeld's roommate and described his friend as "peppy," later saying that Steinfeld's outgoing personality was contagious. Even as the Dukes plugged through the monotonous cadence of practice-game-offseason-training camp, Steinfeld made sure they had their share of fun. "[Leon] kind of just had this grin about him," Jeff Durden later explained. "He was the kid who was probably out a few minutes after curfew, and he wasn't afraid to tell everyone what he had done."

Spring ball was an area where Steinfeld excelled in the art of entertainment. Collectively, the Dukes hated April practice. To the coaches, it was a good barometer for the beginning of summer training camp. But to the players, spring ball meant a month of practice with no games in sight. "It definitely was one of the toughest parts of college football," Magerko admitted. "Everyone is going 110 mph and there's still six months until opening night." Asked in passing one spring how practice was going, Rascati rolled his eyes. "Just trying to get through it," he said.

There was one part of April practice the Dukes enjoyed. After the annual spring game there was an open invitation for every player to attend the Mud Bowl — a keg race between the offense and defense — which generally drew about 30 participants. The event gave the Dukes an opportunity to cut loose at the end of a tedious spring. It was known to get wild, and drew both diehards and casual observers. Davis belonged to the latter group. "I was involved [in the race] one time and one time only," he said. "That was enough for me. 'Wow,' that's all I can say."

The Mud Bowl evolved into a tradition, one of many that Steinfeld was the driving force behind. He and Matt LeZotte also organized group trips to Blue Hole, a natural swimming hole in George Washington National Forest. "A lot of things we did together were Leon's ideas,"

LeZotte said. "Usually it takes one guy to be proactive about something. He was the guy."

The Dukes were creative with their entertainment. D-Hall was a popular venue for outrageous dinner platters, like Burns' brisket-mayo special. The players also hosted an annual talent show at the end of preseason, which Davis could not describe without laughing uncontrollably. "All the rookies had to do an act or a skit or sing," he said. "And the seniors did a show, too. They would get one or two of the freshmen and make them be their chairs or footstools. They'd have cups of water and set them on the freshmen's backs and then leave the stage, and the freshmen would have to get up without spilling it all over themselves."

This, Davis stressed, was not a form of hazing (as some would see it), but a bonding experience. "The talent show was always a good time," Magerko added. "It was a great way to break the ice with the rookies and break the stress of camp." Like Nic Tolley's mission to eat 28 pancakes, the dinner dares and talent shows were part of a time-honored code. Guys (especially guys in college, and especially guys in college lumped together by teams, clubs and organizations) do crazy things in the name of bonding. It's an inexact science — friendships formed through anecdotes of stupid fun.

The Madison coaching staff recognized the need to break mundane work and often gave the players necessary slack when it was needed. The final practice of the season was a treat for the seniors, who would pick an underclassman to ceremonially carry them off the field. "Sometimes this becomes very comical," Sid Evans said, "because you'd always have some offensive lineman selecting a defensive back." But this wasn't limited to the end of the year. "If you came to Friday practices," Matt LeZotte said, "you would have seen us running and acting the fool. I'm talking about linemen running pass routes. We had hat day every once in a while and the guys would come in dressed all crazy. Those days were important. It helped us recharge our batteries."

Steinfeld always seemed to be at the heart of this movement. He once had his hair styled in tight, small braids for no other reason than to give people something to talk about. "No significance at all," he said. Than again, this was Steinfeld and these were the Dukes of 2001-04. They spent so much time together, endured so many lumps on the field, that their camaraderie (not their talent or tradition) was the main thread in the fabric of their success. "Leon had this personality that kept all the kids loose," Schikman said, "and I think that was a big reason why he was an effective leader." Meanwhile, Matthews was more on message, in part because the Dukes did a remarkable job of checking the fun-and-games mentality at the door when it was time to work. "Leon and Magerko both were very strong leaders," he said. "They were positive players who were determined to succeed." Schikman and Matthews had made the same point by emphasizing different attributes.

...

THE DUKES were confident entering 2003 training camp. Most of their starters were upperclassmen and many of the talented underclassmen already had game experience. The offensive line, once a weakness, looked to be a strength. Magerko and Burns were entrenched at guard. And Steinfeld, by now the anchor up front, was poised for a breakout season. "He was dominating," Matthews said. "Heading into training camp he was the best player at his position in the league."

It all came crashing down in a hurry. In August, on the first day the Dukes practiced in pads, and on the first full-contact play of the season, Steinfeld pushed awkwardly off his left leg and partially tore his ACL. "I didn't even hit anyone," he said. Initially it was thought to be a minor injury, but Steinfeld spent the next three weeks out of practice. He rehabbed and made plans to play through the season (even with a damaged ACL a lineman can take short, choppy steps and be effective). Meanwhile, the Dukes erupted into a spontaneous game of musical chairs, with Magerko sliding over to play center, Crowder shifting to guard and Davis entering the starting lineup at tackle.

JMU split its first two games (a 48-6 win over Liberty and a 43-0 loss at Virginia Tech) and on Sept. 9, Steinfeld, wearing a brace for support, returned to practice. He promptly tore his left meniscus on his first day back and was lost for the season. He and Matthews prepared to apply for a medical redshirt, which both believed would be granted. "I knew I was coming back," Steinfeld said. And as the burly center awaited word from the NCAA, the Dukes made due without him. They didn't play poorly in 2003, but they were alarmingly inconsistent. Something was missing. Several players later said that a healthy Steinfeld might have been enough to turn the 6-6 Dukes into a playoff team. "It seemed like we were one guy short the whole season," Matt LeZotte said. "The guys we had did a great job. But something was off."

Even Matthews, usually guarded about speculating, was open about the ripple effect on the line. "I cannot emphasize enough how devastating his injury was," Matthews said. "It took a lot of wind out of our sails."

Steinfeld didn't play a snap in 2003. He was granted the redshirt and returned the following season. He was not as good as he could have been the previous year, but Steinfeld was not an interchangeable part; he was a rare commodity. Steinfeld at 85 percent was better than someone else at full strength. Matthews was thrilled to have him back. "You only have to be at practice for about 30 minutes and watch Leon block to realize how much we missed him last year," Matthews told *Breeze* contributing writer Reid Gadziala that preseason. But it was Durden, in his first Madison training camp, who brought Steinfeld's value into proper perspective. "All the other guys took their lead off him," Durden said. "Leon was the thumb that came over the other four fingers. He made the fist."

The Dukes, as Durden implied, had more punch with Steinfeld in the lineup. Magerko, a solid replacement at center in 2003, shifted back to guard. Crowder returned to tackle and now the Dukes had three 300-pound starters (Crowder, Dunn, Davis) for two tackle positions. The depth, in many cases, was too much for defenses to handle. But JMU's toughness was the true difference. Kicked to the ground for years, the Dukes, by God, weren't going to take it anymore. They aimed to turn the trenches into an all-out war zone. Even practice was a rugged encounter. The coaches often lined up the first-team offense and first-team defense against each other — six linemen plus the tight ends vs. the eight-man front — and the two units simply beat the living hell out of each other. "Those were *battles*," Davis said. "That's just the way we were on both sides of the ball. We were smashmouth."

The Madison offense, coaches believed, was going as far as the line took it. There was an attitude, perhaps even a swagger, developing among the front five. Davis, the starting left tackle and just a sophomore, was entrusted with protecting Rascati's blind side, and set up a pot with his quarterback. "Five dollars for every blind sack I gave up," he said. At the end of the season, three $5 bills were in the pot and Rascati had taken more than 900 snaps from center.

The Dukes believed they could control every game from the line of scrimmage. Steinfeld and Magerko were particularly adamant about dictating the tempo, often reporting back to the coaches that they could run the ball at will. Curt Dudley recalled that in this sense, the two had a remarkable amount of pull when it came to making offensive adjustments. "They'd come back to the sideline and tell Durden or Newsome that they were kicking a defender's butt," Dudley said. "And the coaches would listen to them."

Matthews and Durden loved this mentality. "All good offensive lineman A) want to run the ball and B) want to run the ball," Matthews later quipped. Steinfeld, in particular, was pumped with adrenaline when he sensed the Dukes could out-muscle a defense. He'd rumble to the sideline with Burns and Magerko and tell Newsome to run the ball on every play. Newsome, in an effort to pull Steinfeld back to neutral, kept repeating the same answer. "Calm down," he'd say. "We will."

The JMU running game served many different purposes during the season and moved at an inconsistent pace — largely because the Dukes went through three primary tailbacks. When Fenner got the bulk of the carries, the offense worked like Novocain, featuring power runs inside the tackles that were more effective as the game wore on.

When Banks started, there was the dual threat of using short passes as an extension of the running game, preventing defenses from crowding the box. When Hines was the primary back, however, all bets were off. There wasn't a specific formula. Hines would gain two yards on a zone run to the right, and two plays later, the Dukes would run the same play and he would break loose for 25. The blocking and defensive reaction would be identical; the only difference was that on the second play, Hines made a defender miss. And so the Dukes had to learn to trust their methods. "When you're a physical running team you have to be patient," Matthews said. "Sometimes you're not wildly successful until the second half."

There were times when they weren't successful at all. In the aftermath of the championship, JMU's ability to run the football would be somewhat romanticized, remembered as an unstoppable force. Although there were games when the Dukes were dominant, this was not entirely true. Delaware and Furman, teams that were carbon copies of each other and the Dukes, neutralized the Madison ground attack. Not surprisingly, these were two of JMU's most difficult wins, and the games where the offense struggled most. The Hens held the Dukes to 63 net rushing yards in their battle at Bridgeforth Stadium, yet another reason why Matthews & Co. were thrilled when William & Mary knocked off Delaware in the playoffs. "We really weren't a dominating running team until the end of the postseason," Gary Michael said. "We didn't have a lot of rushing yards at Furman. We certainly didn't dominate at Lehigh."

The latter point was an example of why the numbers weren't reliable. It was widely accepted that the Dukes ran the ball in dominant fashion in their semifinal win over W&M. That night, JMU rushed for three touchdowns and 207 yards on 52 carries. But against Lehigh, a game where the Dukes had a sub-par offensive performance — and a game marked by Hines and Rascati needing seven attempts from the one-yard line to get into the end zone — the stats were nearly identical. JMU rushed for two scores and 207 yards on 50 carries against the Mountain

Hawks. It was a reminder that when it came to success in the trenches, the Dukes were not interested in numbers. They determined effectiveness by the pace and feel of the battle along the line of scrimmage. And against Lehigh, the tempo was all wrong. "No one was happy after the Lehigh game," Steinfeld confirmed. "We knew it wasn't JMU football. It felt like we had lost."

By this point in the season, there was a certain frustration and fatigue setting in that the Dukes had not expected. In the home locker room at Bridgeforth, players and coaches posted goals for the season during training camp. *Win the conference. Win in the playoffs. Win the national championship.* "It always was a bit of a joke," Magerko admitted. "I mean, it's a long season. I don't think we realized how long it could be." Magerko brought up an interesting point. The regular season ebbed and flowed like waves on a beach. It was repetitive and finite. But the playoffs — traditionally games 12-15 on the I-AA schedule — hit like a tsunami. "We actually joked around about it in the locker room," Magerko said. "We said, 'Aw, we'll probably lose this one and get to go home for a late Thanksgiving.' But then we'd win. And at first we'd be all pumped until we realized what it really meant, another week of practice. There were plenty of guys during the playoffs who were saying, 'I don't know if I can take another week of this.'"

By December, the Dukes were in uncharted territory. Mistakes were magnified. In Greenville, Magerko was whistled for a holding penalty at the start of JMU's final drive, setting up first-and-20 at the Madison 16-yard line. "I'm thinking, 'Oh no, I just lost the season,'" Magerko later said. As the Dukes huddled for the next play, Magerko started to apologize. Steinfeld cut him off. "Matt," he said, "shut up and get your head right." An apologetic Magerko was useless and Steinfeld needed his teammate to focus. Two plays later, Rascati completed a 16-yard pass to Boxley and the Dukes were on their way. Rascati, who had been sacked twice and had fumbled earlier in the night, was never pressured on the game's final drive.

Steinfeld's quick reaction in the huddle at Furman was almost uncharacteristic. At this point in his career, he was the clear alpha dog in the JMU locker room. After rotating game captains throughout the season, Steinfeld, Matt LeZotte, McCarter and Townsend held the honors for the duration of the playoffs. Still, Steinfeld's technique for motivation usually was centered on a peppy, positive-thinking approach. In snapping at Magerko, Steinfeld essentially was pulling the fire alarm. "I remember [Matt] apologizing and thinking we didn't have time for it," he later said. "We had to drive down the field. That drive was about us overcoming it all."

...

THE WIN at Furman was a high-water mark for the Dukes. As elated as they were following the national championship, nothing would match their excitement that night in Greenville. The following week's game at William & Mary had the carnival atmosphere of title game in its own right — a de facto state championship between rival schools. By the time the Dukes arrived in Chattanooga they were incredibly loose. The players understood the ramifications of the title game — what it meant to them, the school and the future of the program. But they also understood the need to enjoy the moment.

Early in championship week, Matthews gave his players a night off, and a group, including Steinfeld and Matt LeZotte, decided to explore the downtown nightlife. They went out to a few bars. Here, it's important to note that football players — many of whom are at least 6-feet tall and weigh at least 200 pounds — generally stand out in a crowd. At one bar, the Dukes grabbed a table and a patron (presumably a local) approached them. Steinfeld explained that they were playing in the I-AA championship game later in the week. The patron looked surprised and admitted he had never heard of the event. Steinfeld thought this was odd. Minutes later, backup linebacker Frank McArdle returned to the table from the restroom. McArdle, too, looked puzzled.

LeZotte started looking around the room. "The walls were lime green for some reason," he said. "It was very, very clean; kind of a quiet, social atmosphere with tables in the middle of the room. The lighting was low and there were a bunch of big dudes walking around." McArdle turned to Steinfeld. "Frank asked me if I knew where we were," Steinfeld laughed. "I said no. And then it hit me."

The Dukes unknowingly had ventured into a gay bar, which they thought to be monumentally hilarious. And since they were enjoying themselves, they stayed for a bit. LeZotte, in fact, didn't put it all together until they were leaving. The next day was media day at Max Finley Stadium and Mike Schikman — who had gotten wind of the previous evening's excursion through a reliable source — planned to prank Steinfeld. He pulled the Madison center aside and asked to do a radio interview. Steinfeld agreed and Schikman set up his audio equipment. At this point, the accounts differ. Some people say that Schikman discretely asked Steinfeld if it was true that they had waltzed into a gay bar the previous night. Others insist that Schikman upped the ante and launched into a theatrical introduction. "We're at media day," he is believed to have said, "and I'm here with JMU center Leon Steinfeld, a well-known visitor to gay bars around the greater Chattanooga area. Leon, I hear last night was a totally different experience for you."

Depending on the version of the story, Steinfeld either handled Schikman's innocent query with ease or was caught off guard because he thought the interview was live. According to Schikman, it was the latter. Steinfeld started fumbling with words. "Is that going to be on the radio?" he stammered. Meanwhile, a group of nearby players began laughing uncontrollably. The whole thing was a hoax. "Leon just turned bright red," Schikman later said. "And then he started laughing too. That's how loose the guys were in Chattanooga."

This wasn't necessarily a good thing in the opening quarter against Montana. The Dukes had two yards from scrimmage. Davis, Madison's enforcer up front, looked timid. "That was probably the worst first quarter I've ever played in my life," he later said. "I was hearing it from coach Matthews, coach Newsome and my teammates. I kept thinking, 'I'm not going to be the reason we lose this game.'"

Davis started playing with more aggression. The rest of the line, meanwhile, had focused as the first half came to a close, putting together a cohesive effort on the final drive of the second quarter to give the Dukes a 10-7 lead. In the third quarter, the JMU offense began to take over. "The longer the game went the more they dominated," Matthews said of the front five. And despite giving the lead back after the Banks fumble, the Dukes remained calm. The power game with Fenner was working. "As the game went along you could feel us breaking them down," Magerko later said.

...

THE DUKES set up on the 28-yard line with a little more than seven minutes remaining in the third quarter. The Grizzlies led, 21-17. A physical, sustained drive was necessary. Fenner took a handoff from Rascati on first down and rumbled to the 32 before being dragged down by Nick Vella.

On second-and-six, Fenner got the call again, this time running off right tackle. As Fenner approached the line of scrimmage, Burns pulled from his right guard position and threw a block on an approaching Montana linebacker. Burns nearly ran his man out of bounds and Fenner scooted through the alley for a gain of seven. Just two plays into the drive and the Dukes already were re-asserting themselves up front. "There was an attitude we had been building all game," Davis said. "We knew we were running and they knew we were running. We dared them to stop us."

Rascati brought the Dukes back to the line with two receivers on the near sideline. He turned and handed the ball to Fenner again, and by the time Fenner got his hands on the football the JMU line had driven Montana a full two yards off the line of scrimmage. In the middle, Steinfeld took Montana's Kerry Mullen and stood the 290-pound defensive tackle upright. Steinfeld spun Mullen around before Burns sealed him from the play. Fenner plowed through a huge hole and broke a tackle before being dragged to the ground at midfield.

The push from the JMU line was beginning to eat away at the Grizzlies. The week before, Fenner had gained 106 of his 117 rushing yards in the second half against William & Mary, and with 6:11 left in the third quarter of this game, JMU's battering ram already had 89 yards on 16 carries. Short-term history showed that if the Dukes could run the ball all night they would. Madison was not afraid to become one-dimensional if that one dimension was unstoppable. The Dukes were content to plow ahead. If Steinfeld's overwhelming block on Mullen proved one thing, it was that Montana's biggest defensive player was no match for JMU's most-seasoned hog. "We just kept handing the ball off and letting the line do their thing," Clayton Matthews later said. "You could drive Mack trucks through those holes."

From midfield, the Dukes went back to the right side and sent Fenner off tackle. The five-man orchestra surged forward and drove the middle of the Montana defensive line to the ground. Seeing the line shift to the right, Montana linebacker Adam Hoge moved to intercept Fenner before he crossed the line of scrimmage. As Hoge sidestepped a fallen teammate, Harry Dunn pivoted and stepped forward to intercept. As the two players converged, simple physics took over. Dunn, 6-7 and 325 pounds, eclipsed the 5-10, 250-pound Hoge with a monstrous block. Hoge had made 67 tackles in 2004 but he wasn't getting anywhere near Fenner on this play. Sprung free by Dunn's block, Fenner bulldozed his way upfield and dragged tacklers with him until Shane MacIntyre and Tyler Thomas brought him down at the Montana 37. "They're picking off the linebackers," Rod Gilmore noted from the ESPN booth. "The [Montana] linebackers are getting caught up with the linemen. They're not getting off those blocks and so Fenner is seven yards into the secondary [before anyone gets to him]."

The Dukes had run four running plays in a row, covering 35 yards. They already had 117 rushing yards in the quarter as Rascati brought them back to the line on first down. Madison set up with three receivers and Alvin Banks in the backfield. There was nothing fancy about JMU's gameplan. The Dukes were going to make the Grizzlies stack extra players near the line of scrimmage. And until Montana proved it could slow down the running game, JMU wouldn't stop.

Midnight in Chattanooga | 281

Rascati barked the cadence, dropped back and extended the ball to Banks. As Banks zipped up the field, Magerko steamrolled his defender off the line of scrimmage and then shifted to block Nick Vella. To the left, Davis swatted defensive end Kroy Biermann with a vicious right hand that sent Biermann stumbling into the JMU backfield. With Biermann hopelessly out of position, Banks zipped through a massive hole in the middle of the field, cut behind a block from Nic Tolley and blasted into the Montana secondary.

Banks tore down the field. At the 25 he radically cut to his left and turned cornerback Tuff Harris. completely around. Harris made a frantic lunge and grasped Banks by the facemask but Banks had too much momentum. He stubbornly shook off Harris and motored to the Montana 12 before Torrey Thomas lunged and tripped him with a shoestring tackle. For the second time in the half, Alvin Banks had energized the JMU crowd with an electric run. And with 5:15 to go in the third quarter, the heavyweight fight was on. Neither defense could stop its opponent. The Dukes and Grizzlies were done with trade secrets; they were standing toe-to-toe and swinging haymakers. And the JMU offensive line was hammering Montana's defense into submission. "The way we ran through them," Davis said, "it was like we had a block of cheese and we just kept filing it down."

The Dukes were on the 12 and Banks was still in the backfield as Rascati lined up in shotgun on first-and-10. Rascati faked the handoff to Banks and sprinted for a hole between Magerko and Davis on the left side of the line. As Rascati approached the line of scrimmage, Jamaal Crowder pulled from his right tackle position and sprinted behind the JMU line to lead Rascati upfield. A pulling tackle was a risky play simply because of the sheer distance between Crowder, the last man on the far right side of the line, and the hole, located between the last two men on the left side of the line. But Crowder executed the first part of the play beautifully, reaching the alley two steps ahead of his quarterback.

Crowder turned the corner and put a block on Adam Hoge.

Rascati moved alongside Crowder, lowered his shoulder into Hoge and dragged the Montana linebacker with him before being wrestled to the ground inside the five-yard-line. With blocking, the important things sometimes went unnoticed. Even though Hoge made the tackle, Crowder's block gave Rascati needed leverage and turned a two-yard-run into an eight-yard-run. A review of the game tape showed that Hoge was in perfect position to stuff Rascati at the line of scrimmage until Crowder knocked him off balance. Rascati sacrificed almost 40 pounds against the Montana linebacker. But because he was squared-up and Hoge was not, Rascati was able to muscle over a larger opponent. It would never show up in the box score, but Jamaal Crowder had given JMU an extra six yards of precious real estate.

Back-to-back handoffs to Chris Iorio gave JMU first-and-goal on the Montana two. The eight-play drive had chewed up 70 yards of turf and the frustrated Grizzlies were standing on the goal line with their hands on their hips. The Dukes called on their muscle one more time. Crowder, Burns, Steinfeld, Magerko, Davis and Dunn (in the game as an extra blocker) stepped to the line and planted themselves in place. Tight ends Tom Ridley and Casime Harris completed the eight-man front. Chris Iorio lined up three yards behind Rascati. Fenner lined up two yards behind Iorio.

In a similar goal-line situation earlier in the postseason, Matthews and Durden had stacked the line with eight players and ran Raymond Hines off right tackle. As Rascati barked the cadence and took the snap, the huge Madison line surged forward, slanting hard toward the far sideline and leading Fenner to the right corner. As Fenner took the handoff from Rascati, the Madison line flattened the Grizzlies into the turf. Fenner coasted into the end zone untouched, capping a dominant performance by the JMU offense. The Dukes were back in front. "They looked like baby bulls on that drive," Schikman later said. "There is still no greater image in my mind than seeing the bulls brushing the ground, the heavy mist coming out of their mouths and noses, and just running over Montana in the second half."

David Rabil parked home the extra point, and with 3:25 to go in the third quarter, that swinging pendulum shifted in favor of JMU again at 24-21. As Rabil jogged off the field, the drive stats began to weave through the Finley Stadium pressbox. The Dukes covered 72 yards in nine plays. They did not throw the ball once.

Chapter 17

THE FIELD, which was in poor shape at halftime, was a minefield by the end of the third quarter. Two run-oriented JMU touchdown drives had turned the pavilion-side of the stadium into a pit of sod, dirt and netting. Davenport Field looked as though it had been invaded by an army of gophers.

Maurice Fenner's touchdown run did come with one consequence when Corey Davis (by now certainly not as gentle as he had been at the opening whistle) was called for an unsportsmanlike conduct penalty. Although the touchdown stood, the penalty forced Paul Wantuck to launch the ensuing kickoff from the Madison 20.

In a seesaw battle where neither defense seemed capable of stopping its opponent, the last thing JMU needed was to spot Craig Ochs extra field position. Wantuck's kick was low and tumbled through the air like a wounded bird. It bounced at the Montana 45 and rolled inside the 30, where Levander Segars fielded it and returned it to the 38.

The Montana offense went right back to work with Ochs scrambling for nine yards on first down and Lex Hilliard gaining four on second down, advancing the Grizzlies to midfield. Despite rushing for more than 100 yards five times in 2004, Hilliard had been stuffed by the JMU defense to this point and Bobby Hauck still was searching for a way to get production out of his all-conference tailback. In a one-possession game, an effective final quarter from Hilliard could be enough to give the Grizzlies an edge.

As Hilliard rejoined the Montana huddle, JMU defensive tackle Brandon Beach remained on the ground. Hampered by a torn meniscus, Beach's left knee had been locking up since the Furman game. "It's like sticking a finger in a door jam," he explained. "You can't close the door." The sight of Beach laboring in pain wasn't new. He had been through several leg injuries since his senior year of high school, tearing his right meniscus, left Achilles tendon, left ACL and right ACL from 2000-2003.

Beach had gone from promising talent to forgotten man during this time, playing just eight games and going through two redshirts over a four-year span. "Brandon," Mickey Matthews later said, "was always getting injured early in the season." Perhaps no player on either sideline was more familiar with the operating table than Beach. He sat up on the turf, and with the help of the JMU medical staff, gingerly trotted off the field.

Ochs and the Grizzlies set up shop near midfield. A false start penalty and an eight-yard swing pass to Justin Green put Montana at the Madison 46. Green could have gained more yards had it not been for Sid Evans, who for the second time in the game had broken off the pass rush and tracked down a receiver from behind. "There's Sid Evans again," an impressed Trevor Matich said. "That's a defensive end who rushes the passer and then sprints over to the sideline to make a tackle."

Evans, a 6-foot-1, 260-pound senior from Manassas, Va., was JMU's most-natural defensive lineman and the one of the roster's most-experienced players. Tonight was his 48th college game — of the Madison defensive starters only Townsend and McCarter (with 49 each) had played more. Evans had been a rock in the middle of the defensive line for years, breaking into the rotation as a freshman in 2001 and starting at defensive tackle in 2002 and 2003. His steady presence correlated with the improvement of JMU's run defense at the beginning of the decade. In 2001, the Dukes surrendered 188 rushing yards per game. But in 2004, with the switch to the eight-man front, the Dukes gave up only 87.

He had originally been recruited as a defensive end before moving into the middle, which gave him an understanding of how the line worked. "At tackle, you're in a constant train wreck," Evans said. "You're in the middle of everything. By playing both positions, it gave me an appreciation for each." Evans had cut his teeth during the rebuilding years, but was fortunate to learn under several talented defensive lineman, namely Jerame Southern, Chris Morant and Richard Hicks. Morant, JMU's all-time leader in career sacks, was the A-10 defensive player of the year in 1999. Hicks was team MVP in 2002. Southern, meanwhile, at 6-foot-2 and 200 pounds, was built like a basketball player and was a silent, good-natured locker room leader. He earned first-team all-conference honors in 2003 after making 20 tackles behind the line of scrimmage. "He got great leverage and had a knack for using it against bigger offensive lineman," Evans noted. "At first glance, he didn't have the physical tools of a defensive end, but he was very successful and caused everyone else to take notice."

Evans didn't receive much publicity. He was a sharp student, majoring in JMU's Integrated Science and Technology program with a concentration in biotechnology. Evans was grounded. He wasn't going to the NFL, and while some college players view school as a requirement to stay eligible for football, he thought the opposite. Football was his full-time job to pay for school. Evans was an under-the-radar performer, registering 147 tackles and 4.5 sacks from 2001-03. He recovered a fumble, forced another and blocked a kick. For his first three seasons, he was another cog in the big machine. Evans was dependable, athletic, smart and, at 23, an elder statesman on the roster. But he, like Cortez Thompson and Kwynn Walton, kicked a steady ascent into overdrive during his senior season. "This happens to a lot of guys," George Barlow explained. "They play well their first three years and then have a year where they play great."

For Evans, the improvement came from experience. "Everything kind of clicks," he acknowledged. Shifting back to defensive end didn't hurt, either. The Dukes, attempting to fill the void left by Jerame Southern, moved Evans back to his original position after the 2003 season. The move was logic-based. After bouncing around the roster for two years, Frank Cobbs appeared to have found his niche at defensive tackle. Cobbs, a healthy Brandon Beach and a strong season from Demetrius Shambley, would give the Dukes size in the middle. Meanwhile, Evans would be the veteran presence at defensive end, joining versatile Isai Bradshaw, fast-rising sophomore Kevin Winston and reserve offensive lineman Chuck Suppon.

It was a piece-meal unit of athletic speed rushers, converted linebackers and big bodies. And it worked beautifully. Much of the credit went to the coaching staff, namely Barlow and defensive ends coach J.C. Price. "They set us up for success," Beach said. "Coach Price was big on trust. He gave us a straightforward take on our abilities very early. We all knew where we stood and we had our roles."

Crammed together, the defensive linemen jockeyed for playing time. Winston, on his way to 24.5 career sacks, picked up 4.5 in 2004. Bradshaw, after starting most of the previous two seasons at linebacker, added another 4.5 and 35 tackles. "We knew what to expect from our teammates because we had played those positions," Evans noted. "Isai knew what the linebackers were doing. Suppon knew what the offensive line was doing. That really helped us." Another advantage was personnel management. The Dukes came after teams in waves. Perhaps Price's shrewdest move, Beach recalled, was letting his defensive linemen rotate freely. There was a seven-man group and at least five (Evans, Beach, Cobbs, Winston and Bradshaw) were considered starters. "It's funny," Beach recalled, "because in Chattanooga we had 12 guys in our defensive team photo. We rotated so much that we really had an extra starter on the defensive line."

The middle of the Madison pass rush, Evans noted, was tremendous. Cobbs, a 250-pound weapon of mass destruction, had perhaps the greatest impact of the group, starting 12 games and making seven stops behind the line of scrimmage. He, Beach, Shambley and Suppon contributed 22 tackles for loss — including 14 sacks. Cobbs was a freak athlete with a non-stop engine. Beach, meanwhile, was a bull-rusher who grew more effective as the season progressed. After missing 27 of JMU's 35 games from 2001-03, Beach finally was getting enough reps to improve. For a defensive lineman, playing time correlated to growth, especially when it came to footwork, hand placement and the ability to make adjustments. Beach and Cobbs constantly bounced information to each other. Cobbs was so effective that it was noticeable when he was out of the lineup. He had rolled his ankle before the first William & Mary game and the Dukes were unable to generate pressure. "I think the big thing that day was Cobbs was hurt," Gary Michael agreed. "We had no pass rush."

Evans, meanwhile, had a noticeable improvement in jumping from a hole-clogging defensive tackle to a free-rushing defensive end. He averaged 1.5 sacks per season from 2001-03, but tallied 6.5 in 2004 — tied with Bruce Johnson for second highest on the team. Still, his most notable contributions came in the open field. It was Evans (with help from Johnson) who forced Cedrick Gipson to fumble on the goal line at Furman. And it was Evans tonight tracking down two ball carriers from behind. "How about Sid Evans," Matich had said after Evans caught Heidelberger on a receiver screen in the first half. And now he had done it again, keeping Justin Green short of the first-down marker.

Still, the momentum from Evans' shoestring tackle was short-lived. Ochs quickly brought the Grizzlies back to the line, took the snap from shotgun and dropped back to pass. He pumped, waited for his receivers to break open, and whistled a pass for Heidelberger at the near sideline. As Ochs released the ball, Cobbs slammed him to the turf. But the throw was right on target and Heidelberger caught it at the 16, dragging his left foot in-bounds for a 30-yard gain. "What a catch and what a great pass under pressure by Ochs," Mike Schikman said from the Madison broadcast booth. "He paid the price on that one."

Now deep in JMU territory, the Grizzlies went back to the ground. A draw to Green gained two yards on first down. On second-and-eight, Ochs pitched the ball to Hilliard off right tackle. Hilliard rumbled for the near sideline and hurdled McCarter before Tony LeZotte dropped him near the line of scrimmage. Ochs might be unstoppable but the Montana running game was visibly average against the JMU defense. For the Grizzlies, running the football was becoming an exercise in futility.

Heidelberger's sideline catch had, rather abruptly, turned into third-and-seven at the JMU 14. Ochs set up in shotgun and the Grizzlies stacked three receivers to the far sideline — the same formation they used earlier in the quarter on the Levander Segars touchdown. Ochs took the snap, dropped back to pass and settled into the pocket. As he surveyed the field, Winston broke free and zeroed-in on the Montana quarterback.

Ochs tried to spin away, but Winston wrapped an arm around his leg and grabbed the back of his jersey. With no mobility, no open receivers and a 240-pound anchor fixed to his hip, Ochs frantically spun around to face the line of scrimmage. Cobbs was charging hard. There was no whistle. There should have been a whistle because Ochs was a sitting duck. He flung an incomplete pass as Cobbs buried him into the turf. From the Madison secondary, Tony LeZotte noticed a subtle shift of power taking place along the line of scrimmage. "Our guys were getting more pressure on the quarterback," he later said. "Kevin and Frank were getting to him. Beach too. The defensive line was starting to win the battle."

Beach thought this shift was the product of two things. The Dukes had played on a muddy field the previous week against William & Mary. They were used to poor field conditions. "The bad turf slowed us for a bit," he admitted. "But we were able to adjust." But the second reason was backed by better data. For the entire season, the Dukes had outscored opponents, 286-195, in the first three quarters, a 27-point advantage per period. But in the fourth quarter, that gap spiked to 72 points (135-63). Most of it, Beach argued, was preparation, conditioning and a mental edge — the hallmarks of Jim Durning's offseason strength program. The fourth quarter was Durning time, Beach had said. And with eight seconds left in the third, the Dukes already appeared to have an edge.

For the first time in the second half, the JMU defense had stopped Montana's prolific attack. Now facing fourth down, Hauck sent Dan Carpenter onto the field. It had been a difficult game for Carpenter, who missed a 45-yard field goal in the first half and had battled the bad turf all night. But Carpenter had a strong leg and a field goal would pull the Grizzlies even with the Dukes.

Montana lined up on the right hash and Carpenter paced back, setting up for a 31-yard attempt. The snap and spot were perfect. Carpenter took three quick strides and swung his right leg at the ball. Pieces of dirt and sod flew everywhere as he followed through. The kick traveled low, slicing just over the JMU line and missing badly to the right. Carpenter yanked down on his chinstrap and stared incredulously at the ground. Madison still led, 24-21.

Hours later, Hauck would recall this pivotal moment. Montana now was 0-for-2 in the field goal department — 0-for-3 if you counted the fake field goal attempt in the first quarter. Though it was hard to gauge the impact of the turf, Hauck had one hypothesis: On stable ground, Carpenter, a future NFL kicker, likely would have made his two field goal attempts. He might have made the third, had Hauck decided to attempt it. "The two missed field goals were huge," he later said. As Maurice Fenner plunged into the line to start the next drive, it was easy to believe the Grizzlies could be tied, or even winning. Instead, Montana still trailed by three as the third quarter came to a close.

Chapter 18

THE DUKES opened the fourth quarter on the 21 after Fenner's one-yard gain. On second-and-nine Rascati shoveled a pass to L.C. Baker off left tackle. Montana defensive end Mike Murphy forced Baker to alter his route in the backfield and the 5-foot-7 receiver looped eight yards behind the line of scrimmage, attempting to outrun the bigger defensive end. Baker beat Murphy the corner, crossed the line of scrimmage and reached the 25 before Van Cooper dragged him out of bounds.

Baker's athletic maneuver kept the Dukes out of a third-and-long situation, and Rascati cashed in on the next play, connecting with Ardon Bransford for a first down at the 31. Though Rascati had completed only nine passes all game, seven had gone for first downs.

A draw to Banks and a scramble by Rascati gave Madison another first down. A second scramble by Rascati and a swing pass to Baker moved the Dukes to midfield. The Grizzlies desperately needed to stop the Madison bulldozer and get their offense back onto the field. The Dukes could not pin Craig Ochs, and Montana needed to get the ball back in his hands.

Facing third-and-one, Rascati handed the ball to Fenner, who gingerly approached the line and was up-ended as he crossed into Montana territory by Shane MacIntyre. Fenner fell to the ground at the 49, just enough for another JMU first down. "Very typical of this ballgame for the Dukes," Curt Dudley observed from the JMU booth.

"This is play No. 9 of this drive. They've had a number of very long drives in this ballgame."

A handoff to Iorio and a pass to Tom Ridley brought the Dukes to the Montana 38 and gave JMU its fourth first down of the drive. Montana's defense now was completely off balance. The Grizzlies had been stacking extra players in the box to slow down the running game, and the quick pass to Ridley burned them in the middle of the field. With only two cornerbacks left to cover D.D. Boxley and Ardon Bransford, the Grizzlies were conceding almost every underneath pass route. "They had to respect our running game so much that they were putting nine in the box," Corey Davis later said. "The play-action pass was wide open."

The drive was shaping into a textbook study in balance — one made possible by Madison's earlier touchdown march in the third quarter. By running the ball on every play the previous drive, Jeff Durden and the JMU offense had proven they could steamroll through the Grizzlies. Now they were using that threat tactically.

Rascati handed the ball to Banks on first down from the 38 and Banks gained four yards to the Montana 34. On second down, Rascati faked a handoff to Fenner, rolled to his right and swung the ball out to Ridley at the 30. Ridley spun away from one hit before Mike Murphy brought him down at the 24 for another Madison first down. After completing only four of his first eight throws, Rascati now had converted eight attempts in a row, matching the hot start of his counterpart. And on the Montana sideline, Craig Ochs had gone from star to spectator. Nearly six minutes had lapsed off the clock since the drive started. "Rascati is just filling his role to perfection," Trevor Matich observed.

The same could be said for Ridley, who now had caught three passes — all for first downs — for a team-high 32 yards. He had been one of Rascati's favorite targets all season, catching 27 passes and proving a reliable receiver in the middle of the field. His two catches on this drive had the Grizzlies on their heels as the game slipped past the nine-and-a-half-minute mark.

Perhaps no Madison player had taken a stranger path to Chattanooga than Thomas William Ridley, a standout quarterback and linebacker at Oakton High School, who had been honorable-mention all-state as a senior. This had been his only big season at JMU, thanks to a bizarre college career that included stints at three different schools.

Ridley had enrolled at Madison for the 2000 season. He knew he'd red-shirt, but he also was convinced he'd play quarterback. The Dukes, however, had other plans. "Tom thought he was Johnny Unitas," Matthews later said. "But when we recruited him out of high school we had no intention of having him play quarterback."

After his first few days, it was obvious that Ridley would need to switch positions. The Dukes made plans to shift him to tight end, hoping that his lean 6-foot-4 frame would fill out over the course of his career. Ridley balked, choosing instead to transfer to Averett University, a Division III school in Danville, Va. He played one game at Averett, the 2001 opener, and then, as Ridley later put it, "the team fell apart." Averett finished the 2001 season 0-6 in conference play. The Cougars brought in new uniforms and a new coaching staff for 2002, but by then Ridley was gone again, this time transferring back home to Northern Virginia Community College. "He realized he had made a huge mistake," Matthews later said. "He approached us the following spring and asked if we'd take him back. Certainly we were interested in that. The problem was I didn't know if we'd have a scholarship for him."

The bigger obstacle was getting Ridley eligible. Typically, players transferring schools (unless they are moving to a lower competition level) must sit out a year to comply with NCAA rules. There was a loophole, known as the 4-2-4 rule, which allows players transferring from one four-year school to another to play immediately if they pit stop at a community college and earn an Associate's Degree first. So Ridley went to NOVA, picked up his degree and re-applied to JMU, hoping to crack the football team roster in 2002. "I was told I would be eligible," he later said. "I had a letter from the NCAA stating eligibility. But the compliance department came in and said no."

After sitting out his true freshman season (2000) and playing only one game at a redshirt freshman (2001), Ridley now was forced to miss his redshirt sophomore season as well. It was a frustrating time for the former Oakton standout, who never thought his career would be derailed before it even started. He played his first JMU game in 2003, as a 21-year-old redshirt junior, and caught four passes that season for 54 yards. But Matthews, who had watched Ridley arrive, leave and come back again, was impressed with his new attitude. "Tom showed a lot of perseverance and it was obvious he really wanted to be here," Matthews said. "When he returned, his work was sensational."

By the 2004 season, Ridley had bulked up to 245 pounds. He quickly became JMU's best tight end, displaying good hands and blocking skills. He also had developed into what Durden called, "a true leader," which was surprising, given his lack of tenure on a team filled with upperclassmen. Ridley was very important to the Madison offense, running crossing routes through the middle, sealing the corner on running plays and seamlessly assimilating into the Matthews brand of tough, hard-working football players. Matthews had never wavered on his decision to welcome Ridley back to Harrisonburg. Even after Ridley stubbornly left the program, Matthews believed he possessed desired qualities — work ethic, leadership, football smarts — that were the hallmarks of a productive player.

Ridley was a walking hospital, always nicked, bruised and sore. But he always played, appearing in 27 straight games in 2003 and 2004 (the duration of his short Madison career). He had, Durden later teased, "the body of a 40-year-old," which was funny, given that Durden himself was 39. "Tom would work hard every day and he was like an old man," Durden said. "He'd have a bandage on his knee, his ankle, ice packs on his shoulder, and he'd just go out and give you all he had." This, Durden later explained, was the genesis of Ridley as a leader. He was durable, despite being prone to injury. It was another quality that endeared him to the staff and teammates.

Ridley caught at least one pass in 14 of JMU's 15 games in 2004. But it was the Villanova game, where he caught zero passes and the Dukes had only 11 receiving yards, which stuck out to at least a few teammates. Hurricane Ivan, the sixth-most intense Atlantic hurricane in history, had ripped through the East Coast earlier in the week, dumping several inches of rain in Virginia, West Virginia and Pennsylvania along the way. Road conditions in suburban Philadelphia were awful and the playing surface at Villanova Stadium — a synthetic, AstroPlay turf — was soaked by game day. "These were the kind of games that southern teams hate," Mike Schikman recalled. "And JMU traditionally had problems in bad conditions."

Villanova, ranked No. 5 in the country, was one of the few I-AA schools with unrestricted recruiting because they had access to, as Schikman called it, "the Catholic School market." The Wildcats, behind electric receiver J.J. Outlaw, were heavy favorites, providing, of course, that the game was going to be played at all. Villanova coach Andy Talley approached Matthews shortly before the scheduled kickoff. "He said it looked like it would be clear in an hour or two," Matthews said. Talley offered the Dukes accommodations in the gym (the visiting locker room at Villanova was small and hot) and asked Matthews if he thought the Dukes wanted to try and play. Matthews planned to consult with his coaches, and then changed his mind. "Hell, forget the coaches, I'll talk to the kids," he thought.

Matthews called his seniors into the room, including Ridley, Steinfeld, Jamaal Crowder and Matt LeZotte, and explained the situation. "We were ready to go," Ridley recalled. Matthews asked them what they thought and the result was unanimous. "They got in my face and said, 'Coach, we're playing now,'" Matthews said. The group went to the rest of the team with their decision. Tony LeZotte later would recall it as an important moment of the season. "I remember Matthews asking us what we thought," LeZotte later said. "And Tom Ridley and the seniors immediately saying, 'Hell yeah we want to play.'"

They did play. And they played a physical brand of football that provided a glimpse of the rest of their season, allowing only 91 total yards in a 17-0 win. The conditions were horrible. Schikman invited Kay Matthews into the pressbox to keep dry and Kay couldn't stop cheering. "She was ecstatic," he recalled. "It was such a big game. Our defense came out and beat the living snot out of them. And the posse took care of J.J. Outlaw and beat the heck out of a good Villanova team."

The game would stick out to Matthews and several players. And Ridley, though he only was reacting to a simple question, had — according to LeZotte — shown true leadership. Ridley did not have the track record of many of his fellow seniors — his odd path to Chattanooga cost him several years at the beginning of his career. But Matthews, who tended to be a straight shooter when it came to the value of his players, was blunt in his assessment of Ridley. "We would not have made it without him," he later said.

Ridley has been the main tight end all season. His backup, 6-foot-3, 250-pound Casime Harris contributed 10 catches and a touchdown. The duo combined to give the Dukes solid production, and now, with a little more than nine minutes remaining in the national title game, both were on the field as Rascati brought JMU back to the line on first down.

Madison set up with four receivers and put Rascati in shotgun. Rascati surveyed the field, took the snap and zipped a five-yard slant pass to Harris at the Montana 19. Harris had been split wide to Rascati's left, a location normally reserved for Boxley or Bransford. Most of his catches came on patterns he ran out of the slot or off the line of scrimmage. But Harris wasn't a typical tight end. He was more finesse than strength, a pretty good route runner and definitely more valuable as a receiver than a blocker. The Dukes could use him like an extra receiver because he played like one. And so, by splitting him out wide,

JMU simply was running a four-receiver set, albeit with one wideout who weighed 250 pounds.

This, as Jeff Durden later pointed out, was called "derby," a Rascati favorite that used a fast receiver on the inside to clear out the safety and a bigger target on the outside, lined up on a cornerback. "We used the tight ends wide, which was a mismatch on the corners, and then our wideouts on the safeties, which was a speed mismatch in the middle," Durden explained.

With Harris wide, the Dukes had a considerable height advantage on the far side of the field. Montana cornerback Jimmy Wilson, a 5-foot-10, 175-pound freshman, was tasked with guarding Harris, who caught Rascati's pass and immediately slammed on the breaks at the Montana 20. Wilson wrapped his arms around Harris and Harris tossed him to the ground. MacIntyre hit Harris at the hips and the Madison tight end spun away, breaking free for the JMU sideline. With no blockers to lead the way, Harris instead plowed for the end zone. He dragged Matt Lebsock and Van Cooper on his back for six extra yards — all the way to the Montana nine — before the cavalry wrestled him to the ground. In yet another microcosm of Madison's smashmouth style of play, it had taken almost half of the Montana defense to finally bring Casime Harris to a halt.

In the JMU coaches' booth, Clayton Matthews was floored. "Holy shit," he said. "I never thought I'd see the day that Casime Harris would do that." George Barlow, who had removed his headset, turned to Matthews. "I was just thinking the same thing," he laughed. It wasn't that Harris was soft, Matthews later explained. It was just that Harris, though very athletic for his size, didn't run through people or break tackles often. "He just didn't do that," Matthews later explained. "And to be honest, that was the moment when I thought we would win the game."

The Dukes were less than 30 feet away from taking their second 10-point lead of the half. But things quickly began to unravel. An eight-yard gain by Fenner on first down was wiped away by a holding call on Corey Davis, who, for good measure, followed the play by tossing MacIntyre to the ground like a rag doll. Montana accepted the penalty and pushed the Dukes back four yards. On first-and-goal from the 13, Rascati fired for D.D. Boxley at the goal line and Wilson came over Boxley's back to break up the pass. Boxley popped to his feet, looking for a flag. On the Madison sideline, Mickey Matthews spiked his hat on the turf and began screaming for a pass interference call.

Matthews was still fuming as the Dukes broke the huddle on second down. Rascati faked an end-around to Antoinne Bolton and settled into the pocket. Downfield, Boxley and Bolton ran pass patterns into the end zone. The JMU line held strong but Rascati had no open receivers. He motioned to Boxley, slid to his right and stepped up to throw. Three yards in front of him, Montana defensive tackle Kerry Mullen broke into the backfield and charged at the Madison quarterback.

The sheer mechanics of throwing a football leaves a quarterback completely open to a big hit. Rascati, with his deliberate, over-the-top motion, was exposed as he pumped to throw. No one was open and he heaved the ball through the back of the end zone. A split-second later, Mullen jumped into the air, swung his right arm around and caught Rascati with a punch to the facemask.

The recoil snapped Rascati's head back like a bobblehead doll and sent the Madison quarterback to the ground. The pass landed out of bounds. The penalty flag landed a few yards away from Mullen, who, in the heat of the moment, had completely lost control. "I couldn't believe it," Durden later said. "I kept saying, 'This guy needs to be ejected.' The kid threw a punch and he should have been thrown out of the ballgame. That could have changed everything if he knocked Justin out."

In the Finley Stadium pressbox, writers strained their necks toward the two small corner TV's to catch the replay. On the Montana sideline, a frustrated and stunned Bobby Hauck stared in disbelief before removing his headset and motioning for Mullen to come out of the game. The hit was so surprising that it caught almost everyone off guard. Matthews and Dudley later admitted they didn't see it until they watched film the following day. Mike Barber said the play shocked him. "The game didn't have that flavor to it," he explained. "Sometimes you're sitting in the pressbox and you're waiting for something to happen because you see it building on the field. This wasn't one of those games. At no point was anyone expecting someone to take a shot at Justin."

Instead of third-and-goal from the 13, the Dukes now were awarded a first down at the Montana six. In the JMU huddle, Rascati's emotions had taken over. His normally reserved demeanor had snapped into overdrive after the previous play. Rascati barely realized what had happened; to him it simply was a late hit to the facemask. He wouldn't fully understand until long after the game. Yet he was visibly pumped up, as though he wanted to make the Grizzlies pay for Mullen's costly mistake. "I remember leaving the huddle and thinking I wasn't going to be stopped," he later said.

The Dukes walked to the line and Rascati pointed toward the Montana defense. "You guys just lost the national championship," he is believed to have yelled. And then Rascati boldly cut through the middle and raced into the end zone for his second touchdown run of the night.

Chapter 19

EIGHT MINUTES remained in Chattanooga. Eight minutes left for the Dukes to salt away in their quest for a championship. The defiant Rascati had taken a punch in the jaw but had rebounded to deliver a knockout blow. Mike Barber would refer to Rascati's supposed pre-play message as a moment of folklore. "It's great for mythology," Barber later said. "Did he say it? I could see it. That's sort of the myth of Rascati." And years later, Rascati, never one to boast, but certainly never one to lie, modestly admitted that he "probably said something along those lines."

So Rascati had delivered on his Babe Ruth moment, calling his shot and then blasting a home run. David Rabil's PAT gave JMU a 31-21 lead and the streamers again began floating across the Madison stands. There was a sense of anticipation on the JMU sideline and a nervous energy in the crowd. The Dukes were close. They could taste it.

Only eight minutes to go.

But it was a long eight minutes. As Paul Wantuck lined up for the ensuing kickoff, Craig Ochs again waited his turn on the Montana sideline. Ochs had engineered three quick scoring drives in the game already. The Grizzlies had little doubt he could do it again. The Madison defense, after spending most of the night chasing Ochs and his receivers, needed to make a stand.

Jefferson Heidelberger returned Wantuck's kickoff to the Montana

30, but a holding penalty forced the Grizzlies to start on their own 14. Ochs lined up in shotgun on first down and began the drive by swinging a pass over the middle to Tate Hancock for 11 yards. A nine-yard completion to Jon Talmage and a five-yard pass to Levander Segars gave Montana a first down at the 40. "His passes don't look artistic," Mike Schikman said of Ochs. "They kind of have a float to them. But he knows exactly where his receivers are."

Ochs threw incomplete on first down from the 40, just his sixth unsuccessful pass of the game. On second-and-10 he atoned for the misfire, drilling a pass to Talmage at the near sideline for 25 yards and bringing the Grizzlies back into JMU territory. Less than 40 seconds of game clock had expired on the drive and Ochs again looked unstoppable. If he could keep up this frantic pace, the Grizzlies would be back in the end zone with a little less than seven minutes left in the national title game. And if that happened, JMU's lead again would be trimmed to a precarious three points.

Montana was on a roll again, but a false start penalty on freshman tackle Cody Baylock pushed the Grizzlies back to the JMU 40 and slowed their momentum. On first-and-15, Ochs, facing pressure from Shambley and Bradshaw, sailed a pass over Heidelberger's head for an incompletion. On second down, Ochs was pressured from his right side by Kevin Winston and unloaded a pass over Segars' head in roughly the same spot. Given time to throw, Ochs could pick apart any defense. But after generating little pressure all night, the JMU pass rush finally was getting heat on the Montana quarterback. And the Grizzlies, after successfully carving up the Dukes with short passes and yards-after-the-catch, were being forced to change their strategy. "They're trying to get bigger chunks on the sideline," Curt Dudley observed. "They're trying to preserve the clock."

After covering half the football field in 38 seconds, the Grizzlies suddenly were stuck in neutral. Ochs deployed four receivers on third down. JMU dropped eight defensive players into pass coverage and rushed only three linemen. Ochs settled into the pocket and checked his primary and secondary receivers. No one was open and so Ochs stepped up in the pocket and began running toward the far sideline. He was 15 yards away from the first down marker and had open field in front of him. Ochs stepped around Winston and began to tuck the ball away, aiming for the sticks or the sideline to stop the clock.

He reached neither, as Brandon Beach fought through two blockers and hauled him down near the line of scrimmage. Once an afterthought when it came to the future of the Madison program, Beach, on two bad legs, had put the Grizzlies on the brink of elimination, dragging Ochs to the ground at the JMU 41.

...

THIS WAS not the first time Brandon Beach had surprised people in 2004. His comeback from a 2003 ACL tear — and his injury history — had been widely chronicled during the run to Chattanooga. Beach had injured his right knee as a high school senior in 2000 (exploratory surgery later revealed a torn meniscus). He played the first four games of the 2001 season before rupturing his left Achilles tendon. In 2002 it was another four-game season before a left ACL tear put him on the shelf. And in the spring of 2003, after moving to offensive line, Beach tore his right ACL and took a medical redshirt for the season. "When that happened, the doctor said it probably wasn't in my best interest to play anymore," Beach later told *The Breeze*'s Matt Stoss.

That likely would have been in his best interest, because for Beach, the operating table was becoming an annual destination. "For Brandon Beach, surgery long has discarded its usual adjective of 'elective'," Stoss wrote in January 2005. Beach couldn't stay healthy and the Dukes expected him to take his medical redshirt in 2003 and end his career. "Usually when you give someone a medical scholarship you never see them again," Mickey Matthews said.

Beach, however, was bored without football. And since he often was in the weight room (rehabbing and lifting), he asked Matthews if he could remain with the team as a student assistant. In this role, Beach began working out with his old teammates, finding, to his surprise, that his knees — including his recently reconstructed right ACL — felt strong. Beach changed doctors in early 2004 and was told he could try to play again. He approached Matthews, who subsequently checked with the school's compliance department and learned that recent NCAA legislation allowed a player on medical scholarship to apply for reinstatement.

The application process would take nearly six months, and Beach's career, again, would be in limbo. But it was worth the chance. He felt healthier than ever. And after missing almost three full seasons due to injury, the desire to play was strong. There was a determination (perhaps a stubborn will) when it came to his path back to football. "It had to do with a lot of things," Beach said of his decision to apply for reinstatement, "but the biggest was that I never got a chance to play because of my injuries."

This mentality — of living for the moment, and, if not succeeding, at least *trying* to do something — was front-and-center in the Madison locker room. A big part of it, Beach explained, had to do with Clayton Matthews' accidents. The players never spoke about it, but there was an underlying notion that football, success, even life, was a fragile thing. It was one of the many lessons the Dukes had learned from the events that put Matthews in a wheelchair. Beach, who had missed so much time due to injury, and who also had a close friend who was paralyzed in an ATV accident, understood this reality. "You start thinking," he said. "And you realize that you never want to be the guy who wishes he had tried something. You have to try.

"I didn't want to have that regret."

So Beach applied for reinstatement, spent the spring and summer of 2004 running and working out, and waited for news of his eligibility. He was granted another year in July and then enjoyed his most productive (and healthiest) season at Madison, playing 14 games and finishing with 58 tackles and five sacks. He re-tore his left meniscus during the season and he missed a lot of practice, but Beach slugged through the pain. He wasn't a rallying point for the Dukes (his toughness was admirable but it was not remarkable on this team) but his teammates understood what it took for him to suit up on Saturday. "I don't think you can [overestimate how hard he worked]," Tony LeZotte said. "He was all banged up and he came back from all those surgeries. He showed a ton of toughness."

Beach had a season-high nine tackles against Maine, including a baffling stop from behind on a 44-yard run by tailback Arel Gordon. "This is a defensive lineman with bad legs running down a tailback," JMU equipment manager Pete Johnson recalled with amazement. But Beach saved his best for the postseason, registering 15 tackles and three sacks against Furman, William & Mary and Montana.

His knee hurt like hell, and when the meniscus would balk he would have to pop it back into place on the sideline. Beach would require surgery again in the offseason, but his final games, according to Matthews, were the best of his career. And his final play — a sack of Ochs in the national title game — couldn't have been scripted any better, especially because now Beach was laboring off the field again, gasping for breath and resting his hands on his knees after reaching the sideline.

So snap No. 126 of the national title game would be for all the marbles. Either the Grizzlies would pick up a first down (and in doing so put themselves in position to cut JMU's lead to a single score) or the Dukes would stop them, effectively icing the game. It was fourth-and-16. Montana stacked three receivers to the near sideline and sent Jefferson Heidelberger toward the opposite end of the field. Ochs stood in shotgun and called the cadence. Across the line of scrimmage, JMU dropped eight men into pass coverage.

Ochs backed up to pass near midfield. He had time to throw, but his passing lanes were littered with JMU defensive backs. As the pocket began to break down, Ochs stepped up and launched a prayer for his favorite target. Heidelberger had led the Grizzlies with 1,158 receiving yards in 2004 — almost all of them coming on passes thrown by Ochs.

Now, Montana's championship hopes rested on the chance that the two could link up again.

The pass was underthrown. Heidelberger — covered closely by Clint Kent and Rodney McCarter — had to adjust his route and come back for the football. By adding extra air under the throw and forcing all three players to double back, Ochs inadvertently had created an additional opportunity for the Grizzlies. It wouldn't be a surprise to see a pass interference penalty, especially with three players in the vicinity and the ball hanging in the air as though defying gravity.

At the five-yard line, Heidelberger, Kent and McCarter converged. McCarter had been in front of Heidelberger and had a beat on the ball. "He really just threw it up in the air," McCarter later said. The pass smacked against McCarter's hands. A split-second later, Kent grabbed the ball as well. "I didn't know where he came from," McCarter said. "He just kind of took it out of my hands."

Kent was running as he corralled the ball. Later, McCarter joked that Kent took it away because he didn't trust his teammate. "He'll tell you that he caught it because he didn't think I had good hands," McCarter laughed. As Kent began running away, McCarter, not wanting to be called for an illegal block on Heidelberger, threw his hands in the air.

Kent returned the pass to the JMU 18 before Heidelberger brought him down from behind. It was a bizarre play. McCarter and Kent, two experienced defensive backs, each had made a play for the interception instead of knocking the ball down. The Dukes were getting possession back anyway, and by corralling the interception, Kent actually had cost his team 23 yards of field position. Later, McCarter explained that aside from a time-expiring Hail Mary attempt, it's safer to intercept a pass than to try and knock it down. "If you miss knocking it down, or if you knock it down and it hits off someone else, then they can still catch it," he said. "So there, the safe thing to do is get the interception and secure the ball."

That was explainable. In fact the whole scenario (McCarter catching the ball instead of knocking it down; Kent essentially stealing the ball from McCarter) was explainable — even acceptable for the Dukes, who now led by 10 and had the ball back. But as Tony LeZotte helped Kent off the ground, Kent (in typical Kent fashion) began to skip and dance his way off the field. Then he crossed the line and threw the ball on the turf, drawing an unsportsmanlike conduct penalty. Now he had cost the Dukes 32 yards of field position. Matthews was furious. He screamed at Kent as the Dukes came off the field and Kent, perhaps still on Cloud Nine, walked right past Matthews. "Clint just ignored him and went straight for the defensive team huddle," McCarter later said, laughing.

This sent Matthews further over the edge, and he admittedly was mad at Kent even as the ensuing drive got underway. Kent told McCarter that Matthews would get over it. He would, eventually. But asked two years later about the play, Matthews — sitting in his plush office during summer vacation — suddenly was back on the sideline in Chattanooga, freezing his butt off and watching Kent toss the ball on the ground. "We were only up 10," Matthews said. "It wasn't like the game was over. We had bad position and the game still was in doubt because we were so backed up. I thought we took the upper hand, but I think the penalty took a lot away from it."

So Kent, normally quiet, smart and dependable — a ball-hawking playmaker — had gone a little overboard. Still, JMU had the ball back with 6:30 left in regulation. They had Rascati under center and Fenner and Banks in the backfield. They had the bulls up front. And the bulls didn't care where this drive was starting. They had a one-track mind. They would keep the ball on the ground and, by extension, keep the Montana offense off the field.

They would run until the clock expired and finish the job.

Part VI: Purple Reign

Chapter 20

MATT LEZOTTE stood on the sideline with his arms folded across his chest and a headset hanging around his neck. A black JMU football cap was pulled tightly over his head. It was freezing in Chattanooga — the temperature by now dipping into the low 30s — but the Madison quarterback, like many of his teammates, was wearing short sleeves.

He had not taken a snap in a game since Oct. 30 against VMI, and in the subsequent seven weeks, Matt LeZotte — three-year starter and team captain — had somewhat fallen off the radar. His career, much like the early part of his senior season, had been analyzed, scrutinized, poked and prodded by so many people, and now it quickly, quietly, was fading away.

But not to the people who mattered. The fans would have their opinions and the media would write their stories. But family, friends, teammates and coaches knew the truth. LeZotte had not slipped into the background; he remained at the center of this team and everything it represented. He had held it together when he could have ripped it apart.

Matthew Patrick LeZotte was the third of four children, and thus was accustomed to fighting for his spot on the totem pole. In the LeZotte house, sibling hierarchy promoted a challenging, competition-fueled environment. And so before he became the all-America boy playing the all-America sport, Matt LeZotte first had to become king of his own backyard.

According to Matt, Katherine LeZotte (four years his senior) may well have been the toughest of the four children. A softball player, Katherine instilled fear in her younger brother. Matt knew Katherine's age gave her an advantage, but also knew he would never save face if he lost to a girl — even if it was his athletic, older sister. Likewise, he could never allow younger brother Tony to beat him either. Winning became necessary for Matt because of his position in the family. "Seeing how good Tony was at such a young age made me want to be better," Matt said. " The only thing in the world worse than losing to my older sister was getting whipped by my younger brother. I didn't want him to show me up. The success he had at a young age made me want to become better."

Athletics came naturally for the LeZottes and Matt was no exception. He played basketball, baseball and soccer. He qualified for states in swimming. But football — the sport he watched older brother Jerry play — was his favorite. Like many young boys in Georgia, Matt craved gridiron glory. Unlike many, he found it. And so Matt LeZotte was both common and uncommon. His goals were not unique; his success was.

He attended Westside High School, where Jerry and Katherine had gone before him, and where Tony one day would become a star. Here, LeZotte worked hard to impress Gerald Barnes, who took over as varsity football coach prior to LeZotte's sophomore season in 1997. "I was scared of looking bad in his eyes," LeZotte admitted. "I always wanted to do well."

Barnes needed little convincing. He had watched LeZotte play in church leagues as a kid. He knew Jerry had played at Westside and he was convinced that Matt, with a little work, could be a college-level player. Westside's starting quarterback, Nick Kearns, had just graduated, leaving a big hole on the offense. Kearns, later a defensive back at Georgia Southern, had been an *Associated Press* all-state honoree in 1996 as a do-it-all athlete. He played quarterback, defense and punted. "He could do everything on the field," LeZotte said.

LeZotte modeled himself after Kearns. He wanted to do everything, and Barnes — at the helm of a small program that lacked depth — gave him the freedom to do it. LeZotte punted for two seasons, averaging a shade less than 39 yards per kick. He booted three field goals and converted 42 of 46 PATs. And, of course, he played quarterback, excelling in a simple offense where everything flowed through him. LeZotte ran and passed for 4,582 yards and 46 touchdowns in three seasons as a starter. He was a duel-threat quarterback, usually getting 10 to 12 carries a game — opportunities he welcomed because it gave him a chance to hand out the occasional hit. LeZotte, after all, was a football player first and a quarterback second. He liked the physical aspect of the sport. "I'm not one to shy away from contact," he later said.

His best season at Westside was his last one. As a senior, LeZotte threw for 1,525 yards and 12 touchdowns, and ran for 358 yards and seven more scores. He was named Georgia player of the week twice and earned his own AP all-state honors. His teams, however, were not as successful. Westside was 12-18 from 1997-99. And LeZotte, while productive, did not receive many scholarship offers. He seemed, at face value, to be caught in the middle — a good-sized quarterback with decent mobility and a solid arm at a position where many coaches are looking for game-breakers. The "wow" factor with LeZotte was minimal. He wasn't 6-foot-5; he didn't have tremendous speed; he couldn't throw 70 yards flat-footed.

But he also was productive, tough and smart. Mike Bobo, who played quarterback at Georgia from 1993-97, first met LeZotte at an offseason camp. Bobo, then a graduate assistant, would take a job as quarterbacks coach at Jacksonville State in 2000. He recruited LeZotte and offered him a scholarship. Valdosta State, near the Florida border, also offered LeZotte a full ride.

It was a meeting during his junior year that put LeZotte on the path to JMU. At a winter workout, LeZotte was approached by Mickey

Matthews — at the time a Georgia assistant under head coach Jim Donnan. Matthews was close friends with an Augusta local (and Westside grad) named Ken Hardy. More than a decade after their first meeting, LeZotte recalled it with clarity. "We were going through the ropes and running around a bit," he said. "Coach Matthews asked me to come up to a camp. Then he pointed at my hat."

LeZotte was wearing a Wichita State Shockers hat. Matthews, in typical Matthews fashion, asked LeZotte why a son of Georgia was wearing the hat of school located in Kansas. "He asked why I wasn't wearing a Georgia hat," LeZotte laughed. "I told him I didn't have one and that if he gave me one I would wear it."

Their bond began that day. When Matthews left Georgia for Madison, he kept LeZotte in the back of his mind. The hard-working, personable kid from Augusta had made an impression. So too had the confident coach from Andrews, Texas. LeZotte came to Harrisonburg in November of 1999 to see the school and left very impressed. The coaching staff was caring; the academics were good; the people were great. It didn't hurt that Matthews, knowing LeZotte was a top-flight prospect for his program, had pulled out all the stops. Clayton Matthews — then a star at Spotswood High School — was LeZotte's weekend tour guide. They were cut from the same mold — versatile, smart players and charismatic, fun-loving kids. The two immediately hit it off, forming the foundation of the Matthews-LeZotte family friendship.

That Saturday, the Dukes clinched the A-10 title in front of a packed house. It was the perfect storm for Matthews, who quickly realized the rebuilding project he was walking into. He knew he needed young talent, and fast. LeZotte was one of the first pieces. "Getting a guy like him was big for us," Matthews later said.

When it came time to choose a school, LeZotte told his mom he was going to JMU.

"I would have had a heart attack if you said anywhere else," she said.

...

PATTY LEZOTTE had plenty of opportunity for heartache during Matt's first two seasons at Madison. He and the Dukes, for lack of a better phrase, got their asses kicked. No player epitomized the struggle more than LeZotte. He won the starting quarterback job as a redshirt freshman in 2001 and his reward was a battering ram of abuse — both mental and physical. The Dukes were 2-9 that season. For the first time in LeZotte's life, football was hard and painful. JMU had four freshmen on the offensive line and a rookie quarterback. They were learning an intricate zone-blocking scheme. Most importantly, with 54 freshmen on the roster, Matthews was marching out 18- and 19-year-old kids against 22-year-old men.

The defense (led by Lloyd and Pack) remained stingy. But the offense was a disaster. No one had any experience, so LeZotte became the leader by default. It was a learning curve too steep to handle. Alan Harrison and LeZotte would watch film during that first season and LeZotte would see himself get hit almost every time he dropped back to pass. "Man," Harrison said to his friend, "you got the shit kicked out of you." LeZotte could only nod his head. Matthews, with 30 years of coaching experience, said the beating LeZotte took "was off the scale."

It endeared him to his teammates, who knew how hard he was working to help turn around the program. There never was a lack of support for LeZotte in the Madison locker room. This was important because without a solid support group — and without a tough mental makeup — LeZotte could have become discouraged and ineffective. This might have been his first taste of college football, but the JMU coaching staff was seasoned. "This wasn't their first rodeo," LeZotte later said. And that was a good thing, because even people who had been around football their entire lives cringed during film sessions. "He took a pounding," Clayton Matthews said. "I played three games [in 2001] and I couldn't imagine any more pain. Matt played eight and he was hammered. Unbelievable. During our freshman year, the only games he was healthy were our first and last games of the season."

That opener (a 42-21 win over Elon in his JMU debut) began promisingly enough, with LeZotte throwing two touchdown passes and running for two other scores. But he also hurt his shoulder and played sparingly in the next three games — all losses. In Week 6, the 1-3 Dukes traveled to Philadelphia to play the undefeated Villanova Wildcats, who were the class of the A-10 and boasted stud tailback Brian Westbrook.

In one of the highest scoring games in conference history, the teams combined for 89 points and 912 yards of offense. Westbrook, in the game that launched his run to the 2001 Walter Payton award, rushed for 228 yards and scored five touchdowns. "He made play after play," LeZotte said. "It was the Brian Westbrook show."

LeZotte, however, was just as impressive, throwing for 376 yards. It was a football version of the Gunfight at the O.K. Corral. LeZotte busted his chin early, got stitched up and returned after a few plays. He completed 34 of 58 passes and accounted for four touchdowns — three passing, one rushing — as the Dukes took Villanova into double overtime before falling, 45-44. "Matt torched Villanova," Clayton Matthews said. "If it wasn't for Westbrook, we'd have won that game by 20 points."

Still, every good game seemed to be offset by three bad ones. As LeZotte became the face of the program, he too became the face of its growing pains. It became very difficult to see progress. He threw 10 touchdowns and 20 interceptions in his first two seasons, often under constant pressure. And there existed a cautious relationship between LeZotte and the Madison fans. It became a pleasant surprise to see him get through a game unscathed, especially in 2001, when the Dukes seemed to do nothing right. "It seemed like he always was on his back looking up," Jon McNamara said. "And that summed up that whole season. Every time you thought they could do something right, they would find a way to lose. That team could not get in sync. And the person who paid the most was Matt. He took a lot of physical abuse and he also heard it from the fans.

"The fans that did show up really unloaded on Matt."

The underlying story, however, was that LeZotte (seemingly the cover boy of a struggling program) actually was a main reason the Dukes were somewhat competitive. Fans rarely noticed this, focusing instead on stats and the team's won-loss record. But media members, coaches and teammates knew what LeZotte did for the Dukes. He might have quarterbacked teams with losing records, but without him, things would have been much worse. "You play quarterback and you'll get all the glory and all the blame," Mickey Matthews said. "He took all the blame for a very poor football team and it was very unfair." Clayton Matthews actually went back to the stat sheets and quantified his friend's value. "In 2002 we went 5-7," he said. "If it wasn't for Matt we would have gone 2-10."

It was easy to peg LeZotte as a quarterback who simply did not win. That would be a premature evaluation. Nic Tolley believed LeZotte understood the difference between the finite and infinite parts of his career. What happened on the field lived inside a four-year window of stats, scores and records. But the impact of his time at Madison — the way he carried himself and his role as an ambassador for the program — extended well beyond his playing days. LeZotte always seemed to be the main piece of a rebuilding effort. His Westside teams were 12-18. After he left they went 24-10 over the next three years. His JMU teams were 13-22. From 2004-06 they were 29-9. His coaches pointed out that the teams he left behind were in better shape than the ones he inherited.

This could be seen as coincidence, but LeZotte's teammates didn't buy that rationale. It seemed his resiliency encouraged them to play harder. Part of it was his leadership. LeZotte did the legwork to be successful. There also was his good nature. LeZotte never took himself too seriously. There was a genuine everyman quality to him, often manifesting itself in the form of simple anecdotes. LeZotte, for one, loved the Marching Royal Dukes. On one road trip back to Georgia with Clayton Matthews, LeZotte popped a disc into the car CD player and started jamming out to the JMU fight song.

"Dude, I don't want to listen to that," Clayton whined. "I hear that on campus all the time."

"No way man," LeZotte responded. "I *love* these guys!"

Those who knew him spoke glowingly of him. Classmates and friends knew LeZotte as a rock-solid kid. He was a good student, he loved his school and he was a fierce friend. LeZotte was in Augusta when Clayton Matthews had his first car accident. He was dumbfounded that Clayton — who seemed larger than life — could be paralyzed. LeZotte was scheduled for a follow-up doctor's appointment at the University of Virginia Medical Center for a thumb injury, and when he arrived in Charlottesville, he went to see his friend. "I gave coach Matthews a hug," LeZotte said, "and it was probably the most sincere hug I've ever received."

LeZotte was hell-bent on being the guy who helped turn the Dukes into winners. By 2003 he was one of the more experienced quarterbacks in the A-10 and the team began to turn the corner. After the preseason injury to Leon Steinfeld, it was LeZotte — behind a jumbled, but experienced offensive line — who rallied JMU to its first .500 season since 2000, throwing for 1,753 yards and 13 touchdowns. Steinfeld's injury ultimately was the reason the Dukes did not make a serious run at the playoffs.

Still, there was something missing on the Madison offense. For all the young playmakers (Banks, Fenner, Hinds, Boxley) the Dukes seemed very bland. And LeZotte, despite coming off his best year, was showing signs that perhaps he had reached his ceiling as a player. He no longer was the duel-threat quarterback he was in high school. "I got a bit slower and everyone else got a bit faster," he later joked. The ability to extend plays by scrambling was limited. His progressions (reading receiver routes and coverage during plays) were very systematic — LeZotte made good decisions, but improvisation was not his strength. His accuracy, even at 59.8 percent in 2003, was a touch below the ideal range.

Of course, these were marginal issues. And many of them could be attributed to JMU's Multiple-I, pro-style offense, which relied on the running game, but also called for more traditional pass plays, as opposed to the high-percentage throws of a West Coast or spread offense. Enter Jeff Durden, who, among other things, was hired to open up a conservative attack for JMU's big-play threats. When Durden evaluated the Dukes, he saw a veteran, physical offensive line and lots of young speed at the skill positions. Thus began the first stages of shifting the JMU offense from the Multiple-I to the spread, which called for more horizontal crossing patterns, bubble screens and shotgun formations — all designed to stretch a defense with speed. "It was exciting to see some of the film he brought with him," LeZotte said of Durden. "It also was exciting to see a full-time quarterbacks coach. That had been so-so during my career. A little bit of new is good. I'm not one to shy away from that."

LeZotte openly raved about Durden in spring practice, saying that a fresh gameplan might help the Dukes open the offense. He was very upbeat. For a player who lived by the one-day-at-a-time philosophy, LeZotte perhaps was looking ahead to the 2004 season. With a veteran offensive line guarding his back and a freewheeling play-caller in the coaches' booth, a 2,000-yard, 20-touchdown season wasn't out of the question. Neither was a playoff berth.

As they had done several times in the past, the JMU coaching staff brought in quarterback candidates to challenge for the starting job. This was the way college football worked. You recruit players to replace the players you have. The Dukes had done it in the past with Jayson Cooke, and now they were doing it again. At this point in the offseason (early April of 2004) Justin Rascati was not on the Madison radar. His phone conversation with Matthews and visit to campus wouldn't come for several weeks. LeZotte was the guy. "A lot of people forget this," Durden said, "but I had the whole spring with Matt and we didn't have Justin until the summer. I had six quarterbacks that spring and five weren't good enough."

Four years later, Durden rattled off the names by heart. "Blunt,

Hairston, Cole Shifflett, David Buchanan — there were six quarterbacks here that spring," he said. "And when the dust settled there was Matt LeZotte."

...

OF COURSE the dust didn't settle for long. Rascati signed and he was in training camp that summer, throwing the position into flux. The quarterback competition began that August. LeZotte, for his part, remained outwardly unfazed. He didn't bat an eyelash the day Rascati signed, later saying that he was wondering when the next offseason workout was scheduled for. On the first day of summer workouts, LeZotte walked into the locker room and introduced himself to the Louisville transfer. "I wanted to meet the new guy," LeZotte said. "It was another day at the office. I was going into my senior season and we had goals we wanted to accomplish."

That first goal, however, now was to retain his starting job. LeZotte had to be somewhat irked by the whole situation. For years, Matthews had been trying to upgrade the quarterback position, not just with players to replace LeZotte after he left, but with ones to perhaps displace him while he still was there. Now he had found his most impressive challenger yet in Rascati, who had not been promised the job, but had been promised the chance to compete for it.

But this was LeZotte's world at JMU. He was scrutinized and second-guessed by fans; he was challenged by new quarterbacks; he was pushed to be better by his coaches. "To be honest with you, we probably weren't very happy with our quarterback situation," Matthews later admitted. "Otherwise we wouldn't have been talking to a transfer. On the other side of the coin, we had a lot of time and energy invested in LeZotte."

Matthews hoped the competition would bring out the best in both players. And Durden brought up another good point in noting that Rascati was feeling the heat as well. "You don't want to be a transfer and not play," he said. "So there's pressure on Matt, but at the same time there's pressure on Justin Rascati. So it became a healthy quarterback competition."

Healthy, yes. But it also became a long competition, a close competition and an airtight competition. The two quarterbacks went through a month of training camp without any indication as to who might start. The reps were split. LeZotte and Rascati had equal chances with the first-team offense and Durden charted every throw. They seemed even in arm strength and accuracy. Rascati could scramble better, but LeZotte moved better inside the pocket. As the Dukes inched closer to opening night, Matthews found himself in a precarious situation. "We'd leave practice Tuesday and I'd be convinced that Matt was the best quarterback," he said. "Then we'd go out the next day and I'd come off the field Wednesday and I'd be convinced Justin was the best quarterback. That's really how close it was every day."

Part of the problem, LeZotte thought, was that he and Rascati never were put in a position to separate from each other. The reps were so equally split that whoever was working with the first-team offense on a given day had the upper hand. It was tough to gauge who was better because both players were practically interchangeable parts. Their teammates, careful not to publicly endorse either player, were out of the loop as well. "They were going back-and-forth," Tony LeZotte said. "They would switch snaps with the first team all the time. The coaches never really gave word of who was leading the way. One day it was Matt and the next day it was Justin."

This was everything Matthews had hoped for — and possibly everything he dreaded. He had elevated the play of both quarterbacks. And now he was so split on who should start that even his players were in the dark. Matthews did not want the competition to play out on the front sports page of the *Daily News-Record*, going as far as to make both quarterbacks off-limits to the press. "They wanted us to focus on playing," Rascati later said. "[Mickey] didn't let us talk to [Mike Barber] at all. He didn't want to draw attention to the competition."

By late August, however, it was all anyone could talk about. "Who'll be under center?" was the headline in the August 21 edition. "Mickey: No official starter" ran on August 31, with Matthews repeatedly saying "we don't have a plan" when Barber asked how the coaches were going to make a decision. That quote seemed to sum up the entire situation. Matthews had opened up the position, believing that someone would separate himself by opening day. Now, that idea was out the window.

"You'd like for a No. 1 to emerge dramatically but I don't know if that's going to happen," Matthews admitted midway through in training camp. It hadn't, and now the Dukes had to deal with something they thought they had control over, but was becoming a small circus outside the locker room. "Everyone had a lot of questions," Matt LeZotte said, "and no one had any answers."

Then the small circus became a big one. By opening night, Matthews still hadn't named a starter — though, according to Rascati, he did discuss his plan with both quarterbacks. Matthews told Barber the Monday before the Lock Haven game that he was "going to trot somebody out there to start the game." Surprisingly, the guy he trotted out was Rascati. LeZotte would have been the logical, safe choice if the two quarterbacks really were even. Was this subliminal messaging from Matthews? No, he assured, there was no reason behind his decision to have Rascati start the game over LeZotte. That was followed by this statement from Durden: "I didn't want it to seem like it was arbitrary," he said. And then Durden contradicted himself. "I didn't want them to feel like one of them got picked over the other."

Huh?

By now, the players believed a decision needed to be made. "Either one, whatever coach Durden and coach Matthews decides, that's who we'll be backing up," Nic Tolley told Barber. "I don't think the two-quarterback system works at all." Alvin Banks agreed. "If it starts affecting the rhythm of the game with the offense, then I think they need to pick one," he said. The quarterbacks — and the coaches — thought so, too. They wanted to have a starter by the Villanova game. The problem, they repeated, was neither had pulled ahead. Rascati was

10-of-18 for 136 yards and three touchdowns against Lock Haven. LeZotte finished 8-of-13 for 121 and a score. The Dukes were right back where they started.

Matthews and Durden kept saying that a decision couldn't be made — not yet, at least. But by the second week of the season, that appeared to be a smoke-and-mirrors routine. LeZotte and Rascati had met with Durden before the first game. What they discussed centered on opening night, but LeZotte believed a decision had been made to go with Rascati — not just for the game, but for the season. He later said that he thought the competition really ended at the end of camp. That seemed to tie up a lot of the loose ends (including the decision to have Rascati take the opening drives against Lock Haven). And it corresponded with a slight shift during Week 2. Tolley, ever observant, saw that Rascati incrementally was taking more snaps with the first-team offense. "Though it was never voiced, it was noticed," he later said.

Barber too, noticed this trend. "[Mickey] was very reluctant to name a starter going into that Villanova game," he said. "But it was pretty obvious that Justin was going to be the starter and he was going to be the guy all year. He was getting more reps at practice."

A decision was being made without being announced, Barber thought. Matthews didn't want his quarterbacks talking about the competition and had instructed his team not to discuss it, either. He also asked Barber not to speak with LeZotte or Rascati, fearing that it might turn the competition into a controversy. But Barber, not getting any answers and noticing a possible changing-of-the-guard under center, decided to do it anyway. The Dukes had a bye week between Lock Haven and Villanova. The following Thursday, Matthews said he and Durden had chosen a starting quarterback for Week 2. Rascati took most of the first-team snaps that afternoon, but the team refused to tip its hand. Barber, meanwhile, was interviewing LeZotte (against Matthews' wishes) in preparation for a story on a captain presumably on the brink of losing his job.

Barber's story, "LeZotte: 'I've Given It All'", ran on Friday, Sept.

17, the day before the Villanova game. Matthews was livid. He phoned Barber early that morning. "When I picked up the paper that morning I was not a happy camper," he said. That was an understatement, and one that Barber clarified. Matthews, Barber said, thought the story essentially named Rascati the JMU starting quarterback. And while that wound up being true, it wasn't something Matthews wanted the world to know. His phone call to Barber went unanswered. It was 9:30 in the morning and Barber (after working the night desk at the DN-R until past midnight) was sound asleep.

Unable to talk to Barber, Matthews resorted to screaming at his voicemail instead. When Barber woke up, he played the message, which consisted of an irate Matthews blasting him with obscenities. "He was so angry his words weren't coming out right," Barber said. "He kept saying 'I want those two off-duty' and I think he meant 'off-limits.' His point was he didn't want me talking to Matt and Justin. But that's my job."

Barber waited about an hour before returning the call. That apparently wasn't enough time for Matthews, because he picked up right where he left off. The volume was so loud that Barber had to hold the phone away from his ear. "He called me an effing asshole, over and over and over again," Barber said.

So Villanova weekend got off to a rocky start. Then a hurricane rolled through Philadelphia. Matthews, as expected, gave Rascati the nod at quarterback. He was awful, losing three fumbles on the quarterback-center exchange and completing only two passes all afternoon. Still, no Matt LeZotte, who by now was certain that the ballyhooed quarterback competition officially was over. "That was a game, where, in an open competition, you would have seen the other guy," LeZotte later said.

The Dukes, behind a huge defensive effort, beat Villanova, 17-0, and improved to 2-0. They also, unknowingly, prevented a potential postgame steel cage match between Matthews and Barber. "No joke," Barber later said. "That would have been the worst postgame of all time. There might have been an actual fight."

...

THANKFULLY, THERE was no fight between Matthews and Barber. There was, however, plenty of fight left in Matt LeZotte. He was furious. He had to go from competing against Rascati to supporting him? How the heck was that supposed to work? "It was killing him," Mike Schikman said. "He and I would talk and it would really tick him off big time."

What peeved LeZotte most was the reason (or, more precisely, the lack of a reason) behind the decision. He had met with Matthews — a meeting Matthews later called "the hardest thing I ever had to do in my career" — and the Madison coach told his three-year starter that the Dukes were going with Rascati. LeZotte balked. He wanted to know why and Matthews couldn't give him a straight answer. "It was really hard for him to explain why," LeZotte said. "It might have been a gut feeling from a coach, but I didn't understand why he did it."

LeZotte's senior season was crumbling right in front of him. And he didn't have a clue why it was happening. He was hurt and angry. He had put in a lot of time and sacrifice on bad teams, and now, on the cusp of a winning season, he had been replaced. At this point, barely three weeks into the season, LeZotte was teetering. Even the interview with Barber, which had felt good at first, now felt wrong. "Some things are better left unsaid. I don't know," LeZotte said. "That was still in the stages of where I wanted a shot. If I had a chance to do it again … I'm not sure if I would have changed things."

LeZotte was a mess, in a situation where his season — and with it, the Dukes' season — could have gone one of two ways. He still had power over the locker room, which easily could have fragmented into "camps" endorsing the respective quarterbacks. That would have been disastrous. Though it never became a big problem, Rascati knew there were players — likely upperclassmen — who were angry that LeZotte wasn't starting, not because he was a senior captain, but because they truly believed he was the better quarterback.

At this point in the season, that train of thought was both

unacceptable and detrimental to the team. The competition needed to end; it was beginning to hurt the quarterbacks more than help them. Against West Virginia, Matthews again went back to split playing time. Rascati (11-of-16, 110 yards) played well; LeZotte (2-of-7, 36 yards) did not. Rascati, who grew up watching Doug Johnson and Jesse Palmer rotate at Florida, knew this couldn't work. "It didn't work there and it wasn't working with us," he said. "I was bummed at West Virginia because I had no rhythm at all. They kept pulling me out."

LeZotte felt the same way and knew his opportunity to start was over. The week after the Villanova game, he phoned his close friend from home, Evan Carter, and told him the situation. "Matt," Carter said, "read this Bible verse and call me back." Carter directed him to Psalm 46:10. LeZotte read:

"Be still, and know that I am God."

"That," LeZotte said, "helped me figure it all out. Sometimes it's time to sit back and let something happen and see what comes of it. Evan and that passage helped me be a leader."

Up until that moment, LeZotte had been doing all the right things externally and fighting internally. But after the phone call with Carter, LeZotte understood his new mission. It was his job to be the captain, to be there for Rascati and to keep his team focused. He might play; he might not. But that was out of his control.

What was within his control was the mental makeup of the Dukes. When Rascati made a mistake, LeZotte was the first person he talked to on the sideline. When a teammate needed help, LeZotte was there with guidance. He played very little during the season. A few series against VMI were the final snaps of his career aside from special teams duty. According to Schikman, there were situations where he probably could have played more. Still, the Dukes were winning with Rascati. He wasn't coming out. "Matt was clearly hurt and thought he could do as well," Barber said. "But he never really verbalized that or caused anything."

This was especially important. LeZotte realized that a misstep, a bad quote or the wrong attitude could derail the entire season. Asked what was the most important reason behind the run to Chattanooga, everyone — Matthews, Barber, Schikman, Challace McMillin, Tony LeZotte, Rascati, Durden — mentioned LeZotte's leadership. The most telling description came from Matthews. "Matt could have torn that team apart if he wanted to," he said.

"He chose not to."

LeZotte's role actually grew in many ways, despite the benching. Everything he did was under a microscope in the early weeks of the season. He publicly backed Rascati and worked with him daily on being a better player. He was, Schikman later said, "a good soldier." It wasn't what he wanted to do, but it was what he had to do. "Usually what happens is if you're the guy in danger of losing your job than your tone changes or your body language changes as it starts to slip away," Barber said. "However he did it — and I don't know how, because I would have been extremely unhappy if it was me — Matt was able to maintain that mentality."

In truth, LeZotte was not as cool about the whole situation as he appeared to be in public. He simply swallowed his pride and accepted his place. He became Rascati's mentor and the two, according to multiple sources, actually became friends. "We never had a problem with each other, never got into an argument over the whole thing," said Rascati, who had been the odd-man out in a previous quarterback competition with Stefon LeFors at Louisville. "I've been on the other side of it. He handled it well.

"Without him, I don't think we win the national championship."

It wasn't old-fashioned to say that LeZotte put the team above himself. Rascati, no doubt, appreciated that. Years later, Matthews spoke candidly about a conversation he had late in the year with LeZotte. "The kids all realized how hard it was for him," Matthews said. "They had just voted on playoff captains and he was a unanimous selection. I told him he'd remember that 20 years from now more than he'd remember being the star."

In the national semifinal against William & Mary, ESPN ran a sideline report on LeZotte. He was the media guide cover boy and his jersey was selling in the campus bookstore. He was the team captain and unofficial player spokesman for a group with national title hopes. And he was all of these things even though he wasn't playing. It was remarkable that LeZotte, in losing his starting job, became a stronger leader. He was being recognized, not for his play, but for his character. "He became a man that season," Tony LeZotte later said.

This was his team and these were his boys. It is telling that in nearly every anecdote from that season, LeZotte is involved in some way. In the tunnel, waiting to take the field in Chattanooga, LeZotte turned to his teammates. He, Townsend, Steinfeld and McCarter had just met with Matthews to discuss the opening coin toss in an adjacent room. Now, a few feet from the field entrance, LeZotte spoke, just loud enough for his fellow captains to hear. "I don't care about anything but winning this championship," he said. "You go win this for me."

And then Matt LeZotte and the Dukes raced out of the tunnel. Streamers flew everywhere. Smoke billowed. And the crowd erupted.

Chapter 21

JUSTIN RASCATI opened the game's final drive the same way he had opened every drive in the second half — by giving the ball to his tailback. Maurice Fenner took the handoff and roared through the middle before Torrey Thomas and Nick Vella brought him down at the JMU 18. The nine-yard gain gave Fenner 120 rushing yards for the night on 22 carries, a near carbon copy of his 22-carry, 117-yard performance the previous week in Williamsburg. On the JMU sideline, Tony LeZotte stared at the scoreboard. Five and a half minutes remained in Chattanooga. "Keep that clock going," he thought.

The Dukes came to the line on second down. Rascati surveyed the field over the top of his offensive line and milked the play clock. Finally he called the cadence, turned and handed the ball to Fenner again. Fenner cut up the middle for a gain of seven, good enough for a Madison first down.

Mickey Matthews continued to pace back and forth on the JMU sideline, occasionally breaking stride to adjust his gloves or pull his headset microphone closer to his mouth. He looked fidgety, like a father waiting by the family minivan with nothing left to pack before vacation. It was all on Jeff Durden and the JMU offense from here on out. And Matthews kept walking up and down the sideline, stealing glances at the game clock as it trickled toward the five-minute mark.

Rascati handed the ball to Fenner on first down and Fenner slipped in the backfield for no gain. On second down, the Dukes again called Fenner's number and the big tailback responded with his longest run of the night, sprinting through a massive hole on the right side of the line and blasting into the secondary before Tuff Harris ran him out of bounds at the JMU 49. It was a 24-yard gain for Fenner, who now had 151 rushing yards on the night. "That nine-play drive earlier in the second half I think took an awful lot out of the Montana defense," Rod Gilmore said. "This team has been beat up physically by an offensive line that is a lot bigger and a lot more physical than this small defense can handle."

Inside the Finley Stadium coaches' booth, Clayton Matthews watched the final minutes unfold without expression. His once powerful arms were folded across his chest. A black beanie covered his head. It had been more than two years since Matthews buckled a chinstrap as a football player, but this was his team too. When Rascati dropped back to pass, Clayton imagined himself settling into the pocket. When David Rabil kicked a field goal, Clayton felt himself there. It was a bittersweet moment for him because he wished he could play, but he also was elated that the guys from his class — the seniors — were going out with a bang. These were his friends. He had lived, partied, lost and won with them. He ran wind sprints with them at 6 a.m. more times than he could count. "We're going to win this game," he kept saying. And that was the opinion in the booth. Montana couldn't win anymore unless the Dukes did something stupid.

Now near midfield, the Dukes prepared for the knockout blow. Fenner jogged to the sideline for a breather and Rascati handed the ball to Chris Iorio on first-and-10. Iorio crossed into Montana territory and gained eight yards as the game clock passed the four-minute barrier. The Dukes were back to running the football on every play. They were content to hammer away and eat the clock. "No one really had a blueprint on how to stop us," Durden said. "The minimum thing we wanted to do on that drive was use three minutes."

The Dukes were approaching that goal. Meanwhile, on the Montana sideline, Craig Ochs stared at the field, wondering if he would get another chance. He looked miserable. The Grizzlies had not stopped the JMU ground game at all in the second half, allowing Madison 244 rushing yards in the final two quarters. Ochs had brought Montana back with two quick scoring drives earlier in the half, but now the Grizzlies were running out of time.

Alvin Banks gained two yards up the middle on second-and-two, just enough for another JMU first down. Incredibly, the Dukes had held the ball for all but 1:46 of the fourth quarter. They had scored touchdowns on four of their last five offensive possessions, with each scoring drive covering more than 70 yards. As the teams lined up on first-and-10, the contrast between JMU and Montana was obvious. The Dukes were full of energy; the Grizzlies were exhausted. "At that stage, the JMU offensive line had pounded that Montana defense into submission," Curt Dudley later said. "They just pulverized them from every corner."

Banks hit the middle again for five more yards on first-and-10, giving the Dukes more than 300 rushing yards for the night. On the Madison sideline, Bruce Johnson, Rondell Bradley and Kwynn Walton started throwing their arms in the air. Mike Wilkerson and Rodney McCarter kept stealing glances at the Finley Stadium clock. Raymond Hines stood stoically. Toward the other end of the JMU defensive bench, Isaiah Dottin-Carter sat alone with his hands in his lap. Earlier in the postseason, it was Dottin-Carter's blocked punt that gave the Dukes their first touchdown against Furman — a game Madison eventually would win, 14-13. Now he was just a few minutes away from stepping into history.

Fenner gained a yard on second down, falling forward to the 37. Montana finally had forced the Dukes into third down. With a chance to regain possession, the Grizzlies burned their first timeout.

...

CHALLACE McMILLIN was in his seat, 10 rows up from the 50-yard line, smack in the middle of the mayhem. McMillin had spent most of the day reconnecting with former players and coaches. His family was with him. There might not have been a group that was more deserving of this moment than the trio of McMillin, Dean Ehlers and Ron Carrier, who had overseen the development of the program from its infancy. For McMillin — a former Madison coach — it was especially sweet. Coaching is a fraternity, and so McMillin knew what Matthews was feeling. And Matthews understood what McMillin meant to the Dukes. "Dr. McMillin has purple blood," he once said.

That was evident. There was an overwhelming sense of perspective toward the end of the game for McMillin, the winningest coach in program history. "I flashed back to 1972 and getting started with that first meeting," he said. "There were flashes of different periods — when we started, when we went undefeated, when be beat Virginia."

It all was running through McMillin's head so quickly now. He turned around and saw some of his former players in the seats behind him. "Golly," he said out loud. "This really is something."

The JMU fans were in full party mode as the Dukes broke their sideline meeting. After more than three decades, the Dukes were a few minutes away from closing the deal. Steinfeld and Magerko led the linemen back onto the field for third down. They were caked in mud and sweat. Behind them, Rascati barked the cadence, turned and faked a handoff to Fenner, who hit the left side of the line empty-handed. Rascati wheeled and sprinted for the right sideline and the first-down marker, four yards past the line of scrimmage. The ball-fake caught the Grizzlies completely off guard and Rascati gained a first down before he was touched. Tyler Thomas finally tossed Rascati out of bounds at the 30 after the Madison quarterback gained seven yards. Another JMU first down. "Tick, tick, tick," Cortez Thompson thought. "Keep going."

Less than two minutes remained in the national championship game and the math now became very simple. One more first down would close the book on Montana. Rascati handed the ball to Fenner on first down and Fenner was stonewalled near the line of scrimmage for a gain of one yard. The Grizzlies burned their second timeout.

Geoff Polglase, like McMillin, was in the Madison stands. He was emotionally spent. It had been a long week for Polglase. He had traveled to Williamsburg with his family for the national semifinal and then hosted a holiday dinner party in Harrisonburg the following night. Polglase's son was supposed to go to New York City on Dec. 15 to see the Rockettes for his birthday — a present from his grandmother. That trip was cancelled. "My wife told me there was no way he could miss the national championship game," Polglase said. And so the Polglase family was together in Chattanooga as well. "It's complex for me because I am an alum, because I am a fan, because it is where I work," he said. "But each step of the way it got a little more magical."

The final magic moment for Polglase now was only 110 seconds away. Back on the field, Rascati handed the ball to Fenner on second-and-nine. Fenner plowed forward and gained six yards, forcing the Grizzlies to burn their final timeout with 1:41 left in regulation. Even if the Grizzlies could stop JMU on third-and-three, there wasn't enough time for Montana to rally. Madison's ball-control offense had done its work. They had neutralized the Grizzlies' offense in the most effective way possible: by keeping it off the field. "One more play," Tony LeZotte thought.

Third-and-three. Rascati barked the cadence and handed the ball to Fenner again. Fenner ran hard through the middle behind blocks from Magerko and Iorio. He barreled into Dustin Dlouhy at the 22, and then stormed through the smaller defensive back before going down at the 18-yard line. On third down and three, ESPN's Dave Patsch said, it was rather appropriate that Fenner gained six.

In the JMU grandstand, students began to spill over the bleacher barriers and approach the wall separating the stands from the Madison sideline. They had stormed the field the previous two weeks in Greenville and Williamsburg, and there was no doubt they would storm again. As the clock trickled past the 1:30 mark, more and more fans began to trek down from the upper levels of the stands toward the wall. "There was a lot of hugging right about then," JMU sophomore Brandon Sweeney said. "Who I was hugging, I'm not really sure. It was an experience you can't truly express with words."

As the Dukes broke the huddle, the JMU marching band kicked into "Chant," its ceremonial build-up song. Rascati fielded the snap, dropped to one knee and was covered by Tahir Hinds. Rascati picked himself up, looking surprisingly composed and reserved for the moment. But as the stadium clock passed the one-minute mark, he and the rest of the JMU offense began throwing their arms in the air and yelling toward the Madison crowd.

Hinds, who had rushed back from injury earlier in the season, bathed in the moment. He was a shadow of the player who began the year as JMU's No. 1 receiver and his career would never be the same again. But none of that mattered now. "Had I waited longer I might have gotten healthy by the end of the playoffs," he later admitted. "But this was history. I should not have been out there. I jeopardized my career. But when you're trying to get back onto that field you're not thinking about that stuff anymore. You're thinking about your team. I was on that 2-9 team and they were shouting 'Fire Mickey' and it was ugly out there. There were so many of us still there from those years and we were the guys who kept God and family one and two, school three and football four. That's why I was back on that field."

In the coaches' booth, the celebration, too, was underway. The previous year had been full of curiosity and turmoil, sandwiched between Clayton Matthews' car accidents and Durden's hiring. The game itself had been anxious, especially after the Banks fumble. None of that mattered now, either. "It was tense in there for a good part of the night," Durden later said. "And when we clinched it everyone just started hugging each other. We had gone through a lot of emotion that night and that year. There was a lot of emotion in that box."

The tense moments were over in the coaches' booth, but next door they were just beginning. Mike Barber had been trying all night to get an Internet connection, without success. "Oh my God," he thought. "We just covered the national championship game and we can't get the story out of here."

Barber eventually gave up and wound up filing his content from the hotel later that night. All stories and sidebars were ready. He had nothing left to do but interviews. "At that point — and this is the reason you become a sportswriter — I wanted to enjoy the moment and soak it in," he later said. "The damn Internet wasn't working, but I still wanted to get around and enjoy a cool sports moment." Barber, who always tried to spend the last moments of a game in the middle of the action, quickly made his way out of the pressbox and down to the field.

With 54 seconds remaining, Matthews finally removed his headset and handed it to Pete Johnson. A JMU student in the mid-1980s, Johnson had the longest university tenure of anyone on the Madison coaching staff. He was, in many ways, the keeper of the flame. Johnson served as basketball equipment manager in the 1990s under Lefty Driesell and sang the national anthem at the first home football game after the September 11 terrorist attacks. Now he was trying to enjoy the final countdown while also keeping track of the equipment on the JMU sideline. The students were coming over the wall and they wanted souvenirs. "Helmets, water coolers, cleat cleaners, you name it," Johnson said. "Plus, I'm also trying to protect coach and Mrs. Matthews from getting squashed to death by all the fans."

Mickey Matthews threw both hands in the air as he walked back up the JMU sideline. From his right, Mike Wilkerson came through a crowd of players and drenched Matthews with a cooler of blue Gatorade. Wilkerson slapped Matthews on the back and Matthews wiped the Gatorade off his face, breaking into a huge smile as he turned to face the field. "You never think you'll be in that position," he later admitted. "My first coaching job was at Kansas State and I was getting paid $183 every two weeks. I thought of all the locker rooms I'd been inside — all the long recruiting trips followed by a game the next afternoon. It's never the moment. It's the trip that you remember most."

After weaving her way up the sideline, Kay Matthews finally reached her husband. Mickey lifted her in his arms and Kay broke into a smile that rivaled his. She grabbed her purple cowboy hat with her left hand and swung her free arm over Mickey's back, clutching her husband's victory cigar. It had been 16 months since Clayton's first accident and 13 since the "Fire Mickey" chants. But for one night, at least, the Matthews family was back on top.

Less than 30 seconds remained in regulation. Rascati took the final snap and again dropped to one knee. The Dukes piled across the sideline — some running, some walking, most raising their gold helmets in the air. Mickey and Kay walked arm-in-arm toward midfield, seemingly floating through the crowd, and Kay passed the cigar to her husband. As the clock rolled past the 20-second mark, the first wave of fans made the final leap over the grandstand wall and began sprinting for the mob of people forming at the 45-yard line. "I was 2/3 of the way down and I figured I already should have hit the ground, but I was still falling," Sweeney later said. "That was a lot farther than anyone thought. But to jump that wall was jumping into history."

Inside the Finley Stadium pressbox, Mike Schikman — like McMillin and Matthews — was deep in reflection, even as he described the chaos below. "What the heck can I say?" Schikman wondered. And then he thought about all the conversations with Carrier, Ehlers and McMillin. It had been 34 years since Carrier had first brought up the idea of having football at Madison and that number kept sticking in Schikman's head. As the celebration erupted below him, Schikman exhaled and delivered the final lines of the 2004 season:

"The Dukes come onto the field. The fans come out of the stands. The 34-year-old dream comes true. The Dukes are national champions."

For a few seconds, Schikman and Curt Dudley fell silent and let the noise from below tell the story. The Finley Stadium ticker — now under 10 seconds — was melting away to a thunderous countdown. On his way to the party, Matt LeZotte grabbed Justin Rascati. The backup threw his arms around the starter and the two hugged as they made their way toward midfield. In the stands, the Marching Royal Dukes broke into the JMU fight song and defensive end Isai Bradshaw jumped on top of a bench, faced the band and began waving his arms like a conductor leading an orchestra. As Bradshaw motioned for the music, hundreds of fans continued to pile over the wall. "What a wild ride," Matt LeZotte later said. "You're trying to find everyone you know and everyone you see comes with a memory. There were some guys absolutely balling out there. Everyone saying how we couldn't do it, all the times we came close and couldn't win. It was a surreal scene out there because of what we went through."

By the time the clock reached zero, a large moving body of JMU fans, players and coaches were dancing in the middle of the field. Jeff Durden, having made it out of the coaches' booth and onto the concourse level, eschewed the stands and instead raced down a grass embankment to reach the celebration. His cell phone was ringing off the hook. Fireworks broke overhead, sending the sky into a mixture of color, sound and smoke. "It was bedlam down there," he later said.

Mickey Matthews finally reached midfield, exchanged congratulatory words with Bobby Hauck and turned to answer questions from ESPN reporter Rob Stone. As Matthews and Stone were talking — as the sky was exploding, the marching band was playing and the fans were dancing into the night — *Associated Press* photographer John Russell worked through the congestion and snapped a shot of the mob now taking up almost one-third of the field. The photograph would be plastered all over Virginia the next morning. And when word reached Augusta, Ga., those who knew the boy from Westside High School likely smiled for days. The player on top of the crowd had lifted JMU football to the doorstep of a championship, and it was fitting that in turn, the delirious Madison fans now repaid the favor by lifting him.

Matt LeZotte was crowd surfing.

Epilogue

THE VICTORY party at the Chattanooga Marriott was somewhat exhausting. It was late, the players were tired and most of the Madison fans had scattered to local bars, restaurants or other hotels. It was an odd scene, almost as though the celebration at Finley Stadium was the final act of the title run. "Mickey was supposed to speak," a dazed Jon McNamara recalled, "but I don't think he even showed up." In truth, Matthews did come to the celebration, hoisted the championship trophy and even said a few words. That McNamara couldn't remember any of it was testament to sensory overload. "Bits and pieces come back with clarity," he admitted. "I stood in the stands the entire second half with a hood over my head and my arms crossed. I don't think I spoke to anyone. All of a sudden, I was climbing over the wall. Then, I was at the hotel."

Matt Dougherty, executive director of I-AA football for *The Sports Network*, weaved through the lobby, occasionally being asked to reiterate his initial playoff prediction. Dougherty had picked Southern Illinois to beat Furman for the national title. He was 6-8 during the season picking JMU games — 1-3 in the playoffs. "The joke's on me," he would admit in his weekly column. Still, at least one JMU lineman spent a few minutes teasing Dougherty at the Marriott, casually reminding the sports writer that he certainly was not at a Southern Illinois victory party.

The event was winding down almost as soon as it started. McNamara, exhausted, decided to call it a night. He turned around, started walking out of the lobby and then paused. Something caught his attention. McNamara panned around and glanced toward the corner of the room where Challace McMillin was sitting in a chair, a peculiar smile stretched across his face. "I was just marveling at the whole thing," McMillin later said. "I remember looking around and seeing how many people came out and witnessed where the program came." For McNamara, it was rare insight from across the room to see McMillin, the father of the program, sitting alone in a crowded lobby, soaking it all in.

The 2004 Dukes, as it turned out, would become a precursor — though not necessarily a blueprint for future programs to follow. "We achieved this 2004 championship at a little faster pace than happens at most universities," Linwood Rose told *Montpelier* that spring. By winning three road playoff games and the national title on neutral turf, the Dukes not only made history at their university and within their state, but also at their level of college football.

The victory ceremony in downtown Harrisonburg drew 4,000 people, 20 of which were potential recruits. Despite losing ground in the December recruiting race because of travel, JMU greatly benefited from its championship run, signing what Matthews later called his "best class ever," a group that included defensive lineman Sam Daniels, linebacker D.J. Brandon, defensive backs Phil Minafield and Evan McCollough, receiver Bosco Williams and running back Scotty McGee. On that January afternoon, Matthews received a key to the city. Two months later, he received a new contract, signing a five-year deal that would pay him $175,000 annually plus incentives. In time, that contract would be replaced by another extension, this one raising the base salary to $220,000 with incentives to $280K — doubling the contract he signed prior to the 2004 season. It was a no-brainer for the program, which would average nine wins a year from 2005-08 and annually rank in the top 15 nationally in average attendance.

Of the 23 players the Dukes inked to scholarships in February of

2005, about half would become full-time starters during their Madison careers. Many were high-impact performers. This trend continued, even after the 2004 championship slipped further into the rear-view mirror. The joke among followers of the program was that Matthews could play Mad Libs during his press conference on national signing day, substituting only names and positions, while gushing over the talent of his latest recruiting class. Since his arrival, the JMU coaching staff had been particularly good at finding talent. With a national title under their belts, they began to reach for blue-chip prospects (Daniels, Rockeed McCarter and, later, quarterback Justin Thorpe) with more and more success. Seemingly overnight, JMU became a trendy, sexy destination for high-level I-AA talent and BCS conference transfers. In 2008, Penn State backup quarterback Pat Devlin — the nation's No. 4 quarterback (ranked by Scout.com) coming out of high school — announced intentions to leave Happy Valley, citing hometown Villanova, traditional power Delaware and JMU as his potential destinations. Devlin quickly committed to Delaware — known by many as a haven for transfers — but that the Dukes were even on his short list was impressive in itself.

Matthews still preferred to build from within. His now-completed $10-million athletic performance center didn't hurt. The Dukes, as Jeff Bourne later joked, had to make a last-minute purchase for their new facility — a trophy case. Indeed, people who didn't know anything about the program swore that the Dukes erected their new scoreboard and broke ground on the performance center because they *planned* to win the national championship in 2004. "I can assure you, that was not the designed intent," Curt Dudley later laughed. Still, the coincidence was unshakable. By the beginning of the 2005 season, the glitz and glamour Dukes had signed a five-year deal with Nike for new uniforms and, even after losing 11 starters to graduation, were the preseason favorites to repeat as national champions.

With Rascati, Banks, Fenner, Hines, Boxley, Kent, Tony LeZotte and Ardon Bransford returning, the Dukes were loaded with skill players. Madison's dirty little secret in 2004 was that its best athletes were underclassmen. Magerko and Corey Davis returned on the offensive line, as did backup tackle Harry Dunn. They would anchor one of the best front groups in the country, allowing only 10 sacks all season and paving the way for a ground attack that averaged 234 yards per game.

JMU's title defense began ominously when Boxley, running a hitch route during one-on-one drills in the preseason, caught his ankle on the Bridgeforth Stadium artificial turf and dislocated his right foot. "It was a freak accident. Nobody touched him," Rascati later told Mike Barber. "It's kind of like what they call the turf monster." Boxley would miss two-thirds of the season and catch only eight passes. His absence did not derail the Madison attack, which averaged 35 points per game even without its top receiver, but the freak injury was a sign of turnover, even among the players returning from the title run. Tailback Raymond Hines and receiver Tahir Hinds, key contributors in spurts during 2004, were background players in 2005. Their careers were more like Roman candles than slow-burning flames. Hinds, after pushing himself back onto the field for the 2004 playoff run, was never the same player. Ray Hines, after becoming JMU's first 1,000-yard back since Curtis Keaton in 1999, found himself in familiar territory in 2005, buried on the depth chart behind Banks and Fenner.

The Dukes annihilated Lock Haven, 56-0, on opening night in front of 14,673 fans, the largest season-opening crowd in JMU football history. This too, was a precursor. Madison would outscore opponents 314-75 in its seven wins in 2005, an absurd margin that only magnified the talent gap between the Dukes and most of their foes. But JMU was, for the strangest of reasons, alarmingly inconsistent. The Dukes got cocky entering their second game of the season against Coastal Carolina, an upstart program in only its third season of existence. Months earlier, Coastal head coach David Bennett irked Matthews by agreeing to provide the Madison coach with film from only two games (Matthews wanted to exchange a full season's worth) in preparation for their September tilt in Conway, S.C. Bennett defended his decision, saying that's the agreement he had with every team, and spent the week harping on his team's slim chances against the defending champs. "Them's men," he said. "We got boys going to play men on Saturday." And when Bennett saw Davis (6-foot-4, 340 pounds) and Dunn (6-foot-7, 325 pounds) in person, he was floored. "I quit looking at their offensive tackles. They gave me diarrhea," he said. "I said, 'Lord be with us,' cause they were huge."

Bennett's team however, didn't require help from God. And by the end of the game, it was Matthews who needed the Pepto-Bismol. The Dukes marched into Conway riding a seven-game winning streak on the road. They sulked out with a large helping of crow and their No. 1 ranking in shambles. Coastal quarterback Tyler Thigpen erased a 10-point deficit in the final six minutes. He drove the Chanticleers 93 yards in the final 2:14 for a 31-27 win. The Dukes, if it was possible, had managed to play a mistake-filled game without turning the ball over. Paul Wantuck, filling in for the injured David Rabil, missed a PAT and a 37-yard field goal. Adam Ford, splitting time at cornerback with Leon Mizelle, dropped a sure-fire interception that would have stopped Coastal's game-winning drive. "We were sleepwalking," Rascati later said.

Matthews was fuming. "We're just not a very good football team," he said outside the visiting locker room. "We can't play pass defense, we jumped offsides. ... We're just not very good at all." Meanwhile, Bennett, standing near the end zone, feet away from where hundreds of Coastal students had torn down the goalpost, basked in the monumental win for his program. "The boys did all right," he said as media members and state troopers surrounded him. Bennett's team had fired the first salvo at Madison's title defense and the Dukes had been hit square in the jaw. The boys toppled the man, Barber wrote in the DN-R, and Matthews wasn't happy about it.

Madison rebounded with a vengeance in the following weeks, plastering Delaware State, Hofstra and Maine to climb back to No. 4 in the country and set up an early-season showdown with No. 13

Massachusetts — a game that, at the time, had major conference title implications. Here, on a mud-caked field (it rained the entire week in New England), JMU's season began to unravel.

Tied, 7-7, early in the fourth quarter, an Alvin Banks fumble wiped out JMU's final scoring opportunity. UMass kicked a last-second field goal to win, 10-7, putting the Minutemen in the driver's seat for the A-10 title and knocking the Dukes back into the middle of the chase pack. A week later, on their way to Delaware, the JMU team bus struck a deer on Interstate 81. Was it a bad omen? "Bad for the deer," Matthews deadpanned. Still, the accident was the perfect metaphor. "Danger Lurks For JMU," read the headline in Saturday's DN-R, playing to both the roadside accident and the potential trap game against the 3-3 Blue Hens.

Facing a rebuilding Delaware team that was without a kicking game (the starting place kicker was suspended, the backup had his first kick blocked and the holder left the game with a concussion), JMU surrendered 236 rushing yards to Omar Cuff in a 34-28 loss that now had the Dukes in danger of missing the playoffs altogether. Madison's problems went beyond the scoreboard. The Dukes, it seemed, were snake bit. Midway through the game, Rascati, scrambling for a first down and with open field in front of him, slipped on the turf and fell a yard short of the marker. There wasn't a defender within five feet of him. "That was the difference," Barber said. "The plays they were making in 2004 were being stopped in 2005. Rascati falls down with no one near him? It just didn't make sense."

Indeed, little made sense for JMU in 2005. The Dukes hosted Richmond on homecoming the following weekend, needing to win their remaining four games to stay playoff eligible. In the biggest game of the season, Madison played horribly. The Dukes turned the ball over twice, committed costly penalties, missed a field goal, had a punt blocked and burned all three second-half timeouts in the third quarter. Down, 18-7, Rascati drove the Dukes 90 yards and hit Banks on a 23-yard scoring pass with 5:05 left in regulation. A two-point conversion by Fenner cut the lead to a field goal and set up a final scene that exemplified Madison's topsy-turvy season.

The Dukes defense forced Richmond to punt and JMU got the ball back on its 30 with 1:17 to go. A three-yard pass to Banks, a 10-yard pass to Boxley and a 15-yard personal foul penalty on Magerko left the Dukes exactly where they started. It was an uncharacteristic penalty on Magerko, an All-American who rarely made mistakes. Later, he said he was just playing hard. "I was trying to run downfield and block and I got a late hit. I was trying to knock somebody off the pile 'cause I thought he was still moving." Days later, Matthews couldn't believe the call. "It's close," he told reporters. "[But] I just don't think you need to make that call with 50 seconds left. It's just a really bad call late in the game."

Banished back to the JMU 28, Rascati hit Tahir Hinds on a 19-yard completion, fired incomplete for Brandford, and then, in a play straight out of the 2004 title run, scrambled for 19 more yards to the Richmond 34. Less than 15 seconds remained on the clock. The Dukes, out of timeouts, spiked the football. Rabil had missed from 42 yards away earlier in the game. Wantuck hadn't attempted a field goal since shanking a 37-yard attempt against Coastal Carolina. Neither, Matthews thought, had a chance at making a 51-yarder to tie it, so the game was back in Rascati's hands. He took the snap on second-and-10, glanced at his receivers and then started running to his right, pump-faking throws and weaving down the field, trying desperately to gain yards and stop the clock by reaching either the sideline or the first down marker.

He reached neither. A Richmond defensive back tackled him in bounds at the 27, three yards short of the first down and about five feet from the sideline. As Rascati raced back to the line to spike the football again, the clock ran out. JMU's title defense was over. In the stands, a stunned Madison crowd had trouble comprehending the moment. The Dukes had lost three times already, but all of those had been on the road. It took several minutes for the reality to sink in. In a must-win game, JMU had come up empty. On a must-convert play, Rascati had fallen short. "It was like Superman had let them down," Curt Dudley recalled.

That assessment, fair or not, was accurate. Rascati didn't get seven yards when he needed 10. But, then again, the Dukes didn't give up a 93-yard touchdown drive when they were up by three. And Banks didn't fumble the ball in the red zone with the game in doubt. JMU, through poor execution and bad luck, had lost four games by 16 points, ruining what could have been a dominant season. Statistically, Rascati had been marvelous, completing 69 percent of his passes for 1,822 yards and 17 touchdowns. Banks, in what would be his finest college season, gained 940 yards on the ground and caught 25 passes. He and Fenner combined for 1,851 yards from scrimmage and 20 scores. Clint Kent intercepted four passes. LeZotte was named A-10 defensive player of the year. But it didn't matter. The season was a waste.

The Dukes rebounded to win their final three games against William & Mary, Villanova and Towson to finish 7-4. It seemed like a meaningless feat. It wasn't. In fact, the 30-29 victory over W&M, won on a last-second field goal by Wantuck that cleared the crossbar by inches, would up being the most important play of the season. Without it, the Dukes likely would have gone into a tailspin, finishing at 5-6 (maybe even 4-7) and erasing a lot of long-term equity built by the championship team. Instead, the Dukes ended the season with a solid win over Villanova and a 55-14 thumping of Towson, even earning enough style points to get back into the playoff conversation and crack *The Sports Network* top-25 poll at the end of the year. It might not have saved the season, but Paul Wantuck's first collegiate field goal certainly salvaged the program's momentum.

Still, the Dukes were home for Thanksgiving. And in Matthews' balanced class system that meant a sour ending for many key players, including Isai Bradshaw, Hinds, Dunn, Frank Cobbs, Nick Englehart, Casime Harris, Bruce Johnson, Shambley, Kent, Raymond Hines and Magerko. The 2006 Dukes began spring practice without longtime assistant coach Curt Newsome, who left JMU to become the offensive line coach at Virginia Tech. That February, backup linebacker Reggie Wesby filed assault and battery charges against teammates L.C. Baker, Akeem Jordan and Corey Davis, who, Wesby claimed, jumped him at a house party after he and Baker got into an argument. Baker, Davis and Jordan were arrested and released on bail. The story was slow to leak in the press and Matthews, in much the same fashion that he handled Rondell Bradley's off-field incident in 2004, dealt with it internally. He brushed off the questions surrounding the criminal complaint and, in early March, said Wesby no longer wished to pursue legal action. By the time the four players appeared in court on March 20, the charges had been dropped. Prosecuting attorney David Martin said Wesby told him the incident was a misunderstanding. "It was nothing more than four young college boys got in a fight," Matthews told the DN-R. "That's not the first time it's happened. We've handled it internally. As a football team, we had dealt with it two weeks before it all hit, all went public."

For the Dukes, it was crisis averted. Expectations, after all, were high again. Davis was back to anchor the offensive line. LeZotte, Jordan, Isaiah Dottin-Carter and Minafield returned on defense. Banks, Fenner and junior college transfer Eugene Holloman gave the Dukes a loaded backfield. The Killer Bees — Boxley, Bransford and Baker — were back at receiver.

And of course, there was Rascati, now a senior himself. Perhaps no Madison player hated losing as much as he did. Rascati was 20-6 as a starter, but was eager to get the bad taste of 2005 out of his mouth. "Last year was different. We didn't have the luck like we did [in 2004]," he said before shifting gears. "I put a lot of pressure on myself to do well." Matthews planned to do the same thing, telling reporters that he wouldn't trade Rascati for any player in the country, and more than once saying that the offense would center on his quarterback. After blending in behind JMU's senior leaders in 2004 and enduring a rocky 2005, it was time to see what Justin Rascati was made of.

…

THE DUKES began the season with a false start. Playing on a new field-turf surface that was installed at Bridgeforth Stadium over the summer, Madison trailed Division II Bloomsburg, 3-0, at halftime of its 2006 opener. This wasn't Lock Haven (Bloomsburg was a perennial playoff team) but the Dukes looked flat and uninspired — certainly not like a title contender. Matthews barely spoke to his players at halftime. "You're losing to a fucking Division II school," he allegedly seethed in the locker room. And then Matthews walked out, leaving the Dukes to their own thoughts.

They played poorly for most of the second half as well, until Baker took a screen pass from Rascati and raced down the sideline for a 52-yard touchdown. JMU added a late score by Fenner to win, 14-3, and survive what would have been an awful early-season loss. The following week, in a battle between the previous two national champions, the Dukes again struggled on offense in a 21-10 loss at Appalachian State. The defense, however, was stingy, surrendering only 236 yards and briefly knocking Mountaineers quarterback Trey Elder out of the game. His replacement? A skinny dread-locked freshman named Armanti Edwards.

At 1-1, the Dukes were where they needed to be. But they weren't happy. Matthews, in a message that seemed to take place every year in late September, preached the need to open up the offense. The Dukes had a bye week and then hosted Northeastern in their A-10 opener on Sept. 23. It was show time for JMU and the Dukes delivered. Holloman, replacing both Banks (injury) and Fenner (fumble problems) atop the depth chart, took a handoff on the second play of the game and sprinted 74 yards for a touchdown. Later in the quarter, Rascati and Baker hooked up on a 71-yard scoring pass and the rout was on. The Dukes won, 52-14, kicking off a seven-game winning streak in which they averaged 39 points per game.

From late September through early November, the Dukes beat every team they faced by at least 12 points — including a 42-23 rout of No. 1 New Hampshire. Rascati, as Matthews had promised in August, was the focal point. He completed 76 percent of his passes over this stretch, running and throwing for 14 touchdowns and playing himself into contention for the Walter Payton award. The Dukes capped the streak with a 44-24 dismantling of Delaware in their last home game of the regular season as Rascati (211 yards passing, three touchdowns), Holloman (171 yards rushing) and Boxley (70-yard touchdown reception) provided entertainment that rivaled the post-game fireworks show.

This was the year of the big-play Dukes and Jeff Durden loved it. Holloman, a more explosive version of Raymond Hines, finished the season with 1,085 rushing yards and had four games in which he reeled off a run of at least 50 yards. Four of Baker's eight touchdown catches were from at least 40 yards out. Banks, despite missing four games and posting a career-low rushing total, found the end zone eight times. But the Dukes played defense, too. Jordan, the runner-up for the Buck Buchanon award, had 140 tackles. LeZotte and Dottin-Carter added 82 and 81, respectively. Kevin Winston had 11 sacks. It was, perhaps, Matthews' most balanced team at JMU. By the end of the regular season, even after a shocking 21-20 loss at Villanova that cost the Dukes the A-10 title, JMU was in a small group (along with Massachusetts and Montana) capable of challenging Appalachian State for the national title. The Mountaineers, after dropping their season opener at I-A North Carolina State, had been challenged only twice during the season, a 14-7 win over Wofford and a 27-20 win in double overtime against Georgia Southern. Appalachian State was 10-1, and Edwards, after taking over for Elder during the JMU game, was the read deal, topping 3,000 all-purpose yards as a true freshman.

The FCS playoff system is an imperfect science. The top four teams are seeded; matchups are determined by geographic proximity, conference affiliation (teams from the same conference can't meet in the first round) and — outside of the seeded teams — sealed bids are used to determine home games. "Getting one of those seeds," Barber said, "makes a world of a difference in the playoffs." The Dukes had blown their chance at a seed by losing to Villanova. Still, their 38-3 rout of Towson in the season finale gave them a 9-2 overall record and a 7-1 mark in conference play. UMass, at 10-1 overall, earned the A-10 automatic bid and the No. 3 seed. Appalachian State and Montana (10-1) were ranked No. 1 and No. 2. Gateway Conference champion Youngstown State (9-2) earned the No. 4 spot.

That left four other automatic qualifiers: Mid-Eastern Athletic Conference champion Hampton, Ohio Valley champion Tennessee-Martin, Patriot League champion Lafayette and Southland Conference champion McNeese State. Eight at-large qualifiers — JMU, New Hampshire, Montana State, Coastal Carolina, Southern Illinois, Illinois State, Eastern Illinois and Furman — rounded out the field. Of 15 potential opponents for JMU, four were located within a geographic radius that eliminated major travel: Hampton, Lafayette, Youngstown and Appalachian State. A JMU-Hampton matchup, pitting two Virginia schools at Bridgeforth Stadium, seemed likely.

In fact, a home date with Hampton was expected. But the Sunday after their 35-point win over Towson, the Dukes received startling news. They were going to Youngstown. The geographic argument was passable, yet something was wrong with the matchup. The Dukes, the fifth or sixth best team in the 16-team field, were traveling to play the No. 4 seed in the first round. Meanwhile, Hampton, out of the MEAC (traditionally one of the weaker FCS conferences), was hosting New Hampshire, a team the Dukes hammered on the road in October. This wasn't 2004, where a low bid cost JMU a home game. The Dukes had been screwed. New Hampshire goes to Hampton and JMU goes to Youngstown? Matthews was baffled. "I'm stunned," he said after the selection show. "Someone smarter than me is going to have to explain that one to me. … How can you seed New Hampshire over us? [Because] that's really what they've done."

Matthews then went a step further, hinting that he believed ESPN, which was airing the JMU-Youngstown game nationally, had influenced the bracket to get a more desirable matchup for its primetime slot. The selection committee denied this hypothesis, saying the matchups were put together before the network made its decision. Still, something didn't feel right. "The game is a very peculiar matchup for James Madison," Dougherty wrote for *The Sports Network* "[They] appeared to be in position to play a regional contest against Hampton and would have been a logical candidate for a home game with an impressive overall resume … what did Youngstown State and James Madison do to draw the wrath of the committee?"

Predictably, New Hampshire took care of Hampton, jumping out to a 34-21 halftime lead and holding off the Pirates for a 41-38 win. And predictably, JMU and Youngstown State — two teams that could have been playing each other in the semifinals — staged a battle worth remembering. Despite the daunting trip, the Dukes, with their stingy run defense, matched up well with the Penguins, who loved to run the ball with bruising tailback Marcus Mason. But Mason, a Payton award finalist who rushed for 1,496 yards in the regular season, was nursing an ankle injury and the Dukes would hold him to 72 yards on 26 carries, his lowest output of the season.

Youngstown State struck first, driving 84 yards on the game's first drive to take a 7-0 lead. The Dukes answered quickly. Freshman Scotty McGee, in what would be a preview of his electric career, took the ensuing kickoff up the near sideline, veered back across the field and stumbled into the end zone untouched for a 99-yard touchdown to knot the game at 7-7. The Dukes took a 14-10 lead on a touchdown run by Rascati, but JMU fizzled in the second quarter. Youngstown State took a 17-14 lead on a halfback pass and turned a Rascati fumble into a field goal for a 20-14 edge.

David Rabil's 37-yard field goal pulled the Dukes within three at halftime, and in the third quarter, JMU began to pull away. Rascati hit freshman tight end Mike Caussin in the back of the end zone for a 24-20 lead. After a Youngstown punt, the Dukes drove to the Penguins' 27-yard line, where, on the first play of the fourth quarter, Rascati scrambled into the end zone to put JMU up by 11 with 14:52 left in the game.

The teams traded punts on the next two possessions. Down 11 and with 10:36 left in regulation, Youngstown quarterback Tom Zetts quickly drove the Penguins to another touchdown, hitting T.J. Peterson on a six-yard scoring pass and then connecting with Peterson again on a two-point conversion to pull the Penguins within three. Still, the Dukes, with Holloman, Banks and Rascati all running effectively, were eight minutes away from escaping Ohio with a win. Madison started the ensuing drive on the 27, and, after a nine-yard run by Holloman, Banks delivered what appeared to be the knockout blow, rumbling 43 yards down the near sideline to put the Dukes deep in Youngstown territory. JMU kept the ball on the ground. Holloman gained four yards and then was stopped for no gain. Rascati picked up five on third-and-six, bringing up fourth-and-one from the Youngstown 12-yard line.

The Dukes burned a timeout with 4:44 left in the game. A field goal would give them a six-point lead. A first down almost certainly would take another minute or two off the clock. Matthews, a defensive-minded guy who also had a bit of a gambler's swagger, wanted to get the yard and go home. He looked at Rascati and his big offensive line (Vernon Eason, Scott Lemn and Mike Parham all weighed between 285 and 295 pounds; Davis and Terrence Apted were 340) and decided he wanted to win the game right then and there.

Rascati took the snap and plunged forward, churning over the line of scrimmage and reaching the ball across the imaginary barrier. He had enough for the first down. The Dukes were going to run out the clock. They were going to win another road playoff game. The pile of players broke up and the referee placed the ball inside the 12-yard line. Rascati stood with his hands on his hips, staring at the ball as game officials brought out the chains for a measurement. "We certainly thought we had the first down," Matthews said after the game. "We thought it was a bad spot."

The Dukes were five inches short.

Rascati walked across the line of scrimmage, glaring at the spot and the referee, still staring with his hands on his hips. He couldn't believe it.

The Penguins were alive. Three plays later, on third-and-15 from his own seven-yard line, Zetts connected with Peterson, who outjumped JMU defensive back Evan McCollough for a 30-yard gain. Two completions, a pass interference penalty on McCollough and a three-yard run by Mason put the Penguins on the JMU 30. Zetts then hit Peterson again for seven yards to the 23. It was Coastal Carolina all over again. The Dukes, airtight against the run, slowly were being burned through the air. It was the Achilles heel for the Madison secondary, which lacked ball-hawking playmakers. The Dukes were strong, but there wasn't a Clint Kent among them. McCollough was a true sophomore, McGee was a redshirt freshman and Minafield was a converted safety. The JMU secondary had intercepted only five passes in 2006, compared to 17 in the previous two seasons. Sitting in the JMU section with his father, Jon McNamara, now an alum, felt like he was watching a train wreck in slow motion. McNamara had been in Conway, S.C. a year earlier, on assignment for *The Breeze*. He felt like throwing up. "Not again," he cringed.

The Penguins went back to Mason, who rushed for seven, 10 and five yards on three consecutive carries — his most effective spurt of the game. Youngstown State, after being left for dead 10 minutes earlier, was a yard away from taking the lead. The Dukes burned a timeout with 1:15 left. On second-and-goal, Mason zipped into the end zone to put the Penguins on top. Across the field, Rascati glanced at the clock. One minute, 12 seconds remained. Madison trailed by four. The Dukes were out of timeouts.

JMU still had a chance. Baker and Boxley were big-play threats and Rascati was never out of it — his comeback wins against Maine and Furman two years earlier proved that much. McGee raced the ensuing kickoff to the JMU 34 and Madison began its final drive with 60 seconds left in the game. Rascati hit Baker for eight yards and Baker got out of bounds to stop the clock. A 12-yard run by Rascati gave the Dukes a first down at the Youngstown 46. More than 40 seconds remained — an eternity considering the circumstances. Then Baker dropped a pass on first-and-10 and Boxley — usually sure-handed — dropped another one on second down. Rascati fired incomplete for Baker on third-and-10 and the Penguins burned a timeout. The Dukes were down to their final play.

Rascati lined up in shotgun on fourth-and-10 with five wide receivers and 19 seconds left on the clock. He fielded the snap and dropped into the pocket, then stepped up and pump-faked with 15 seconds to go. His receivers were covered, and now Rascati — displaying what Matthews called his only negative trait — was running for the first down, trusting his legs more than his right arm. Running to his right, Rascati crossed the line of scrimmage on an angled path. Like his failed attempt against Richmond in 2005, he was hunting for the first down marker and the sideline. Rascati reached the sideline hashmarks and drove his body forward. He was hit from the front and the side, falling forward and out of bounds at the Youngstown 38, two yards short of the marker.

For the second time in two years, JMU's season ended with Rascati trying to make a play. But while his scramble against Richmond was a figurative finish to Madison's title defense, this one was a literal ending. Rascati's career was over, as were those of Banks, Fenner, Davis, Boxley, Bransford, Jordan, Dottin-Carter and Rabil. Though they all had been key contributors to JMU's current run of success (a 29-9 record from 2004-06) they had progressed at different speeds, and so this core group of players never reached a collective peak. Dottin-Carter and Jordan grew steadily before having breakout senior seasons. Banks and Fenner were high-impact performers, averaging a combined 1,568 rushing yards per season from 2003-05 before tumbling to 527 yards in 2006. Boxley, after a breakout 2004 season, caught only 21 passes the rest of his career. Meanwhile, Bransford, Davis and Rascati were strong, healthy performers every season. Bransford, the least celebrated of the

Killer Bees, was the most consistent, catching at least 20 passes and scoring at least three touchdowns in each of his final three seasons.

It certainly felt like the end of an era. Of the active players for the 2004 national title game, only LeZotte, Baker, Antoinne Bolton, Nick Adams, Marvin Brown and Adam Ford remained. There was something bitter about the loss in Youngstown because the Dukes were perhaps the only playoff team who had a chance at beating Appalachian State on the road. Madison's physical, run-stopping defense and powerful offense was the only known recipe to win in Boone, where the Mountaineers had won 24 straight entering their first-round playoff game against Coastal Carolina. The trick to winning at "The Rock" was to keep the ball away from Appalachian's high-octane offense, something none of their playoff opponents in Boone were able to accomplish. By blowing an 11-point fourth quarter lead in the opening round, the Dukes had given ASU a clear path to Chattanooga. The Mountaineers won their three home playoff games by 17, 21 and 25 points, thrashing Youngstown, 49-24, in the semifinal. A week later, they out-muscled Massachusetts, 28-17, for their second straight national title.

The Dukes, meanwhile, were left to stew. Rascati, who finished the Youngstown game 14-of-24 for 145 yards and a touchdown — and ran for 93 yards and two more scores — was seething, darting off the field as soon as the game ended. He was not present at the post-game press conference. It was, Mike Barber believed, the first time the senior quarterback had not met with the media after a game. "On a surprisingly warm night in northern Ohio, nobody was cooler than Tom Zetts," Barber wrote. And nobody was hotter than Justin Rascati, who screamed at a referee after the spot on fourth down and did not speak to the media for another two days. Critics argued that Rascati was bitching about the call and placing blame for the loss. That didn't make sense, especially considering his track record. Later, Rascati said that Gary Michael, noting how hard the loss had been, had pulled him back from the press conference. That made more sense, given Michael's deft ability at handling the needs of both player and media.

"It's hard to explain," Rascati said years later. "But that loss was probably one of the hardest things I had to deal with in my life." Rascati wasn't a sore loser; he just hated to lose. Perhaps the outburst of emotion was the result of something the usually composed quarterback never prepared himself to face.

Maybe, in that moment, Justin Rascati simply didn't know how to deal with the end.

...

PUBLICALLY, MATTHEWS prepped Madison fans for the start of a new era, pointing to the Dukes' inexperience and brutal early-season schedule as an indication that 2007 might be a rebuilding year. After three straight seasons of openers against Division II schools, JMU would begin 2007 on the road against Butch Davis and I-A North Carolina. A home date with New Hampshire was to follow, and it wasn't hard to think the Dukes could be 0-2 out of the gate. Privately, however, Matthews had confidence that this Madison team could set the foundation for another title run. Everyone was worried about the post-Rascati era except those closest to the program. They knew that for all his qualities, Rascati did not have the athleticism of his successor. "Mickey loved Justin," one team staff member said, "but he thought Rodney Landers was the best player in the country. Mickey was drooling over Landers."

Ironically, the Dukes had locked up Rodney Landers — now a redshirt junior — on one of Matthews' worst days as a head coach. Landers had been on his recruiting visit the day Matt LeZotte and the Dukes were drummed by Northeastern in the final game of the 2003 season. Still, he chose Madison as his college destination, in large part because the Dukes were giving him a chance to play quarterback. Landers had been recruited by several Division I-A programs as a defensive back, but he wanted to stay under center. Matthews, surely noticing Landers' prodigious talent, complied.

As Rascati's backup in 2005 and 2006, Landers had played sparingly. But his rushing totals were off the charts. He averaged 8.86 yards per carry. Rascati was a great quarterback who could run. Landers was an exceptional running back who could throw. The Dukes tweaked their offense, adding designed runs and option plays to center the offense on Landers. He was the most dangerous player on the field and Matthews wanted the ball in his hands all the time. Landers was a bruising player. He, like Rascati, weighed 220 pounds, but Landers looked like he was chiseled from marble. In 2005, during his redshirt freshman season, Landers was on Madison's punt return team as a blocker. That season, against Maine, L.C. Baker fielded a kick at his own 43-yard line and streaked up the JMU sideline. A Maine defender was closing in for the hit when Landers, who ran the 40-yard dash in 4.6 seconds, came into view and leveled the defender with a shoulder to the chest. In the Madison stands, a JMU fan started laughing. "That," he announced, "was our backup quarterback."

The block was a glimpse into the future for Landers — a downhill, powerful athlete. While Armanti Edwards was a speedy, elusive runner at quarterback, Landers was physical. "Armanti is like a receiver with the ball; he'll run around you and run past you," Appalachian State coach Jerry Moore told *USA Today* in 2008. "Rodney will just run over you."

The Rodney Landers Show, however, got off to a rocky start. Starting a game for the first time since his senior year of high school, the heralded quarterback and his teammates were overwhelmed in Chapel Hill. The Dukes gave up a 65-yard touchdown pass on the third play from scrimmage. Landers then fumbled away his first snap as a starter. Punter Jason Pritchard had two kicks blocked. JMU trailed, 21-0, at the end of the first quarter, on its way to a 37-14 loss. It was a sobering game for the Dukes, who expected to contend against a traditionally weak I-A opponent. Even worse, the game came on the back end of Appalachian State's 34-32 shocker over Michigan. Overnight, the Mountaineers went from being the two-time defending I-AA champions to America's favorite underdog story.

Of course, Appalachian State was nobody's underdog at the I-AA level. Its win over the Wolverines merely reinforced its dominance. With 22 straight wins over I-AA opponents and now an historic victory over one of the nation's most storied programs, the Mountaineers were the new — in fact, the only — national brand name in their football subdivision. Meanwhile, the Dukes, owners of a 29-9 record from 2004-06 — the Mountaineers were 32-9 over the same stretch — now simply were known as "the last team other than Appalachian State to win the I-AA championship." It wasn't exactly a ringing endorsement. Still, under Matthews, the Dukes were 0-4 against I-A teams and had been outscored 172-24 in those games. And since mainstream media was only paying attention to I-AA football when one of its teams knocked off a I-A squad, the Dukes were resigned to play second fiddle.

Matthews did not like facing I-A teams. To him, it was a risk to his players and did nothing to help a team that played in I-AA's toughest conference. From 2004-08, the A-10 (which shifted to the Colonial Athletic Association in 2007) sent at least two and as many as five teams to the playoffs. Playing against a I-A team was a paycheck game for the Dukes. Though Matthews would never admit it, followers of the program believed he simply wanted to get in and get out with a healthy team. Indeed, the offensive gameplan often was bland in these I-A contests. Perhaps it was opening day rust, but maybe the Dukes also didn't want to show their entire playbook in a game that meant little to their postseason chances.

Landers, despite his opening-night jitters, did not play terribly. He threw for 100 yards and a touchdown and ran for 71 yards and another score. But he threw two interceptions and did not look comfortable in the pocket. Indeed, Landers looked better when he was throwing on the run, something Durden noticed and planned to implement as the season progressed. The 23-point loss in Chapel Hill was not a precursor to the season, just another false start. The Dukes rebounded to win their next six games, pasting New Hampshire, VMI, Coastal Carolina and Villanova at home before gutting out road wins at Northeastern and Rhode Island. Landers, as Matthews predicted, was an alpha force on offense. He ran and passed for 369 yards against New Hampshire, added 292 total yards against Coastal and torched Villanova with a 300-yard passing effort. Over this stretch, Landers combined for 15 running and passing touchdowns and tossed zero interceptions. Against Rhode Island, his 242 passing yards and 166 rushing yards paved the way for a 44-point outburst.

Landers was not Rascati, fans had feared, but now it was clear that he might be even better. The Dukes were 6-1 and ranked in the top 10. And they were doing it without Eugene Holloman, who had torn cartilage in his right knee early in the New Hampshire game and was out for the season. But despite Madison's 4-0 record in conference play, Holloman's injury created a disastrous domino effect. He and Landers were expected to be the workhorse runners in JMU's spread-option attack, which ran the ball 73 percent of the time. Without Holloman, the Dukes were forced to plunge into their reserves at tailback, leaning heavily on redshirt senior Antoinne Bolton, redshirt freshmen Griff Yancy and Jamal Sullivan, and even activating stud recruit Scott Noble, a 205-pounder from Baltimore, who was supposed to sit out the 2007 season.

The quartet performed admirably. Noble scored four touchdowns on only 24 carries. Yancy, Bolton and Sullivan rushed for 1,504 yards and 19 scores. They combined to be a solid supplement to Landers, who, through injuries and his own physical dominance, rapidly was becoming a one-man show. The Dukes were banged up. L.C. Baker, who caught 46 passes the previous season and had a strong start to 2007, tweaked first his left, and then his right hamstrings midway through the year. He missed four games and caught only seven passes after Sept. 29. LeZotte, JMU's Iron man, had a pin surgically implanted in his injured left wrist during Madison's bye week and played the rest of the season with a cast on his left hand. Still, there was no stopping LeZotte, who finished the season with 95 tackles, pushing his career total to 416. "Tony just goes," Bolton told the *Daily News-Record*. "He's like one of those 18-wheelers. You've got one flat tire on an 18-wheeler, that joint just keeps on trucking. Tony just keeps trucking."

The Dukes, likewise, were trucking — perhaps laboring — toward another shot at that elusive automatic bid to the playoffs. They had averaged 38.5 points per game during their six-game streak, but the floor was about to collapse. JMU hosted Richmond on homecoming. The Spiders, after making the playoffs in 2005 and struggling in 2006, were back in full force behind a swarming defense and tailback Tim Hightower. They had no problem playing physical football, and on a sun-splashed afternoon in Harrisonburg, the Spiders bit the Dukes, jumping out to a 17-0 lead in the first half and holding Landers to a pedestrian 79 rushing yards.

JMU fought back, however. A long touchdown pass from Landers to Bosco Williams and three field goals by place kicker Dave Stannard made it a one-point game with six minutes to go. The Dukes forced the Spiders to punt and Landers took over on the JMU 34 with 2:03 left in the game. A completion to Rockeed McCarter and runs by Bolton and Landers moved JMU to the Richmond 44. On first-and-10, however, Landers tried to thread a pass to Bolton on the far sideline and his throw was picked off by Stephen Howell, ending the comeback. A week later, the Dukes dropped another close one, 37-34, at Delaware, and now they were 6-3, one loss away from missing the playoffs for the second time in three years.

The frustration was palpable. Omar Cuff, in what was becoming a common occurrence, ripped JMU for 167 all-purpose yards and three touchdowns. Meanwhile, the Dukes had somehow lost a game in which they received a combined 343 rushing yards and four scores from Bolton and Yancy.

It was a baffling scene in Newark. With Baker out and a cast on LeZotte's left hand, Landers was pressed into punt return duties. Yancy, who averaged 10.1 yards per carry, fumbled late in the game (this was becoming an ugly habit among the young tailbacks) and killed an important drive. And Landers, who had been so efficient throwing the ball (91-of-125 in JMU's first seven games) suddenly was firing with the accuracy of a malfunctioning Gatling gun. Against Richmond and Delaware, two fellow playoff contenders, Landers was a disastrous 13-of-36 for 168 yards and two interceptions. Later, despite his quarterback's grace and honesty in front of the camera, Matthews made Landers off-limits to the press.

The high-powered JMU offense was one-dimensional. Madison couldn't throw and lacked a go-to tailback. Yancy was running through people, but didn't protect the football. Bolton was sure-handed, but at 5-foot-7, he couldn't take the pounding. Baker appeared finished and LeZotte was playing with one hand. The Dukes were a mess.

Fortunately for JMU, the final two games set up nicely. In Williamsburg, Landers and Yancy torched a bad William & Mary defense for six touchdowns in a 55-34 shellacking of the Tribe. A week later, Scotty McGee took the opening kickoff 100 yards for a touchdown to jump-start a 23-13 win over Towson in the regular season finale. The Dukes were 8-3 and Landers was back on the upswing, rushing for 171 yards against W&M, 150 against Towson, and throwing the ball efficiently in both games.

Selection Sunday was a bit of a formality. The Dukes knew where they were going. As fans and experts toggled through the seeded teams at Northern Iowa, McNeese State, Southern Illinois and Montana, a showdown was brewing in Boone between JMU and Appalachian State. The Mountaineers looked vulnerable at times during the season. They lost at Wofford, 42-31, in late September. A month later, Georgia Southern went into "The Rock" and ended ASU's 30-game winning streak at Kidd Brewer Stadium. The Dukes took a measure of optimism in these games. Wofford and Georgia Southern had ball-control, run-oriented offenses. And the Mountaineers were suspect on defense. They struggled against Wofford's option attack and were burned by duel threat quarterbacks Jayson Foster (Georgia Southern) and Renaldo Gray (Furman) during the regular season.

Still, these were the Mountaineers. They had Armanti Edwards,

Kevin Richardson and Dexter Jackson, all explosive players with big-play potential. They also had that win over Michigan in their hip pocket. Jackson, a 5-foot-10 speedster from Dunwoody, Ga., was a nightmare to cover. He caught only 30 passes all season, but seven went for at least 40 yards. Landers, who injured his ankle against Towson, skipped practice on Tuesday and hobbled around for the rest of the week. He was questionable as late as Friday afternoon. But on game day, Landers told Matthews he was ready. Matthews had not been shy about his team during the season. He thought the Dukes were championship caliber and that turnovers were the only reason for their daunting task in the opening round. He had a point. The Dukes had a simple plan and everyone knew it. They would run the ball right at the Mountaineers, milk the clock, and keep Edwards off the field for as long as possible. For the Dukes, it was the only blueprint to win in Boone.

For 52 punishing minutes, the Dukes executed that blueprint to perfection. They swarmed Richardson, harassed Edwards and held the mighty ASU scoring machine in check. They ran the ball at will. Edwards still got his yards (he'd finish with 132 on the ground and 126 through the air) but Landers was just as good, running for 129 and passing for 124. Meanwhile, the JMU offensive line was taking the game away from Edwards and deciding the outcome in the trenches. The Dukes ran for 312 yards. They scored on a fake field goal. They held the ball for more than two-thirds of the game. And they led the two-time defending champions, 27-19, with 7:31 left in the fourth quarter. "We were running at will against them," Matthews told reporters after the game. "We just didn't think they could stop us."

Champions, however, have a unique way of surviving. The Mountaineers, held scoreless for the entire third quarter, used a nine-play drive and a Julian Rauch field goal to cut the Madison lead to 27-22 with 4:41 to play. The Dukes took over on their own 23 and tried to bleed out the clock. They ran Sullivan into the line three times and the freshman tailback gained nine yards, setting up fourth-and-one at the JMU 32-yard line with 2:06 left. Though Durden, now in his fourth season as offensive coordinator, called most of the plays, this — like Fenner's goal-line plunge in Chattanooga and the failed Rascati sneak in Youngstown — was a decision for Matthews. The ninth-year Madison coach didn't hesitate. "If we make a first down, the game is over." he thought. Matthews was convinced the Dukes were better than the Mountaineers. "The only way they can beat us is if their quarterback beats us," he had told reporters earlier in the week, "and we've got to keep [Edwards] off the field." To Matthews, Armanti Edwards was dangerous no matter where he had the ball. On the JMU sideline, LeZotte implored his coach to ice the game. "We were getting the yards so we thought we could get the yard," he said after the game. "I was yelling at coach to tell them to go for it."

The Dukes went for it. Landers lowered his head, charged up the middle and was stuffed at the line by Appalachian State tackle Anthony Williams for no gain. Replay showed that the Dukes missed a block. Regardless, the Mountaineers had the ball back. With 1:35 to go, they faced fourth-and-three at the JMU 25. For a second time, the Dukes were one play away. Edwards calmly hit backup tailback Devon Moore for 20 yards and a first down. On the next play, Edwards scampered into the end zone for a 28-27 lead. The Rock was in frenzy and the Dukes, after playing brilliantly for more than three quarters, were on the wrong end of the score with 1:10 to go in regulation.

As if two fourth-down plays and a touchdown with 70 seconds left wasn't enough, the Dukes and Mountaineers staged a roller-coaster final minute. McGee raced the ensuing kickoff back to the Madison 29, and Landers, on the drive's first play, connected with Bosco Williams for 36 yards down the right sideline. Back-to-back runs by Landers and a JMU timeout brought up third-and-one at the ASU 26-yard line with 42 seconds left. This time the Dukes went to Sullivan and the freshman darted into the secondary for 17 yards. Landers spiked the football, and with 27 seconds left, the Dukes had second-and-goal at the Mountaineers' nine-yard line. "It's not how you start, it's how you finish, man," Antoinne Bolton had told the DN-R during the week. And now the Dukes appeared ready to finish the job.

On second-and-goal, Landers handed the ball to Sullivan up the middle. It was the last offensive play Matthews planned to run. He was going to kick on third down and Sullivan's carry had as much to do with the clock (ASU had only one timeout remaining) as forward progress. Stannard, 12-of-14 on field goal attempts during the regular season, was perfect from inside 30 yards. Weeks later, Matthews admitted that the right move was to have Landers kneel the ball in the backfield and set up a game-winning chip shot. That play was commonly called "bulls-eye" by the Dukes. But Sullivan (12 carries for 67 yards and a touchdown) had been so good in the second half that Matthews felt comfortable giving him the ball. Even if Sullivan was stopped for no gain, Stannard would be looking at a 26-yard field goal in the final seconds.

Sullivan took the handoff and plowed into the left side of the line, gaining yards, bleeding the clock and moving the ball into the center of the field. As Sullivan approached the six-yard line, ASU defensive end Gary Tharrington swept an arm out. "I was hoping to get an ankle or something to trip him up," Tharrington later told reporters. Mountaineers linebacker Jacque Roman also closed in and ASU safety Corey Lynch barreled into Sullivan, who fell forward and then rolled to his left, empty-handed.

"The ball is loose!" Mike Schikman screamed over the air. And in that second every Madison fan — from the East stands at Kidd Brewer Stadium, through Harrisonburg, Richmond, Washington D.C. and all the way to upstate New York — stopped breathing.

Sullivan popped up, dazed, and then scrambled toward the sideline. He was way behind the lead pack of players chasing the ball, which had bounced and rolled to the ASU 10. JMU tight end Marvin Brown and ASU safety Pierre Banks were the first to arrive. "I took off towards it," Banks later told *The Watauga Democrat*, "but it felt like my legs were heavy or something. I was moving in slow motion." Brown and Banks reached the ball at the same time. Banks shoved Brown and the

Madison tight end rolled over the fumble. Banks hooked his right arm around the ball, stood up and lifted his arms in the air. There were 22 seconds left in the game. "I just picked it up," he said, "and by the grace of God, we moved to round two."

Sullivan's fumble was the third turnover of the game for the Dukes. Earlier in the afternoon, tight end Mike Caussin had fumbled away a completion on the ASU 21-yard line that Roman returned deep into JMU territory. That play was a 14-point swing. This one marked the end of the Dukes' season. "It was kind of like a blank moment," Roman later told reporters. "It's like when you see a car going fast and then go past you and get into an accident. It happens so quick and so fast it's to the point you don't know until after it happened." To Roman, the entire play bordered on the surreal, especially considering the magnitude of the victory. Appalachian State's quest for another title was intact. The Mountaineers were alive.

The Dukes, meanwhile, were numb. It was perhaps the most gut-wrenching loss in program history. JMU had dominated the two-time defending champs. The Dukes gained more yards, earned more first downs and owned a 2-to-1 advantage in time of possession. They had fewer penalties and converted 15 of 24 plays on third and fourth down. But it wasn't enough. And the bitter taste lingered. Landers walked off the field with his hands on his hips. Matthews shook hands with ASU coach Jerry Moore and then quickly retreated to the visiting locker room. Later, he would bark at Barber and *Daily News-Record* reporter Matthew Stoss regarding the availability of his players. NCAA regulations required that locker rooms be open to the media after playoff games. Matthews didn't care. The Madison locker room was closed. Only Matthews and his two captains (LeZotte and Bolton) spoke to reporters. Matthews was crushed and he deflected the blame away from Sullivan. "It wasn't that kid's fault," he kept repeating. "We were going to kick it on third down. It's a bad coaching decision by me. We should have kicked it. I've been doing it 30 years. It's not fair for that kid. I should never have put him in that position."

Three weeks later, Appalachian State completed its three-peat with a 48-21 romp over Delaware in Chattanooga, establishing the first true dynasty of the newly named Football Championship Subdivision. Meanwhile, back in Harrisonburg, a calmer Matthews stood by his decision on fourth-and-one, and again blamed himself for the final play. "As low as everyone is right now, and I understand that, believe me, wherever you are, it doesn't compare with the devastation we have at our place," Matthews said of his team. Then, in the middle of his final press conference of the 2007 season, Matthews was overcome by his emotions. He covered his face and left the room to compose himself.

It was hard to remember Matthews being hit so hard by one loss. He used the word "embarrassed" when describing Madison's meltdown against Richmond in 2005 and was visibly angry after the Youngstown game in 2006, but now, sitting in a chair and answering questions, Matthews looked defeated. He had wisely taken the blame for the loss in Boone, keeping Sullivan away from the cameras and shining the light on himself instead. But some JMU fans, now expecting more from the Dukes than playoff appearances, took the opportunity to hang Matthews out to dry. Those message boards, so instrumental to the growth of the fan base in 2004, became an outlet for frustration in the days after the 2007 season ended. Some people wanted Matthews to be fired. Others wanted to keep him but thought he made questionable decisions during the game. Defenders, meanwhile, ripped the instigators.

The JMU fan base was angry. And this was over a team that had lost three I-AA games by a total of five points. Years earlier, after the 2003 season, Matthews casually reminded people of the difference between a I-A coach and a I-AA coach when it came to expectations. "I was 6-6 and people were saying I should be fired," he said. "In I-A, if you're 6-6 then you're bowl eligible." The Dukes weren't bad — they weren't even mediocre. They were very good, perhaps even great. Matthews led JMU to a 37-13 record, three trips to the playoffs and one national championship from 2004-07. Yet after one questionable call and a late fumble, he was a marked man. "He took a team to the playoffs and stood toe-to-toe with the best team in the country," one reporter remarked. "And he did it all *without* his top running back."

The absence of Holloman, the most sure-handed of all the JMU tailbacks, likely cost the Dukes a shot at making a run in the playoffs. Matthews went further, saying that Holloman's knee injury "cost us the national championship." But because he had been injured so early in the season, Holloman was granted a medical redshirt by the NCAA. Landers was returning, as was most of the Madison offense, and now JMU's 1,000-yard man would be back for 2008 as well.

The only question was: Would Matthews join them?

...

MICKEY WAS not on the hot seat. Other than Frank Beamer, he probably had the best job security in the commonwealth. In fact, he and Jeff Bourne began renegotiating his contract shortly after the New Year. But success has its price. Matthews had been floated around as a potential candidate for the head coaching job at Marshall a few years earlier. In February of 2008, another rumor started spreading. Matthews, it appeared, was on the short list — perhaps even the leading candidate — to become the first head coach at the University of South Alabama, a state school located in Mobile, which had a timeline to begin competing at the club level in 2009 and progress to I-A by 2013.

At first, the opportunity seemed weak. South Alabama wouldn't play its first game for 18 months and wouldn't reach I-A for five years. By then, Matthews would be 60 and perhaps thinking about retirement. And his situation in Harrisonburg was ideal. His daughter, Meredith Anne, had recently given birth to Mickey's first grandchild, Jackson. Baby No. 2 was on the way. Plus, Matthews was a cemented figure at JMU. He was poised to become the winningest coach in program history and the school had just released preliminary plans to expand Bridgeforth Stadium to 25,000 seats by 2012. "The House that Mickey Built," some people cracked, but those claims were not far-fetched. "Matthews," one person close to the program remarked, "is working his way toward having a statue built for him on campus. Why on earth would he leave this place so he can get his head kicked around as the inaugural coach of a transition program?"

All good points. Still, South Alabama presented Matthews with two things JMU simply could not match. The first was an opportunity to become a Division I-A coach by his 60th birthday. The second was money. Matthews was making nearly $280,000 a year at Madison (including incentives) and the university likely couldn't go much higher. But the South Alabama job and Matthews seemed like the matching of a square peg and a round hole. For one, Matthews, at 55 years old, wasn't a young hotshot coach anymore. Then there was the transition. Many people close to the program believed Matthews would be miserable if he was stuck coaching a losing team. And South Alabama was going to lose a lot in its first seasons. Still, the opportunity to build his own program — with his son at his side — likely was a strong selling point. "When you are building a program from scratch it's yours," Jon McNamara later said. "You get to pick the house, the kitchen and stock the cupboards. He had carte blanche."

Though the Dukes had been down this road before, Matthews had never been in demand like this during his Madison tenure. Rumors usually fizzled quickly. This one, however, brewed. And Matthews kept things close to the vest. Speculation ran rampant. "Matthews is gone," an intern close to the program said. "He's flying down for a meeting." A dozen new threads devoted to Matthews and South Alabama popped up on the Madison message board of CAAZone. com between February 10 and 12. They ranged from informational (Matthews and South Alabama?) to opinionated (Football Replacement Candidates) to worrisome (Latest from DNR: Not looking good) and finally delusional (Coach not under faculty email address). Meanwhile, confusion reigned on campus. "At this point," Curt Dudley told one reporter, "you probably know as much as I know."

On Tuesday, Feb. 12, there was a reported offer — five years at $350,000 annually — and that night, the Dukes received messages from their assistant coaches, calling for a Wednesday morning meeting at the

Plecker Center. "Right then, I thought, I was like, I don't know what to think," defensive tackle Sam Daniels told the DN-R. Meanwhile, rumors were circling that South Alabama was sending a plane to pick up Matthews and his wife on Wednesday afternoon to fly them to Mobile. The writing was on the wall. "Is Matthews Going?" read the headline in Tuesday's DN-R. It certainly was a real possibility. "That's when I was getting a little worried," Holloman admitted.

Matthews met with his assistant coaches at 7:30 the next morning and then immediately stepped into a briefing with his players, who had crowded into the conference room at the Plecker Center. Both meetings were closed to the media. About a minute after Matthews entered the room, Barber reported, his players began applauding.

Matthews was staying.

Later, he said family trumped money in his decision. "In many ways, it was going to be fun starting a program. Hiring secretaries. You get to order the pencils, order the pads," he admitted. "But Virginia is my home." Two weeks later, he and Bourne agreed to a contract that would extend Matthews through 2012 and raise his base salary by almost $50,000 a year. And aside from family ties, Matthews had a juggernaut returning in 2008. "We have the most returning players we've ever had," he told reporters. "I'm sure we'll be preseason No. 1, or in the top two or three, going into the season. Our best players are our young players. Obviously, we've got it going here. We're on a roll."

This statement brought things back to neutral in Harrisonburg, where the Dukes had been somewhat displaced by the South Alabama situation. JMU was revving for another title run. For the players, the 2008 season began in November of 2007, after Jamal Sullivan's lost fumble in Boone. The Dukes, it was clear, were on a mission.

...

THAT MISSION, however, did not include another stomping to open the season. For the second year in a row, the Dukes ventured to Tobacco Road for a game against a weak I-A program with a new coach. And 12 months after Butch Davis and North Carolina slammed

JMU, 37-14, David Cutliffe and Duke drummed Madison, 31-7. It now was official — at least according to critics — that a Matthews-led JMU team would never beat a I-A opponent. The 23-point loss in Chapel Hill was bad, but it was excusable given JMU's inexperience at premier positions. And the Tar Heels were a .500 program in 2004 and 2005 before collapsing in 2006. But Duke? Duke! The Blue Devils were 1-23 over the past two years. They were shut out by Richmond in 2006. But against JMU, they looked like world-beaters. Being blown out by Duke in the second half (it was 14-7 at the intermission) was a disaster. Landers' wobbly interception to open the third quarter was unwatchable. Losing like that, as far as the fans were concerned, was an embarrassment.

A potentially big season was in danger of going down the tubes in a hurry. The middle of the Madison schedule was loaded. There were conference games against UMass, Richmond and Villanova. And, of course, there was the Sept. 20 showdown at Bridgeforth Stadium with Appalachian State — the back end of JMU's home-and-home deal with the Mountaineers that began in 2006.

It was popular opinion that the Dukes would be fortunate to make it through September with a 3-2 overall record. But they rebounded nicely from their loss in Durham, bombing North Carolina Central, 56-7, and then running away from No. 3 UMass, 52-38. The game against the Minutemen was a slugfest. The two CAA teams combined for 866 yards. Landers rushed for 206 by himself and McGee had 196 yards on punt and kickoff returns. No one, it seemed, played defense. "I'm sure both defensive groups made enough mistakes to fill the Farmers' Almanac," Matthews told reporters after the game.

This was a huge win for JMU because the Minutemen — not the Dukes — were preseason favorites to win the CAA. Still, to many fans, the victory merely set up a rematch with the No. 1 Mountaineers, a game the entire Madison community had been anticipating since the previous Thanksgiving. ASU again was loaded with downfield talent (CoCo Hillary, Ben Jorden, Brian Quick) and a stable of young tailbacks. Edwards, just a junior, had been roughed up in the season opener against LSU, but he remained the most dangerous I-AA player in the country.

And the No. 5 Dukes? They had a human battering ram (Landers), a home run return man (McGee) and a pass rush that would finish the year with 34 sacks (the second-highest in the conference). Meanwhile, Holloman, after having a second surgery in March to clean up scar tissue in his repaired right knee, had gotten out of the gate slowly because of a bruised thigh. He was falling down every time he tried to accelerate and actually sat out the UMass game. Holloman would be available against Appalachian State but his effectiveness was another matter. This was Super Bowl week at JMU and the growing rivalry between the two programs had spread to mainstream media. "James Madison gets another shot at Appalachian State," read the headline in Wednesday's *USA Today*. And for what it was worth, the Dukes were confident. They thought they were the best team 10 months earlier in Boone and nothing had changed. "We're going to put on a show," the usually reserved Landers told reporters. "I feel that we have the best team in the country. I'm not going to sit here and lie and say I don't feel that way. I think we have the best team in the country."

The fans — at least those wearing purple — had to agree. The Dukes were going to win this game. Somehow, they would slow Edwards and hammer his receivers and knock the mighty Mountaineers off their perch. It had nearly happened the previous fall and now it was time to finish what they started. This easily was the biggest regular-season home game in program history and 17,163 people crammed into Bridgeforth Stadium to watch it unfold. As Dixon Wright prepared to kick off for JMU, the crowd was in frenzy.

And then the Dukes fell apart.

Landers threw a pick on JMU's first offensive play. Backup punter Andy Smith shanked two kicks. Appalachian State started three drives in Madison territory. Edwards scrambled for 17 yards on third-and-11. Stannard missed a 44-yard field goal at the end of the second quarter.

At halftime, the Mountaineers led, 21-0.

The Dukes had 66 yards of total offense in the first half. Edwards, by comparison, had 97 by himself on the ground. ASU, 12-3 all-time vs. Madison, was on its way to a rout, and the JMU fans were floored. They booed the Dukes loudly as they came off the field. "We didn't do a good job, I guess, handling the moment in the beginning of the game," Landers later told reporters. "You can want to beat somebody so bad that you over-think some things, and you take yourself out of the game. I think that's what we did in the beginning."

Matthews, who usually meets with his coaches before the team at the intermission, this time went straight for his players. "I thought I needed to regroup everyone," he later said. The head coach was businesslike, sources inside the locker room later told Chris Simmons. Matthews was adamant that there was a lot of football to be played.

It was an extremely one-sided conversation, and the Dukes responded with their greatest second-half comeback in Mickey's tenure, a fitting start to a wild 2008 season. McGee, already with a punt return for a touchdown on the season, fielded the second half kickoff in front of the Madison goal line and raced through the Mountaineers' defense for a 99-yard touchdown that jolted Bridgeforth Stadium back to life. Five plays later, after an ASU punt, Landers darted through the middle for a 62-yard score. A Mountaineers' field goal made it 24-14, but on the ensuing JMU drive, Landers faked a run, pulled back, and hit Yancy on a 35-yard touchdown strike to pull the Dukes within three.

It was a tale of two halves, and the Dukes were winning the final act. Darrieus Ramsey, who quit the team earlier in the season, asked to come back, and was allowed to return only after his fellow seniors gave Matthews the green light, intercepted Edwards on the second play of the fourth quarter to give the Dukes a short field. Landers ran and passed Madison to the ASU 24, bringing up fourth-and-one. Here, on a play they had failed to convert 10 months earlier in Boone, the Dukes gave the ball to Yancy, and the big tailback powered through the right side for six yards. Two runs by Landers and an ASU facemask penalty put the Dukes on the four. On the next play, Landers faked a run to the right and pitched the ball back to the left for Holloman, who raced untouched into the end zone. The Dukes led, 28-24, with 10:48 to play and Bridgeforth was in bedlam.

Appalachian State began its next drive with three quick first downs, marching all the way to the JMU 24-yard line. The Mountaineers ran a play for Robert Welton on first-and-10. Welton scrapped and clawed his way down the sideline for another first down, but as he fought for extra yards, JMU freshman linebacker Jaime Veney ripped the ball from his arm. The fumble was recovered by defensive back Gerrin Griffin at the JMU 13. Ten plays later, after a big third-down reception by Mike Caussin and a 47-yard run by Holloman, Landers plunged into the end zone from a yard out to give Madison a 35-24 cushion. It was eerily fitting that the Dukes would take and hold the lead by converting a fourth-down play and then forcing a fumble, since that's how the Mountaineers had beaten them the previous season.

Appalachian State added a late touchdown and a two-point conversion to close to 35-32, but the Dukes recovered the ensuing onside kick. On fourth down with 12 seconds left, Matthews — not wanting to give the Mountaineers a chance to return a punt, and certainly not wanting to turn the ball over on downs — called for a quick kick. Landers lined up in shotgun, fielded the snap and got off a high punt that bounced and rolled to a stop at the ASU 16-yard line as time expired. The stands emptied and the fans rushed the field, and for the second time in five seasons the Dukes had knocked off a defending national champion at Bridgeforth Stadium.

Madison jumped to No. 2 in *The Sports Network*'s September 22 poll and took over the top spot the following week when No. 1 Richmond lost at Villanova. A 24-10 win over Maine was followed by a 56-0 thrashing of Hofstra, and by Oct. 6, the 5-1 Dukes were sitting in the driver's seat. Two road games — at Richmond and at Villanova — were all that separated JMU from deciding the conference title in Harrisonburg.

But these also were the toughest road games on the CAA slate. Richmond, behind all-world defensive ends Lawrence Sidbury Jr. and Sherman Logan, boasted one of the strongest defenses in the country. The Spiders had beaten the Dukes the previous season in Harrisonburg and had stymied Landers. But this rivalry, growing stronger every season, had been one of give-and-take. The home team had not won since 2003 and the Spiders, who drew small crowds and played in cavernous University of Richmond Stadium, often surrendered home-field advantage to a massive flock of JMU fans. On this day, the paid attendance was 16,151, buoyed by a Madison contingent that took up the entire west end of the stadium.

The teams, ranked No. 1 and No. 5 in the country, hammered each other from the start. They combined for 670 yards and 69 points, each playing an aggressive, but smart, brand of football. The Dukes, keenly aware of Richmond running back Josh Vaughan, employed the same tactic they used the previous season against Tim Hightower. It was silly to think they could stop a great running back; instead the Dukes aimed to make him earn every inch. Vaughan, on his way to 1,884 yards in 2008, gained 94 on 23 carries. The Spiders, meanwhile, made Scotty McGee priority No. 1. They practiced specialty kicks all week and aimed to keep the ball out of his hands. Richmond coach Mike London was adamant about turning the electric return man into a non-factor.

The lead changed hands for the fifth time on Richmond quarterback Eric Ward's three-yard touchdown run that put the Spiders up, 24-20, with 10:49 left in the fourth quarter. A 40-yard Stannard field goal trimmed the lead to one, but Richmond reclaimed momentum with a Vaughan touchdown run to go up, 31-23, with less than four minutes to play.

The Dukes were running out of time. They were running well, and would finish with 226 yards on the ground, but it was a joint effort between Holloman, Landers, Yancy and Sullivan. Now, they needed a jailbreak, or at least a few runs into the secondary. JMU began its next drive on the 37 and went to work. An 11-yard run by Yancy and five-yard run by Yancy moved the Dukes across midfield. Yancy fumbled the second carry, but the ball was recovered by JMU lineman Dorian Brooks. Landers then completed an eight-yard pass to freshman Kerby Long to put the Dukes on the Richmond 38.

On the next play, Landers lined up in shotgun and ran a draw up the middle. He darted around a pair of defenders, ran through another and powered his way for 22 yards. The tide was shifting. Richmond called a timeout, and with 2:08 to go, the Dukes had a first down on the 16. Landers and Holloman gained three and five yards, respectively, on the next two plays, bringing up third-and-two from the eight-yard line. Holloman, the most sure-handed JMU running back, had been in the game since Yancy's fumble. He still was not 100% healthy, and never again would be the breakaway runner he was in 2006. But he was reinventing himself as a forward-falling back who gained tough yards. The Dukes were methodical in the red zone, usually running sprint options through Landers. Occasionally they also used a play-action pass to Caussin. Landers lined up in shotgun and handed the ball to Holloman, who squeezed through the line and fell into the end zone to pull JMU within a two-point conversion of tying the game. The Madison sideline erupted. A year earlier, Landers had been flustered and had thrown a bad interception against Richmond late in the game. This time, his judgment and execution had been sound.

After burning a timeout, the Dukes came back onto the field and lined up in a pro-style set with Landers under center. This was noticeable only because JMU rarely had used the formation since 2006. As Landers ducked under center, the Dukes sprung their trap, with Holloman, Yancy and tight end Charlie Newman going in motion to the right side and Landers pacing back into shotgun. Landers took the snap, sprinted to the right and flipped a pass to Yancy, who caught the conversion as he fall across the end zone sideline. "They were too concerned about trying to box me in on the run, I guess, and I just floated it out there," Landers later told reporters.

The Dukes and Spiders were tied with 59 seconds left in regulation.

Richmond began the next drive on the 28 and with two timeouts. A 14-yard pass from Ward to Eric Grayson netted a first down. Then the Spiders began moving in reverse. A three-yard completion, an incomplete pass and a false start penalty brought up third-and-12. Then Ward was sacked by J.D. Skolnitsky for a six-yard loss. The Dukes called their final timeout, and Richmond, facing fourth-and-18, was in a precarious situation. The Spiders were going to have to kick to Scotty McGee.

Brian Radford's first two punts of the game had been returned for a total of zero yards. The first had been downed. McGee had fielded the second and had been tackled immediately. Still, London was taking no chances. He wanted this punt angled toward the far sideline, away from McGee. On the opposite end of the field, Matthews huddled with his special teams unit. Priority No. 1 was fielding the punt cleanly and getting into good position to kick a game-winning field goal. But as the Dukes prepared to take the field, Matthews looked at McGee. "If you hit the gash, go ahead and take it," he said.

Radford's punt was not angled. It was not very high, nor was it deep. It was everything he didn't want it to be: flat, short and right down the middle. McGee fielded it at the 31 and began moving to the right. The funnel was directly in front of him and McGee darted for the sideline, picking up blockers as he crossed midfield with 10 seconds remaining in the game. Rockeed McCarter was in front of him and McCarter shielded McGee from three Richmond defenders as the diminutive returner approached the 30. Matthews had been thinking field goal. But now the clock was ticking and McGee was running and there was no one between him and the end zone. On the Madison sideline, Landers was floored. "I didn't think they'd kick it to Scotty," he said. Landers, in fact, barely saw the play. He was on the headset talking to Durden about a plan for overtime. As it turned out, he wouldn't need it.

McGee crossed the goal line with one second remaining.

JMU led, 37-31, on its way to a 38-31 win that emboldened the Dukes and, simultaneously, devastated the Spiders. "On that particular occasion we wanted the ball placed in a different area," London later told reporters. Still, he had to be fuming. At 4-3 overall, after close losses to JMU and Villanova and a 16-0 defeat at Virginia, London's boys were facing elimination games the rest of the season. "It's 'We, ours and us.' It's not one individual," he later told the *Richmond Times-Dispatch*. "If you want to point fingers, you can point fingers at me for saying, 'Hey look, we're not going to kick it to him,' and then I guess in an attempt not to kick it to him, we unfortunately kicked it to him."

The Dukes, at 6-1 overall, now had beaten two top-five teams in dramatic fashion, leading to a belief that this Madison team had an extra gear it could go to when necessary. It wasn't designed intent, but the Dukes seemed to enjoy the pressure. "When you make plays to win late it becomes a habit," Matthews later said. "Winning is no accident."

True, but it was a slippery slope. At some point, the Dukes would find themselves in a hole too big to climb out of, right? In the midst of the Richmond comeback, JMU had lost senior linebacker D.J. Brandon to an ACL tear, leaving the Dukes with a thin line of underclassmen in the middle of the defense. They couldn't keep playing with fire like this. But after stirring wins against Appalachian State and Richmond, JMU also appeared to be riding a wave of good fortune. The following game at Villanova, the Dukes trailed the Wildcats, 19-17, with 1:01 left in the fourth quarter. Landers (25 carries, 133 yards) had been running at will, but the Madison offense, aside from two long touchdown passes, had been flat. Villanova, 5-1 overall, was one of the most balanced teams in the country. The Wildcats used a two-quarterback system and at times also ran plays using direct snaps to receiver Matt Szczur. Today, the plan was working beautifully. Szczur, quarterback Chris Whitney and tailback Aaron Ball had combined for 233 rushing yards, and Villanova was 61 seconds away from knocking the No. 1 Dukes out of the driver's seat in the CAA.

Landers and the Dukes took the field for the final drive of the game. It was raining in Philadelphia and the wind was gusting up to 25 mph. A completed pass, a sack and a spike to stop the clock turned first-and-10 into fourth-and-10 at the JMU 34. Then the Dukes caught a break, when Holloman — running a pass pattern out of the backfield — found a soft spot in the Villanova defense and caught a 15-yard pass as he slipped to the ground near midfield. A 13-yard run by Landers, an eight-yard pass to McCarter and a false start penalty left the Dukes on the Villanova 35 with 4.3 seconds left in the game.

A field goal attempt was out of the question. Stannard, automatic from inside 40 yards in his career, would be facing a 52-yarder into the wind. So the Dukes did the only thing they could do. They sent Landers and the offense out to attempt a Hail Mary pass. The Dukes lined up Marcus Turner, Bosco Williams and McCarter to the right side of the line and ran all three up the field. Landers' pass was high and dropped into a crowd of players in the back of the end zone. McCarter jumped. "It was coming down and I was going to go get the ball," he later told Mike Barber, "but there was a defender right in front of me."

Actually, there were three defenders. One of them, linebacker Osayi Osunde, swatted a hand at the pass and batted it into the helmet of safety Darrel Young. The ball caromed into the air and landed in the arms of Bosco Williams for the game-winning score.

Another unbelievable play had capped a remarkable comeback. "The miracle on the Main Line," Clayton Matthews later quipped, speaking to Villanova's location along the old Pennsylvania Railroad path. But these wins, jokes aside, bordered on the surreal. The Dukes had beaten Appalachian State on a 21-point second-half comeback, had toppled Richmond by scoring 15 points in the final 59 seconds and now had bounced Villanova on a deflected Hail Mary as time expired. "In a matchup of the last two Colonial Athletic Association teams without a conference loss, No. 7 Villanova proved beyond it doubt that it is a title contender," Barber wrote in the *Daily News-Record*. "JMU showed — once again — that it may be a team of destiny."

Even the players — usually guarded when talking about fate and football — admitted to being stunned at their late-game success. "It definitely crosses your mind when stuff like that happens," Sam Daniels told Barber. But Mickey Matthews was sticking to facts. "Great athletes make big plays at the end to win," he said. "I've been on both sides. And right now our kids believe they're going to make the plays to win it."

Things were measurably easier after that. The Dukes hammered Delaware, 41-7, and clinched the CAA title with a 48-24 win over William & Mary. They finished the regular season with their annual drumming of Towson, bombing the Tigers, 58-27, and bringing more fans into Johnny Unitas Stadium than the home team. The Dukes had accomplished their first mission. They were 10-1, undefeated in I-AA play and the unquestioned No. 1 team in the country. No bid snafus this time. No questionable seeding or first-round dates with the defending champs. The road to Chattanooga was going through Harrisonburg, where the Dukes were 26-3 since the beginning of the 2004 season.

Their mettle and luck would be tested in the postseason. An opening-round date with Wofford set the tone for a brutal playoff run. The Terriers featured an option-based offense, which the Dukes historically struggled against. They also rarely punted, instead preferring to attempt fourth-down conversions. If Wofford was within five yards of a first down, there was a good chance it would run a belly-option instead of punting the ball away, essentially turning the entire field into four-down territory.

True to form, the Terriers battered the Dukes on the ground, rolling up 301 rushing yards. JMU took a 28-14 lead just before halftime, but Wofford fought back, scoring on consecutive possessions early in the third quarter to knot the game at 28. The Dukes led, 31-28, with a little more than nine minutes left in the game when Wofford, after stalling at the JMU 40-yard line, faced fourth-and-six. Not surprisingly, the Terriers went for the first down (they were three-for-three in this department on the afternoon) and handed the ball to bruising fullback Dane Romero. The 220-pounder, who had scored all four Wofford touchdowns, barreled into the line and was met by safety Pat Williams and linebacker Vidal Nelson, who brought him down inches short of the first down marker.

From there, the Dukes went back to their old standbys, Landers and Holloman, who milked 5:44 off the clock and churned out four first downs on a 59-yard drive to the Wofford six-yard line. On third-and-goal Landers broke three tackles and powered into the end zone to put the Dukes up by 10. They survived a final Wofford score to hang on for a 38-35 win and a spot in the NCAA quarterfinals — their first playoff win since 2004. For Landers, the final score was a defining moment in a season of defining moments, thought Chris Simmons. "His well-wrapped wrists and well-muscled legs accounted for four touchdowns," Simmons wrote, "none more Landers-esque than a bullish 6-yard run with 3:21 left that gave Madison a 10-point lead against a potent Wofford team that ran at will against JMU's defense." Weeks later, Simmons would have a more concise way of putting it. "This was the iconic TD of the senior quarterback's career."

The Dukes weren't just thriving under pressure; they seemed emboldened by their ability to do so. The following week brought a rematch with Villanova — perhaps the most dangerous team in the country — and another heart-stopping finish. The Dukes watched an early 14-0 lead evaporate by halftime, but rebounded to take a 24-14 advantage entering the fourth quarter. Then they faltered, giving up two quick scores and bumbling on offense as Villanova rallied to take a 27-24 lead with 6:54 remaining. After struggling in Philadelphia earlier in the season, the Dukes now had failed to bury the Wildcats when they had the chance. As it had against Coastal Carolina, Youngstown State and Appalachian State in the past, Madison had blown a second-half lead and all the momentum that came with it.

Enter Landers, who by now was entering folklore territory with his ability to put a team on his back. He ran and passed the Dukes to the Villanova 46, where, facing fourth-and-two, JMU was staring its own mortality in the eyes. Landers had not been stopped on the ground all afternoon, rushing for 129 yards thus far. Everyone in the stadium knew he was keeping the ball, which is why the Dukes instead pitched it to Yancey off right tackle for 22 yards and a first down. Runs by Holloman, Yancey and Landers netted two more first downs. With 1:46 remaining, Madison, still down by three, was on the one-yard line.

Landers intentionally fell on the ball on first down, bleeding more time off the clock and forcing the Wildcats to burn a timeout. On second-and-goal, he powered through Villanova safety John Dempsey for the go-ahead score. "If I was really, had a lot of, whatever … I would have told him not to score on second down," Matthews said at the press conference. "I had a lot of confidence in the offensive line and Rodney, obviously, like everyone does."

Stannard's PAT gave the Dukes a 31-27 lead, and the Wildcats, after missing a PAT of their own earlier in the quarter, now needed a touchdown to stay alive. They picked up a pair of first downs on the ensuing drive and were on their own 41 when Chris Whitney — after playing brilliantly all afternoon — made his first mistake of the game, overshooting his intended receiver in the middle of the field. The Dukes, playing back in the secondary, were ready for it. Whitney's throw fell into the waiting arms of Marcus Haywood to preserve the win and send JMU into the national semifinals for the second time in five years.

The opponent, fittingly, would be the Montana Grizzlies.

…

MEANWHILE, ON the other side of the FCS playoff bracket, Northern Iowa, the most decorated program never to win a title, would host Richmond in the second semifinal — a game publicized perhaps because of the team that wasn't playing more so than because of the teams that were. Appalachian State, with its untouchable quarterback, steeped pedigree and 13-game postseason winning streak, had been blitzed out of its own stadium by Richmond the previous week. The Mountaineers' quest for a four-peat was over, lost in a seven-turnover haze of mistakes. And the Spiders, left for dead after their October meltdown against the Dukes, now were riding a seven-game winning streak, punctuated by a 33-13 win in Boone against the three-time defending champs. Richmond was peaking at the right time, and an all-Virginia final was possible — if the Spiders could get past Northern Iowa.

The Dukes, on the other hand, seemed like a lock for Chattanooga. They now were 28-3 at Bridgeforth Stadium since 2004 and Montana was a pedestrian 4-3 in the playoffs from 2005-08. The Grizzlies had been bounced in the first round in 2005 and 2007, defeats that had sliced into their mystique. And although Montana was 13-1, this was somewhat of a rebuilding year in Missoula. The Grizzlies had replaced 14 starters from the 2007 team. The Dukes, in most circles, were 7-10 point favorites.

That Montana had been present at the beginning of JMU's championship era was fitting because now the Grizzlies sought to end it. Both sides were extremely confident entering their frigid Friday showdown at Bridgeforth. Montana, perhaps more than any team in the country, would not be intimidated by a hostile sellout crowd. Its fans were loud; its players were seasoned. The Grizzlies, for all the rebuilding talk, had been riding a wave of good football. This was nothing like the Montana team that had been steamrolled by JMU in the second half of the 2004 title game. That team had been built around finesse, timing and a stud quarterback. This one was much more physical, anchored by a massive offensive line, a tough tailback and a stingy defense that had allowed 61 points over its last six games.

JMU, meanwhile, had the home crowd, a 12-game winning streak and the unstoppable force in Landers, by now arguably the best run-pass threat on the planet. That was the comfort point for Madison fans. A game could go horrifically bad. It could spin out of control. It could get ugly. But Landers, now known as "Superman" — and in smaller circles "God-ney" — by the Madison faithful, was the one FCS player who could own a game by himself. Landers would be dominant tonight, the JMU fans agreed, and if he was dominant, the Dukes could not be stopped.

This faith was tested early, however, because the Dukes had all kinds of trouble from the start. Down, 7-3, with 4:59 left in the first quarter, Scotty McGee fumbled a Montana kickoff at his own 15, leading to a quick score and a 14-3 advantage for the Grizzlies. It was 14-10 after a Holloman touchdown and a Montana missed field goal when Landers, after marching the Dukes down the field, fumbled the ball away deep in Grizzly territory with 4:36 left in the half. After turning the ball over 12 times in its first 13 games, JMU now had two turnovers in the first 25 minutes of the national semifinal. And though they were moving the ball at will, the Dukes could not get out of their own way. "That's something we haven't done all year, turn the ball over," Landers later told reporters. "We couldn't take care of the ball."

The Landers fumble yielded a Montana punt and JMU took over on its own 47-yard line with 2:54 remaining in the first half. A four-yard run by McGee and a five-yard run through the middle by Landers brought up third-and-one at the Montana 44. Despite the fumble, and despite completing only one of his first four passes, Landers indeed had been unstoppable on the ground, piling up 84 rushing yards on 17 bruising carries. He now had carried the ball 491 times in the past 26 games and had rushed for more yards (3,043) than any Colonial player in 2007 and 2008. And now, with 2:20 left in the first half against Montana, Rodney Landers was not getting up. He was on the ground, grabbing his right ankle.

For a few horrifying minutes, everything stopped inside Bridgeforth Stadium. "My heart sank into my stomach when I watched him limp off the field," said Brandon Sweeney, by now president of the Graduate Duke Club. "We knew the best chance we had of winning that game was Rodney." A numbing sequence of events began to unfold that the Dukes, their fans, and their seemingly indestructible quarterback never believed would happen. Landers, with help from a trainer, slowly walked off the field. The student body, frozen, bundled and petrified, gave him a light cheer, imploring his return. Backup quarterback Drew Dudzik pumped a few warm-up throws and entered the game. Dudzik had not played a significant snap in his college career. Yet here he was, thrust into the middle of a wild playoff game on national TV, expected to replace the most dominant offensive player in school history.

He made things interesting, running for 16 yards on three carries to put the Dukes on the fringe of Stannard's field goal range. But then, with less than 30 seconds left in the half, Dudzik threw a pass over Patrick Ward's head and the ball fell into the waiting arms of Montana cornerback Andrew Swink — Madison's third turnover of the night.

The Grizzlies took their 14-10 lead into the locker room. With Landers in doubt and the Dukes on the ropes, Bridgeforth Stadium was a scene of frozen misery. Landers had not been down long and had walked off the field under his own power. Most of the crowd probably expected him to return in the second half. Some recalled that Landers had been questionable with an ankle injury heading into the Appalachian State playoff game the previous year, only to play every snap. What they didn't know was that Landers had been dinged up entering the Montana game. He already was playing on a sprained right ankle and had re-aggravated it on his final run of the first half. "I didn't want to hurt the team by going out there and trying to play through an injury that I knew I couldn't give 100 percent," he later told Mike Barber.

When the second half started, Superman was nowhere to be found. He eventually emerged from the locker room, walking slowly up the JMU sideline and looking far less imposing than usual. It took a few minutes to realize why. And then it became clear that Rodney Landers' night was over. He wasn't wearing pads.

So it was Dudzik's show from here on out. If the Dukes were to engineer their fifth comeback win of the season, the backup from Centreville would lead the way. And there were some who remained supremely confident. JMU trailed 3-0 in the turnover department and had lost its best player, yet the Dukes were down by only four points. "I didn't expect a downgrade," Sweeney recalled, "maybe something different, but not a downgrade. The possibility of Drew starting that playoff game in 2007 didn't faze me and neither did this. He had been a good quarterback his entire life."

True, but Dudzik also appeared powerless to rescue a team that was collapsing around him. Marc Mariani returned the second-half kickoff to the Montana 44-yard line and seven plays later the Grizzlies were in the end zone on a touchdown pass from Cole Bergquist to Chase Reynolds. Then Ward, receiving a short ensuing kickoff, fumbled the ball away at the JMU 34 (Madison's fourth turnover), leading to another Bergquist scoring pass and a 28-10 lead for the Grizzlies with 8:14 left in the third quarter. Dudzik hadn't taken a second-half snap and the four-point deficit had ballooned to 18 in less than six minutes.

With Landers out of the game and the Dukes self-destructing, Montana was threatening to turn the national semifinal into a runaway. A 27-yard sprint by Holloman and an acrobatic 10-yard touchdown run by Dudzik pulled Madison to within 11 at 28-17. But the momentum was short-lived. The Grizzlies countered with a seven-play, 60-yard scoring drive of their own to go up, 35-17, with one quarter to go. The Dukes were in desperation mode now. Their quest to win the national title was in serious jeopardy.

JMU slowly moved down the field on its next drive, taking nine plays to reach the doorstep of the end zone. They sent Holloman and Dudzik into the middle and both were repelled short of the goal line. On fourth-and-one they tried Holloman to the right side, and backfield penetration blew up the play for a two-yard loss. "That's it," one frustrated JMU fan said from her seat in Section 6. "This game is over."

It was hard to argue with that logic. Montana was up 18, with the ball and only 11 minutes to go. And Bridgeforth was a glass-eyed tomb. This was the first nationally televised game in the stadium's history and 15,976 fans had packed the house. They were silent now, worn down by the cold weather and JMU's poor play. And though Dudzik had provided a shot of adrenaline with his third-quarter touchdown run (in which he nearly was tackled, placed a hand on the ground to keep his balance and then zipped into the end zone), he also had shown that he could not duplicate his predecessor. Dudzik, at a listed 195 pounds, was not a goal-line runner — that role was reserved for the 220-pound Landers. And Holloman, though a fine tailback, was no battering ram either. The fourth-down attempt should have gone to Landers. But he was done and the Dukes, it seemed, were about to follow him out the door.

Then the Grizzlies made their only mistake of the night. After taking over on downs at the three-yard line, they failed to go anywhere and were forced to punt from inside their end zone. Long snapper Kevin Klaboe zipped the ball high over punter Ken Wood's head for a safety, giving the Dukes two points and the ball. Now trailing, 35-19, JMU suddenly was in a two-possession game again, and the Dukes responded with their quickest drive of the night — a six-play, 57-yard burst down the field that took just 2:12 off the clock. A 29-yard pass from Dudzik to Kerby Long on fourth-and-eight put the Dukes deep in Montana territory. Two plays later, Dudzik sprinted through the middle for an 18-yard touchdown run to bring Madison within 10 at 35-25.

Bridgeforth, silent only moments ago, had been boosted back to life, and the Dukes lined up for a two-point conversion to pull within one score. They set up in a pro-style formation and then shifted personnel, flooding the right side with backs and receivers. It was the same formation they used against Richmond. Dudzik paced back into shotgun, took the snap and rolled to his right. Nobody was open, and so Dudzik slammed on the breaks and cut back toward the center of the field, racing for the end zone and launching himself in the air at the two-yard line. He stuck the ball out, was hit first at the legs and then the shoulders, causing him to front-flip on the goal line and crash down inside the one. The attempt had failed. The Grizzlies began celebrating.

And then Mickey Matthews asked for the officials to review the play.

Because the FCS semifinal was broadcast by ESPN, the use of instant replay to verify calls was permissible. This, in itself, was ridiculous because video review did not exist in FCS football. Still, Matthews and Bobby Hauck were allowed to ask for a replay if they didn't like the call. That the Dukes were asking for a review was as much posturing as it was hope. They were down 10 with less than seven minutes to go and desperately needed the points. Matthews was out of bullets.

Dan Woolridge, the lead official in the replay booth, and referee Jerry Frump of the Missouri Valley Conference, reviewed the play and saw that Dudzik, in stretching the ball forward at the apex of his leap, had broken the goal line with a sliver of the ball. "After further review, the ball broke the plane of the goal line," said Frump, raising both hands in the air to signal a successful conversion. Matthews did the same.

The Dukes, down 18 with 11 minutes left in the game, had trimmed the lead to eight with 6:10 remaining. Their defense forced the Grizzlies into a fourth-and-two situation on the ensuing drive after a long pass from Bergquist to Mariani also was reviewed and overturned by replay. Bridgeforth was in bedlam, a stirring combination of hope and disbelief. Both calls could have gone either way. After winning four games in dramatic fashion during the season, it seemed a higher power was working to give the Dukes one more shot. The Madison students spontaneously began flapping their arms like birds (in homage to the movie "Angels in the Outfield") as a signal that the Dukes were receiving help from above. In the middle of this group was Corey Davis. In the section to his left was Cortez Thompson. Elsewhere in the stadium, Leon Steinfeld looked on.

Ken Wood lined up near his own 30 and Scotty McGee bounced on the balls of his feet inside the JMU red zone. The arm flapping gave way to a ruckus chant ("SC-OTTY, SC-OTTY, SC-OTTY!") for the electric return man. McGee had brought the Dukes back before. Could he do it again? Wood's punt was straight and McGee fielded it at the 17, drifting one way and then cutting back the other way, attempting to loop behind his blockers for a big return. McGee rarely did this. He was sacrificing field position in the hopes that he could spring one loose. He ended up losing three yards and an illegal blocking penalty pushed the Dukes back another seven. It was McGee's worst return of the season.

Dudzik, trailing, 35-27, now faced the final hurdle of quarterback immortality. The Dukes had 93 yards to cover, 2:06 left in the game and two timeouts. The drive began with promise. A 14-yard run by Dudzik, a three-yard run by Holloman and a timeout put the Dukes on the 24 with 1:42 remaining. A 16-yard shovel pass to Holloman and an 11-yard completion to Marcus Turner crossed Madison into Montana territory with more than a minute to go. "I don't think they really missed a beat with that backup quarterback," Montana defensive tackle Craig Mettler later said. Dudzik, truthfully, had been fabulous since his second-quarter interception, completing 6 of 10 passes for 70 yards and rushing for 88 yards on 12 carries.

An incomplete pass for Turner and a holding penalty pushed the Dukes back to their own 41. Two more incomplete passes brought up fourth-and-20 with 57 seconds left in the game. JMU burned its final timeout. On the verge of losing control all night, the Dukes had reached their breaking point. But they had found strange ways to come back all season and a conversion on fourth-and-20 late in the game — though nothing short of a miracle — wasn't as far-fetched given Madison's flair for the dramatic.

The Dukes spread receivers out to both sides of the field and Dudzik settled back into the pocket. His protection was very good. The Grizzlies rushed four and dropped seven in pass coverage. Dudzik bounced, pumped and stepped up to throw. To his right, Rockeed McCarter drove downfield, cut right and angled toward the JMU sideline. Dudzik's throw was perfect and McCarter caught the ball at the Montana 40, falling forward and rolling to the 37 for 22 yards and a JMU first down. "A completion to the far side," ESPN's Bob Wischusen yelled from the broadcast booth on the opposite end of the stadium.

McCarter's back was to Wischusen and the Madison student section, which now was in utter chaos. The Dukes were alive again, they all thought, even as McCarter completed his spin and stretched his arms out, the ball rolling harmlessly on the turf in front of him.

"No," Wischusen quickly corrected himself.

"McCarter dropped it."

...

THE DUKES were done, ousted from the playoffs for the third straight year in a game that came down to the final minute. This time, however, unlike the comeback wins engineered by Youngstown State and Appalachian State, Madison had no one to blame but itself. The Dukes handed the game to the Grizzlies, losing the turnover battle, 4-0, and spotting Montana two gift touchdowns. And yet, despite fumbling the ball away three times, despite throwing an interception in the red zone and getting stopped on fourth-and-goal, and despite playing the entire second half without their star quarterback, the Dukes had been within 59 yards of tying the game.

This, of course, was of no consolation to a Madison team that, to a man, still believed it was the best in the country. The Dukes were furious about playing such sloppy ball against a team they should have beaten by two scores. "Unending frustration for JMU," read the headline in Monday's *Daily News-Record*, and there was no doubt about its accuracy. In his post-game interview with Mike Schikman, a bitterly angry Matthews was in disbelief. "I've never seen that before," he said. "We didn't even punt."

Still, it was the Grizzlies, not the Dukes, who were heading to Chattanooga. They would play Richmond, a 21-20 comeback winner over Northern Iowa. The Spiders, the fourth different CAA program in five years to reach the championship game, had completed their half of the all-Virginia bargain. Richmond played the kind of game against Montana that the Dukes should have played. The Spiders were physical and relentless, and they dismantled the overachieving Grizzlies from the start, winning, 24-7, in a game that wasn't as close as the final score indicated. The Madison coaching staff, which earlier that week had pulled the names of its seniors off the depth-chart bulletin board (the first step toward 2009), suddenly had company atop the Virginia FCS landscape. Richmond, behind first Dave Clawson and now Mike London, owned a 7-2 record in three playoff trips from 2005-08, including a national championship.

The Dukes no longer could say they were the only Virginia program with a national title. They only could boast of being the first. The next year, playing for the first time with a roster that had zero ties to the championship team, JMU tumbled. Dudzik suffered a season-ending injury and the Dukes finished 6-5 — missing the playoffs, falling out of the final top-25 poll for the first time since 2003, and enduring their longest losing streak in seven years.

Author's Note

THIS TOOK a long time to write — much longer than I originally planned. The idea for *Midnight in Chattanooga* actually began four years ago, in July of 2006. I spent that summer at home in New City, N.Y., where BMWs and Lexus SUVs grace the roadways and everyone has a parent, relative or friend who works in Manhattan. It was the last summer of my childhood. I had a diploma in one hand, a Bud Light in the other and I was itching to do something big before I had to worry about 401(k) plans and my health insurance premium.

Sometime in the middle of the summer, my friend Ian threw a cookout that most of us recall with hazy memory. It's a little fuzzy but I can tell you we drank a lot of beer, grilled a lot of food and spent the majority of the weekend creating an alcohol-themed version of the Olympics in Ian's backyard. Around 2 a.m., my friend Chris, who had the reputation for being a bit of a partier, was entertaining the crowd with a crazy story from college. Chris, while not the most gifted storyteller, has incredible material to work with because he's absolutely nuts. He finished his story with a big punch line that sent half the crowd into laughter (and half into absolute shock) and then he celebrated by tumbling into Ian's pool — full beer in hand.

When Chris emerged from the water, I tossed a towel his way and asked him if his story was true. Chris laughed and said, "Jim, someday I'm going to have a great story to tell. But I'll never be able to remember it. So be ready to write a book on all our lives. We'll tell our stories and you can write it."

I had built the reputation for having an outstanding memory for random facts and jargon over the years. To this day I can recite almost every line from "Old School" and I can tell you the names of every math teacher I had from eighth grade until the end of college. I have a photographic memory of sorts, and it makes me a great resource when you consider how much alcohol the average American consumes between the ages of 17 and 23.

Anyway, I don't know if what Chris said set off a neuron bomb in my brain and I don't know if I decided to write a book at that very second, but from the lawn chair on Ian's patio, it sounded like a pretty good idea. And lets not forget I had nothing else going on. I was working at a summer camp and sleeping until noon every weekend. Time certainly was on my side.

I haven't started writing that memoir about our lives. But less than a month later I sat down in the den at my parent's house and started putting together an outline for a book on Mickey Matthews and the 2004 James Madison football team. I'm not an expert on anything, but I figured I knew a bit about the program. I had been fortunate enough to cover the Dukes as the sports editor of *The Breeze* from 2004-05 and I had a good relationship with a few of the players. Plus, Mickey hadn't verbally berated me, so I figured I was in good standing with the Madison coach.

At the end of the summer, I moved to Arlington, Va., and began a portion of my life that would span two jobs, three apartments, six trips to the Department of Motor Vehicles and two presidents. The one constant was this project. I'm not sure why I started this book, but I've always wanted to finish it. And since I don't really know where the idea came from I'll attribute it to Chris Dapolito, a friend whose best idea came when it was least expected. Thanks buddy.

...

MICKEY MATTHEWS is perhaps the only source I've worked

with who leaves me perplexed before, during and after interviews. Since the day I first met him, I've been convinced he knows me. And I'm also certain he has no clue who I am.

I remember the first time I met Matthews. It was August 2004, my first day covering JMU football for *The Breeze*, and I showed up to practice wearing khaki shorts, New Balance sneakers and a baseball T-shirt from the University of Maine. I had a cousin who attended Maine and sent me the shirt when I was in high school. It was worn in, faded and frayed. It also was my go-to shirt regardless of the occasion. I was a sophomore.

Like the dumb kid I was, I never put two and two together. I was New York born and bred, and to me, the only connection between Orono, Maine and Harrisonburg, Va. was that they were roughly the same distance (in complete opposite directions) from my parents' house. So it came to be that on a hot August afternoon, the naïve sports editor of *The Breeze* confidently walked up to Mickey Matthews and introduced himself, while wearing a shirt emblazoned with the logo of one of JMU's conference rivals.

"I'm James Irwin," I said to Matthews with an extended hand.

I should have added, "and I'm an idiot."

Matthews observed me from two feet away, introduced himself and shook my hand. We pivoted away from each other and stood, side-by-side, facing practice. Three minutes passed, and then Matthews, still staring at his players, muttered under his breath.

"We're going to have to get you a new T-shirt, boy."

I turned flush red and smiled as though I was facing my executioner. I knew what he meant immediately. For a second, Matthews looked dead serious.

"Oh shit," I thought. "He's going to kill me."

I had thought my days as an intimidated athlete were over. But in that very moment I was 14 years old again, running foul poles at practice on my travel baseball team. I looked at Matthews, convinced he was throwing me out of practice. He glanced at me and flashed a quick smile, his way of saying I was off the hook. Then he turned his attention back to practice and walked away.

Seasoned football coach 1, cocky student reporter 0.

Thankfully, I was able to make a more positive first impression the second time around. I had been somewhat timid around Matthews until my final year as a student reporter. Looking back, I probably should have enjoyed it more. I'm sure Matthews thought it amusing that a green, 19-year-old kid thought he could get juicy material out of a veteran coach who dealt with real media on a daily basis. Not only was I incapable of breaking news, I wasn't confident enough to ask tough questions. Admittedly, Matt Stoss (assistant sports editor) and I were winging it with our football coverage. That I acted like I knew what I was doing probably only made my efforts look more ridiculous.

Still, Matthews was a fine host for my efforts. He gave me an exclusive tour of the Athletic Performance Center in the spring of 2005 and, dare I say, actually seemed to enjoy having me around. This was easy street for him. I was writing positive stories about his championship-winning football team and boosting his exposure within the JMU community. Looking back, I should have asked Matthews to hire me as his personal press secretary. I'm sure the pay would have been better.

In any event, I found that my stories were predictable, bland and uninspiring. Two years later, before he and I sat down for our first interview for *Midnight in Chattanooga*, I explained that in order to capture the essence of this story, I would have to push hard and ask tough questions. I had grown as a reporter (or so I thought) and I was prepared to write a blunt, honest account of the growth of JMU football. Matthews seemed to appreciate the heads up, which was both a declaration of the project's depth and a warning that I was going to dive into some uncharted waters. Mickey and I, after all, did not have much of a track record and I wanted to prepare him for the nature of my questions.

He understood, and perhaps looked forward to this arrangement, and agreed to address all topics. In that moment, I became a better reporter and this project became authentic. And so this book would not have been possible without the cooperation of Michael C. Matthews, who was gracious throughout the process and gave me all the access I required. Thanks for not kicking me out of practice, Mickey. I really appreciate it.

This book (much like the championship season) would not have been possible without the events that took place from 2000-2008 at James Madison University. And *Midnight in Chattanooga* never would have happened without the help of many people who provided me with more information than I thought possible.

My colleagues in the media — Mike Schikman, Curt Dudley, Gary Michael, Chris Simmons and Mike Barber — provided me with enough insight to write an encyclopedia on JMU football. Their information was incredibly helpful and their efforts greatly appreciated.

JMU assistant coaches Jeff Durden, Ulrick Edmonds and George Barlow were willing to take time out of their busy schedules for multiple interviews. Many JMU football staff members, including Pete Johnson, also were gracious with their time. A special thanks to Tammy Jordan and Patty Dorfer in the football office for helping me schedule interviews and track down former players. Your help was invaluable.

Thanks to Geoff Polglase, Jeff Bourne and Linwood Rose for sharing their stories and endorsing my efforts. University general counsel Jack Knight and media law professors Roger Soenksen and Dona Gilliam were very helpful on all legal questions. Both Susan Shifflett and Johlene Hess saved me hours of time and effort by sifting through archived copies of *The Breeze*. Mike Carpenter's stats on JMU ticket sales and attendance figures were very valuable, as were the contributions of University of Tennessee-Chattanooga sports information director Jeff Romero and Greater Tennessee Sports & Events Commission vice president Scott Smith.

My gratitude to Brad Edmondson, Ashley Sumner and Brandon Sweeney for their facts, figures, knowledge and anecdotes. And to Stephen Lackey, who braved the elements on a frigid January night to take the perfect cover photograph for this book. There is — in my mind — one iconic image when it comes to the success of JMU football, and Stephen captured it beautifully.

A special thanks to my friends from home in Rockland County, N.Y. Also to my parents, who always told me I'd do something like this. I often brag to people about how lucky I am to have wonderful friends and family. Although none of them are associated with this story, I'd like to think they are very much responsible for it being written.

My sincere gratitude to Jon McNamara, who served as a source, editor, project manager and sounding board for more than three years while *Midnight in Chattanooga* was in production. At times, I honestly believed that he wanted this story to be written more than I did. When this project overwhelmed me, Jon helped to clarify it. When I thought the writing was bad, he found the right way to get me back on track. And, most importantly, when I thought something was great, Jon wasn't afraid to tell me if I was wrong.

Thanks also to Dr. Challace McMillin, who was gracious, insightful and penned a wonderful forward that perfectly captures the essence of this project. Dr. McMillin has been connected to JMU football since its infancy and he was the perfect person to introduce readers to this story.

Of course, this book never would have been written without the cooperation of former players. More than 30 were contacted and more than 20 were willing to tell their stories. My thanks to all of them, especially Clayton Matthews, Justin Rascati, Matt LeZotte, Tony LeZotte, Raymond Hines, Trey Townsend, Rodney McCarter, David Rabil, Cortez Thompson, D.D. Boxley, Tahir Hinds and Nic Tolley, each of whom sat for multiple interviews either in person, over the phone or via e-mail.

A special thanks to my college roommates, Matt Fenzel, Reid Gadziala and Dave Connor, who traveled with me to Chattanooga for the I-AA championship game. Also to Blaine Hastings and Adam Regula, who met us at Matt's house in Louisville, caravanned down to the game and spent the night on the floor of my hotel room, drunk and exhausted with joy. And to Phil Janney, Tyler Burton, Matt, Reid, Dave and the rest of the crew who traveled with me to Williamsburg a week earlier for the semifinal game against William & Mary. We danced on that rain-soaked field and partied into the early hours of the morning as though nothing else mattered. I always will associate those two weekends with you, and they were among the most exhilarating experiences I had as a student at James Madison University.

Finally, to alumni, students and fans who gathered together and watched Madison's 2004 playoff journey in bars, restaurants, houses and apartments scattered across the country. And to all the JMU fans who traveled to games, tailgated and threw streamers in Bethlehem, Greenville, Williamsburg and Chattanooga. You lived this story. And I hope you've enjoyed reading it as much as I enjoyed putting it together.

Works Cited

Barber, Mike. "Clayton's Career Over." <u>Daily News-Record</u>, 2 Aug. 2003.

Barber, Mike. "Louisville QB Headed to JMU." <u>Daily News-Record</u>, 28 April 2004.

Barber, Mike. "Ironman Tony." <u>Daily News-Record</u>, 24, Aug. 2006.

Barber, Mike. "Furman Familiar To Mickey." <u>Daily News-Record</u>, 30, Nov. 2004.

Barber, Mike. "On To The Semis." <u>Daily News-Record</u>, 6, Dec. 2004.

Barber, Mike. "JMU Sees Banks As Home-Run Threat." <u>Daily News-Record</u>, 16, Aug. 2003.

Barber, Mike. "JMU Banks On Tailback." <u>Daily News-Record</u>, 2, Sept. 2003.

Barber, Mike. "Who'll Be Under Center?" <u>Daily News-Record</u>, 21, Aug. 2004.

Barber, Mike. "Mickey: No Official Starter." <u>Daily News-Record</u>, 31, Aug. 2004.

Barber, Mike. "JMU Won't Go With Two QBs." <u>Daily News-Record</u>, 7, Sept. 2004.

Barber, Mike. "LeZotte: 'I've Given It All.'" <u>Daily News-Record</u>, 17, Sept. 2004.

Barber, Mike. "Furman Familiar To Mickey." <u>Daily News-Record</u>, 30, Nov. 2004.

Barber, Mike. "Dukes Roll On." <u>Daily News-Record</u>, 11, Dec. 2004.

Barber, Mike. "Boxley To Miss Weeks." <u>Daily News-Record</u>, 25, Aug. 2005.

Barber, Mike. "Mickey Questions Team." <u>Daily News-Record</u>, 12, Sept. 2005.

Barber, Mike. "Danger Lurks For JMU." Daily News-Record, 22, Oct. 2005.

Barber, Mike. "Sloppy Dukes Fall Hard." Daily News-Record, 31, Oct. 2005.

Barber, Mike. "Mickey Wanted Leaders." Daily News-Record, 1, Nov. 2005.

Barber, Mike. "JMU Player Drops Charges." Daily News-Record, 21 March 2006.

Barber, Mike. "More Rascati Magic In 2006?" Daily News-Record, 20 April 2006.

Barber, Mike. "Dukes Relegated To Road." Daily News-Record, 20, Nov. 2006.

Barber, Mike. "Youngstown State Ends James Madison's Football Season." Daily News-Record, 27, Nov. 2006.

Barber, Mike. "No Stopping LeZotte." Daily News-Record, 16, Nov. 2007.

Barber, Mike. "Dukes Fumble It Away." Daily News-Record, 24, Nov. 2007.

Barber, Mike. "4th And Done For JMU?" Daily News-Record, 27, Nov. 2007.

Barber, Mike. "Is Matthews Going?" Daily News-Record, 12, Feb. 2008.

Barber, Mike. "Family Trumped Money In Matthews Decision." Daily News-Record, 14, Feb. 2008.

Barber, Mike. "JMU Hold Off Massachusetts, 52-38." Daily News-Record, 13, Sept. 2008.

Barber, Mike. "Dukes Top No. 1 Appalachian State." Daily News-Record, 22, Sept. 2008.

Barber, Mike. "McGee Dukes Stun Richmond." Daily News-Record, 11, Oct. 2008.

Barber, Mike. "Dukes Stun Villanova On Final Play." Daily News-Record, 25, Oct. 2008.

Barber, Mike. "Unending Frustration For JMU." *Daily News-Record*, 15, Dec. 2008.

Behr, Steve. "Defensive play of 2007?" *The Watauga Democrat*, 23, Nov. 2007.

Coulson, David. "Hysteria builds for App State/JMU." *The Sports Network*, 17, Sept. 2008.

Dougherty, Matt. "JMU Title Highlights 2004 Season." *The Sports Network*, 22, Dec. 2004.

Dougherty, Matt. "Playoff Selections: Treasures for Montana." *The Sports Network*, 19, Nov. 2006.

Gadziala, Reid. "Steinfeld, Magerko to anchor veteran front five." *The Breeze*, 23, Aug. 2004.

Gardiner, Andy. "James Madison gets another shot at Appalachian State." *USA Today*, 17, Sept. 2008.

Graham, Martha Bell. *Madison Century*. Virginia Beach, Va. Donning Company Publishers, 2007.

Hilton, Fred. "First Football Game." *Madison Century*. Virginia Beach, Va. Donning Company Publishers, 2007. *Centennial Celebration*. 2009. James Madison University.

Hite, Michelle. "National Champions!" *Montpelier*, Winter 2005.

Irwin, James. "Dukes face tall task at Furman." *The Breeze*, 2, Dec. 2004

McNamara, Jon. "Dukes make due with cuts." *The Breeze*, 15, April 2004.

NCAA Division I-AA Football, Delaware at James Madison. Mike Schikman and Curt Dudley. JMU nTelos Sports Network. WSVA, Harrisonburg, Va. 6, Nov. 2004.

NCAA Division I-AA National Championship Game. Mike Schikman and Curt Dudley. JMU nTelos Sports Network. WSVA, Harrisonburg, Va., 17 Dec. 2004.

NCAA Division I-AA National Championship Game. Dave Pasch, Rod Gilmore and Trevor Matich. ESPN, Bristol, Conn., 17 Dec. 2004.

NCAA Division I-AA National Semifinal. Bob Wischusen and Brock Huard. ESPN, Bristol, Conn., 12, Dec. 2008.

O'Connor, John. "UR NOTES: Recovery mode is week's first step." Richmond Times-Dispatch, 14, Oct. 2008.

Orton, Kathy. "JMU Edges Villanova in Quarterfinals." The Washington Post, 7, Dec. 2008.

Rose, Linwood. "Linwood H. Rose Inauguration Address." James Madison University, Harrisonburg, Va. 17, Sept. 1999.

Schikman, Mike. Interview with Mickey Matthews. JMU Football Postgame Show. JMU nTelos Sports Network. WSVA, 12, Dec. 2008.

Schlabach, Mark. "Matthews determined to lead a productive life." ESPN.com, 27, Sept. 2006.

Simmons, Chris. "For Rascati, Dream Lingers." Daily News-Record, 9 Nov. 2007.

Simmons, Chris. "Dukes Move Up In Pecking Order." Daily News-Record, 8, Nov. 2004.

Simmons, Chris. "Did One Call Alter Madison's Season." Daily News-Record, 13, Dec. 2007.

Simmons, Chris. "Style, Grace, Guts — And An Amazing JMU Victory." Daily News-Record, 21 Sept. 2008.

Simmons, Chris. "For Landers, It's All In The Wrists." Daily News-Record, 30, Nov. 2008.

Simmons, Chris. "Still Amazing." Daily News-Record, 13, Dec. 2008.

Stoss, Matt. "McCarter's kick-blocking ability adds to his value." The Breeze, 11, Nov. 2004

Stoss, Matt. "Beach shelved by surgeries." The Breeze, 13, Jan. 2005.

About the author

James Irwin is a 2006 graduate of James Madison University. The New City, N.Y. native covered the 2004 JMU football program as the sports editor of the Madison campus newspaper, *The Breeze*, and as a freelance reporter for the Harrisonburg *Daily News-Record*. He currently is the sports editor of *The Washington Examiner*.

Made in the USA
Middletown, DE
28 November 2017